THE PRACTICE OF REFORM IN HEALTH, MEDICINE, AND SCIENCE, 1500–2000

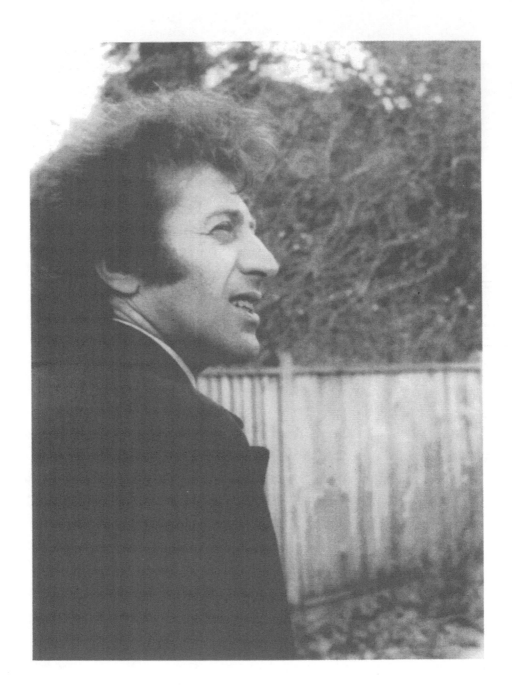

The Practice of Reform in Health, Medicine, and Science, 1500–2000

Essays for Charles Webster

Edited by

MARGARET PELLING
University of Oxford, UK

SCOTT MANDELBROTE
University of Cambridge, UK

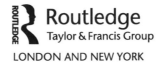

Routledge
Taylor & Francis Group

LONDON AND NEW YORK

First published 2005 by Ashgate Publishing

2 Park Square, Milton Park, Abingdon, Oxfordshire OX14 4RN
52 Vanderbilt Avenue, New York, NY 10017

Routledge is an imprint of the Taylor & Francis Group, an informa business

First issued in hardback 2019

British Library Cataloguing in Publication Data
The practice of reform in health, medicine, and science, 1500–2000 : essays for Charles
   Webster
   1. Medicine – Great Britain – History 2. Medicine – Europe – History 3. Health care
   reform – Great Britain – History 5. Medical care – Great Britain – History 6. Science –
   Great Britain – History
   I. Pelling, Margaret II. Mandelbrote, Scott III. Webster, Charles, 1936–
   610.9'41

Library of Congress Cataloging-in-Publication Data
The practice of reform in health, medicine, and science, 1500–2000 : essays for Charles
Webster / edited by Margaret Pelling and Scott Mandelbrote.
       p. cm.
   Includes bibliographical references and index.
   ISBN 0-7546-3933-9 (alk. paper)
   1. Medicine—Great Britain—History. 2. Medicine—Europe—History. 3. Health care
reform—Great Britain—History. 4. Medical policy—Great Britain—History. 5. Medical
care—Great Britain—History. 6. Science—Great Britain—History. I. Webster, Charles,
1936– II. Pelling, Margaret. III. Mandelbrote, Scott.

   R486. P73 2005
   610'.94—dc22

                                                                    2005015471

ISBN 13: 978-0-7546-3933-6 (hbk)

Contents

Notes on Contributors

JONATHAN BARRY joined the University of Exeter in 1985 after three years as Charles Webster's Research Assistant for his official history of the NHS at the Wellcome Unit in Oxford. He is now Senior Lecturer in History and Head of the School of Historical, Political and Sociological Studies. He has published extensively on urban and cultural history and the middling sort in early modern England, especially Bristol and the south west. He is currently working on several projects on the socio-cultural history of religion, witchcraft and medicine in the south west c.1640–1800.

VIRGINIA BERRIDGE is Professor of History at the London School of Hygiene and Tropical Medicine, University of London. She is head of the History Group and of the newly established Centre for History in Public Health. Her research interests range from smoking, illicit drugs, alcohol and HIV/AIDS, to the recent history of public health. Her publications include *Opium and the People: Opiate Use and Drug Control Policy in Nineteenth and Early Twentieth-Century England* (2nd edn, Free Association Books, 1999); *AIDS in the UK: The Making of Policy 1981–1994* (Oxford University Press, 1996); *Health and Society in Britain since 1939* (CUP/The Economic History Society, New Studies in Economic and Social History, 1999); and *Poor Health: Social Inequality Before and After the Black Report* (Frank Cass, 2002).

LINDA BRYDER is Associate Professor in the Department of History, University of Auckland. Her first book, *Below the Magic Mountain: A Social History of Tuberculosis in Twentieth-Century Britain* (Oxford University Press, 1988), was based on her D. Phil. thesis supervised by Charles Webster. She is currently researching the history of the National Women's Hospital, Auckland. Her most recent publications include *A Voice for Mothers: The Plunket Society and Infant Welfare in New Zealand 1907–2000* (Auckland University Press, 2003).

ANTONIO CLERICUZIO is Associate Professor of History of Science at the University of Cassino. He is the author of *Elements, Principles and Corpuscles. A Study of Atomism and Chemistry in the Seventeenth Century* (Dordrecht, 2000), and co-editor of *The Correspondence of Robert Boyle* (6 vols, London, 2001).

PIETRO CORSI is Professor of the History of Science at Paris 1 University, Panthéon-Sorbonne, and Director of Studies at the Ecole des Hautes Etudes en Sciences Sociales, Paris. He is author of *Science and Religion: Baden Powell and the Anglican Debate, 1800–1860* (Cambridge, 1988), based on a D. Phil. thesis supervised by Charles Webster, and *Lamarck. Genèse et enjeux du transformisme 1770–1830* (Paris, 2001).

ROBERT CROCKER completed his doctorate on Henry More under Charles Webster at Oxford in 1986. Since then he has taught European and Australian history at Flinders University, and history of architecture and design at the University of South Australia. He recently published a revised version of his thesis entitled *Henry More, 1614–1687: A Biography of the Cambridge Platonist* (Dordrecht, Kluwer, 2003).

MORDECHAI FEINGOLD, a Professor of History at the California Institute of Technology, has written extensively on early modern intellectual history and the history of science. His most recent book is *The Newtonian Moment: Isaac Newton and the Making of Modern Culture* (Oxford University Press, 2004).

PENELOPE GOUK is a Senior Lecturer in History at the University of Manchester. She is currently writing about changing medical explanations for music's effects on human nature between the Renaissance and the Enlightenment. She is editor of (with Helen Hills) *Representing Emotions: New Connections in the Histories of Art, Music and Medicine* (Ashgate, 2004), and of *Musical Healing in Cultural Contexts* (Ashgate, 2000); and author of *Music, Science and Natural Magic in Seventeenth-Century England* (Yale University Press, 1999).

HOWARD HOTSON is Professor of Early Modern History and Director of the Centre for Early Modern Studies, King's College, University of Aberdeen. His monographs include *Johann Heinrich Alsted 1588–1638: Between Renaissance, Reformation and Universal Reform* (Oxford, 2000), which derived from a D. Phil. dissertation supervised by Charles Webster.

LAUREN KASSELL is a Lecturer in the Department of History and Philosophy of Science and Fellow of Pembroke College, Cambridge. She is the author of *Medicine and Magic in Elizabethan London: Simon Forman, Astrologer, Alchemist, and Physician* (Oxford University Press, 2005), and several essays on the history of medicine, astrology, and alchemy in early modern England.

COLIN KIDD is Professor of Modern History at the University of Glasgow. Current interests include the intellectual status of race during the early modern and modern eras, and the role of the Union in modern Scottish political thought. He is the author of *Subverting Scotland's Past* (Cambridge University Press, 1993) and *British Identities before Nationalism* (Cambridge University Press, 1999).

JANE LEWIS is Professor of Social Policy at the London School of Economics. She has written widely on the history of social policy and on gender and welfare state restructuring. Her most recent books are: *The End of Marriage? Individualism and Intimate Relations* (Elgar, 2001) and (with Kathleen Kiernan and Hilary Land) *Lone Motherhood in Twentieth-Century Britain* (Clarendon Press, 1998).

SCOTT MANDELBROTE is Fellow and Director of Studies in History at Peterhouse, Cambridge, and a Fellow of All Souls College, Oxford. His publications include: (with Jim Bennett) *The Garden, the Ark, the Tower, the*

Temple: Biblical Metaphors of Knowledge in Early Modern Europe (Oxford, 1998); *Footprints of the Lion: Isaac Newton at Work* (Cambridge, 2001); and (as editor) *Newton and Newtonianism*, Special Issue of *Studies in History and Philosophy of Science* (September, 2004).

MARGARET PELLING is Reader in the Social History of Medicine at the University of Oxford and a Fellow of St Cross College. Her M. Litt. thesis, later published as *Cholera, Fever and English Medicine 1825–1865* (Oxford, 1978), was completed under Charles Webster's supervision. Until 1998 she was Deputy Director of the Wellcome Unit for the History of Medicine in Oxford. Her recent publications include *The Common Lot: Sickness, Medical Occupations and the Urban Poor in Early Modern England* (Longman, 1998); *Medical Conflicts in Early Modern London: Patronage, Physicians and Irregular Practitioners, 1550–1640* (Oxford University Press, 2003).

ANNE MARIE RAFFERTY is Dean and Chair in Nursing Policy at the Florence Nightingale School of Nursing and Midwifery at King's College, London. She holds degrees in Nursing Studies (B. Sc. (Soc. Sci.)) from Edinburgh University; M. Phil. (Surgery) from the University of Nottingham, and D. Phil. (Modern History) from the University of Oxford under the supervision of Charles Webster. Her research interests combine history, health services and workforce issues. Recent publications include (with J. Buchan) 'Not from our own backyard? The United Kingdom, Europe, and international recruitment of nurses', in M. McKee, L. MacLehose, and E. Nolte, eds, *Health Policy and European Union Enlargement* (Open University Press, 2004), pp. 143–56; (with S. Gunnarsdottir) 'Designing the working conditions in the health care sector', in McKee, et al., eds, *Human Resources for Health in Europe* (forthcoming).

JOHN STEWART is a Principal Lecturer in the Department of History, Oxford Brookes University. His most recent book is *Taking Stock: Scottish Social Welfare after Devolution* (Bristol, The Policy Press, 2004), and he has also published articles in journals such as *Medical History*, *Scottish Historical Review*, and *Historical Research*.

STEFANO VILLANI (Genoa 1968) is Lecturer at the University of Pisa. He wrote his Laurea thesis on Gerrard Winstanley under the supervision of the late Professor Onofrio Nicastro (University of Pisa). In his Ph.D. thesis (Scuola Normale Superiore, Pisa) 'Uomini, idee, notizie tra l'Inghilterra della Rivoluzione e l'Italia della Controriforma', he investigated the reactions of Italian culture and society to the English civil wars. He has worked extensively on Quaker missionary activity in the Mediterranean. His publications include *Tremolanti e Papisti. Missioni quacchere nell'Italia del Seicento* (Rome, Edizioni di Storia e Letteratura, 1996); *Il calzolaio quacchero e il finto cadì* (Palermo, Sellerio, 2001); and an edition of *A True Account of the great Tryals and Cruel Sufferings undergone by those two faithful servants of God Katherine Evans and Sarah Cheevers: La vicenda di due quacchere prigioniere dell'inquisizione di Malta* (Pisa, Scuola Normale Superiore, 2003).

JOHN WELSHMAN is currently Senior Lecturer in Public Health in the Institute for Health Research at Lancaster University. His research interests are in the history of public health and social policy in twentieth-century Britain. He is currently working on the history of the concept of the 'underclass'; on tuberculosis, 'race', and migration; and on resource allocation and hospital building in the early National Health Service.

Preface

'For the Improvement of all Things'

Histories of medicine and science are histories of political and social change, as well as accounts of the transformation of particular disciplines over time. The essays in this volume consider the effect that demands for social and political reform have had on the promotion of human health, and on the theory and, above all, the practice of medicine and science. Beginning in Reformation Europe, they follow this theme through the Scientific Revolution and the Enlightenment to the present day.

The eighteen essays by an international group of scholars provide case studies, covering a wide range of locations and contexts, of the successes and failures of reform and reformers in challenging the status quo. They discuss the impact of religious and secular ideologies on ideas about the nature and organization of health, medicine, and science, as well as the effects of social and political institutions, including the professions themselves, in shaping the possibilities for change and renewal.

The Practice of Reform also addresses the afterlife of reforming concepts, and describes local and regional differences in the practice and perception of reform, culminating in the politics of welfare in the twentieth century. The authors build up a composite picture of the interactions of politics and health, medicine, and science in western Europe over time that can pose questions for the future of policy as well as explaining some of the achievements and setbacks of the past. Such a picture necessarily includes obstacles or resistance to change, problems of implementation, and alternatives which were never wholly accepted.

In addition, what we hope for this book is that it should demonstrate something positive about the state of scholarship in the history of science and medicine, interpreted in the broadest sense. It is convenient to use the term 'social' to describe this kind of interpretation, provided that 'social' is taken to include political and economic history and the technical content of scientific ideas. Our collective view is that this subject area belongs in the historical mainstream, and should be both intelligible and relevant to generalists. Accordingly, some of our contributors would define themselves not as historians of medicine or science, but as social or intellectual historians. There are, nonetheless, specific interests or approaches which we all share. As an aim, such a policy of integration is hardly new, but it has proved much harder to achieve than to state. We hope that this volume provides substance rather than mere aspiration. If it does, this is a tribute to Charles Webster, to whom it is dedicated. Its publication date marks the thirtieth anniversary of the first edition of Webster's *The Great Instauration*, the classic work on the seventeenth-century political and scientific revolution, for which he is perhaps best known.

Although we have included a bibliography of Webster's publications, this cannot be regarded as complete, because Webster is still actively writing and publishing. For similar reasons, we do not see it as appropriate at this point even to attempt a biographical sketch, interesting though that would be. Intellectual and personal histories are of course linked, as Webster's own life and work abundantly show, but our emphasis here is on the intellectual side as manifested in the evolution of the social history of medicine and science during the more than 30 years of Webster's influence to date.

However, as a glance at the bibliography will confirm, Webster's influence is not confined to the history of medicine and science. He made an equally early commitment to the history of education, and did much both to enliven this subject area and to raise its intellectual status. Education is arguably as essential to the improvement of health and well-being as it is to political reform, and Webster gave serious attention to twentieth-century health education as well as to the notable reforms of education and educational institutions proposed by the Puritans and their sources of inspiration such as Comenius. Less obvious, and less recognized, are Webster's contributions to economic history. These include not only his consistent alertness to the importance of economic factors in the politics of welfare, but also major themes in *The Great Instauration* and related work, which have perhaps been obscured by the attraction of the nexus of religion and science. As far as possible, we have tried to represent these normally distinct areas of interest in the essays that follow.

Our list of contributors is far from including all those scholars whose work is appropriate to our theme, or who would have wished to participate. A few were asked who could not contribute; others later found they had to withdraw. These remain with the volume in spirit if not in print. Obviously the project had to be limited to a feasible size: we make all necessary apologies for the effects of this. We adopted a rough criterion which we think reflects Webster's own lifelong commitment to teaching and assisting younger scholars: all those represented here were either at one time students of Webster or feel that they owe him a debt in terms of personal influence or guidance. This necessarily excludes representatives of Webster's own generation whom we know would have liked to be involved. Again, for practical reasons, our contributors are all professional historians, or experts in social policy for whom historical writing is essential to their approach. We know that a number of Webster's students chose instead to follow careers in administrative, political, or health-related environments, and we fully recognize both how significant their academic experience may have been, and how fruitful the link between historical training and non-academic vocations can be. We hope that those taught or influenced by Webster who did not become historians will also feel that their interests are represented here.

As the bibliography indicates, much of Webster's published work focuses on England or Britain. The choices this represents may have had more to do with circumstance than with preference. Those taught by Webster remember a constant emphasis on the wider European dimension, and projects which he initiated, like the Cambridge History of Medicine series, included subjects outside Europe and America at a time when this was uncommon. His studies of early modern subjects, including *The Great Instauration*, were very much concerned with the effects on this country of influences from abroad. In his work on the National Health Service (NHS), particular attention was paid to the regions and to Scotland and Wales. The contributions in this volume reflect this, as well as the special (but not unique) receptivity to Webster's work shown by Italian scholarship. We regret not having any contributions from northern Europe, especially the Netherlands and Scandinavia.

In spite of interdisciplinary and integrative trends, of which we would like to present this volume as an example, much historical writing remains compartmentalized, and publishers' preferences echo these habits of mind. We are grateful to Ashgate for allowing us the scope to recognize, in terms of chronological coverage, both the true breadth of our subject matter, and the unusual nature of Webster's achievement. Webster taught and supervised theses on all periods from the late middle ages onwards, and his authority on subjects between 1500 and 1700 is equalled by his grasp of nineteenth-century intellectual and religious controversies and of the voluminous history of twentieth-century welfare. The comparative absence in his bibliography of studies on the period between 1700 and 1800 would have been filled by a major prosopographical and political project on the British voluntary hospital movement which had to be abandoned before completion. This was intended to focus on contrasting visions for hospitals and dispensaries, particularly as influenced by Enlightenment ideas and religious dissent. His continuing interest in Paracelsianism, especially in its changing religious and political dimensions, has produced work showing its relevance over a wide chronological range, an object lesson in how to pursue a set of ideas over time without lapsing into simplifications about linear development. We have tried here, in particular, to meet two challenges offered by the example of Webster's work and teaching: to avoid being constrained by artificial boundaries and chronologies, while at the same time providing investigations in depth which respect the priorities and beliefs of the period in question.

Nonetheless, many find it puzzling that Webster, having made such an impact with *The Great Instauration*, should have moved so wholeheartedly into the apparently very different territory of twentieth-century welfare. We can only offer our own interpretations of this, which have helped to shape the title and contents of the present book. First, there are perhaps certain continuities in terms of the influence and long-term evolution of Protestantism. Secondly, Webster certainly contemplated a companion volume to *The Great Instauration*, dealing with the afterlife of revolutionary schemes for reform. However, he disliked the period after the Restoration, and, although the debt of Enlightenment thinkers to the Puritan reformers was very considerable, the history of the second half of the seventeenth century in England was essentially one of failure and disappointment in terms of radical politics. The British National Health Service, by contrast, offered an opportunity to investigate political ideals as they were put into practice. Although there is little direct resemblance between mid-seventeenth-century England and twentieth-century Britain, it could be argued that there are affinities in terms of the impulse to investigate and improve the health and well-being of the bulk of the population. The NHS was not only planned, but established as one of the most important institutions in modern British society. This is in spite of the limitations and political shortcomings on which Webster has dwelt at some length. As we hope this volume also shows, an interest in reform, in principle as well as practice, needs to be accompanied by an equal commitment to realism and respect for evidence. That the collection's end date is well into the latter half of the twentieth century pays homage to Webster's belief, not only that historians have a role in making sense of the recent past, but that history (short of crude utilitarianism) has functions and responsibilities in guiding future policy.

The epigraph to this preface translates a Latin tag adopted from Comenius, and used by Webster in 1987, in a report summarizing the first fifteen years of existence of the Oxford Wellcome Unit from which he was shortly to resign as Director. The sentiment expressed is, we think, characteristic: 'it is to be hoped that stability and success will not be attained at the cost of commitment *de emendatione rerum*'.[1] In Webster's own case, this is certainly true.

A final point: those taught or influenced by Webster remember not only his intellectual quality and ability to inspire, but also his warmth, generosity, and seemingly inexhaustible support, especially for those not likely to be helped by anyone else. For those of us interested in personality, none is more interesting, more complex, or more humorous than his. It therefore seems very odd to refer to him, as we do in this book, as 'Webster'. We have adopted this as being the accepted academic style.

We owe grateful thanks to the contributors for their consistent enthusiasm and support, including comments on this preface; to John Smedley, of Ashgate, for his patience and his receptivity to the project; to All Souls College, Oxford, and in particular Humaira Erfan Ahmed, who made the whole project possible by producing camera-ready copy; to Andrew Cleland at Peterhouse, Cambridge; to the staff of the Bodleian Library, Oxford, the University Library, Cambridge, and the Codrington Library at All Souls College; and to Derek Dow, who provided the index. The photograph used for the frontispiece was taken in Oxford by Margaret Pelling shortly before *The Great Instauration* was published. The illustration on the dustjacket, which echoes that used for the first edition of *The Great Instauration*, is from the title-page of the second edition of Comenius's *Orbis Sensualium Pictus* (1659) and is reproduced by permission of the Codrington Library. The illustration of an alchemical laboratory from *Amphitheatrum sapientiae aeternae*

1   *Wellcome Unit for the History of Medicine* [Report] (Oxford, 1987), p. 6.

by Heinrich Khunrath, 1609 (shelfmark R.1.9.Med.) is reproduced by permission of the Bodleian Library.

M.P.
S.H.M.

Chapter 1

The Instauration of the Image of God in Man: Humanist Anthropology, Encyclopaedic Pedagogy, Baconianism and Universal Reform

Howard Hotson

On 16 April 1599, the Silesian pedagogue Melchior Lauban delivered an oration to celebrate the 'instauration' of the gymnasium in Goldberg (Złotoryja), in the Silesian county of Liegnitz.[1] Lauban began by reflecting on the ultimate purpose to be served by the refounded school, which he identified as a second and still more important 'instauration': the 'instauration of the image of God in man'.[2] The image of divine perfection in which mankind had originally been created, he recalled, was in large measure lost in the Fall. Man's spiritual gifts had been lost completely, while his natural gifts – through which he once ascertained the inward natures of all created things, named and exercised dominion over them, and perfectly understood the laws and duties of his own life within human society – had been deplorably weakened. No aspect of human nature had escaped this corruption; but the faculties of intellect, will, and language still set mankind above the rest of creation, and within these faculties Lauban detected a basis upon which reconstruction could begin. 'Within the human mind there still sparkle certain slender rays of its pristine light': the basic principles of logic, mathematics, physics, and ethics. The great dignity and necessity of schools, in his view, derived from the key role

---

1   Melchior Lauban, 'De stulticia naturalia, eiusque per virgam eruditionis exstirpatione ex Proverbior. c. 22. v. 15'; in Lauban and Johann Feige, *Illustris Scholae Goldberg-ensis Instauratio* (Liegnitz, 1599), esp. sigs Q1ᵛ–S3ᵛ.
2   The Latin phrase – *instauratio imaginis Dei in homine* – is gender-neutral. The prototype of the *imago Dei in homine* in the mind of Lauban and his contemporaries, however, was masculine (Adam, rather than Eve); the proposal to restore that image through a humanist or encyclopaedic education was directed at individuals, rather than the human race as a whole; and the individuals intended to benefit from this Latinate education were, in practice if not in principle, predominantly male. Gender-specific terminology is therefore employed in the text when other expressions would be inaccurate, anachronistic, or cumbersome.

they played in nurturing and combining these basic principles to help restore the shattered image of God to fallen man. Through daily instruction and exercise in arts and sciences, the principles of speech and reason could be rekindled, the will trained to love the honourable and hate wickedness, the affections subjected to the guidance of reason, external manners refashioned with elegance and charm, and, in short, individual men restored to perfection and rendered ready to assume the duties of civil life. While human diligence could contribute nothing to the restoration of man's spiritual gifts, strenuous effort could in part repair the natural gifts; and God in his mercy had established 'literary workshops' in which this 'instauration of the divine image in us can well begin'. This was the ultimate purpose of education; and having outlined these principles, Lauban concluded his oration by outlining regulations and curricula for the Goldberg school designed to serve these ends – arrangements recounted at length in the *Leges Scholae Goldbergensis* appended to the oration.

The conception of the school as a workshop for restoring the image of God in man was by no means unique to Lauban. It seems in fact to have been quite widespread in central European Reformed pedagogical writings in precisely the period in which Lauban wrote. The year after this Goldberg oration, Otto Casmann – rector in Stade and one of the founders of the central European Reformed pedagogical tradition – devoted an early chapter of a programmatic treatise to the role of philosophy in restoring perfection to human nature.[3] The following year, the Hermetically inclined Hessian physician, Rudolph Goclenius the younger, expressed similar notions in celebrating the foundation of another Reformed school in Budingen (in the Wetterau county of Isenburg) in 1601.[4] Two years later still, in 1603, the notable political theorist in nearby Herborn, Johannes Althusius, developed the idea in the introduction and conclusion of a panegyric on the utility, necessity, and antiquity of schools, which was repeatedly published as an appendix to his famous *Politica*.[5] In 1606 his colleague, the irenical philosopher and theologian, Matthias Martinius, expounded the *topos* in the preface to a work pioneering

---

3 Casmann, *Philosophiae et Christianae et verae...modesta assertio* (Frankfurt am Main, 1600), pp. 21–30: 'An Philosophia hominis naturam et perfectionem procuret et instauret'.

4 Rodolphus Goclenius, MD, *Oratio de scholarum necessitate et doctrina, pro apertura et fundatione Scholae Budingensis* (Hanau, 1601), pp. 5–8. The elder Rudolph Goclenius also alludes to this scheme, for instance in his *Partitionum dialecticarum... libri ii* (2nd edn, Frankfurt am Main, 1598), book 2: *Praxis logica*, p. 12.

5 Althusius, 'De utilitate, necessitate et antiquitate scholarum admonitio panegyrica', first published in the *Politica* (Herborn, 1603), pp. [2][1]–48; more accessible in the third edition: *Politica methodicè digesta* (Herborn, 1614; facs. edn, Aalen, 1981), pp. 969–1003, esp. pp. 970–2, 1003. For commentary see Gustav Adolf Benrath, 'Johannes Althusius an der Hohen Schule in Herborn', in Karl-Wilhelm Dahm, Werner Krawietz, and Dieter Wyduckel, eds, *Politische Theorie des Johannes Althusius* (Berlin, 1988), pp. 89–107: pp. 99–107.

Herborn's tradition of encyclopaedic pedagogy.[6] And during these years, as we shall see shortly, others from this close-knit Reformed academic community were developing the idea still more systematically as the foundation of that encyclopaedic tradition.

Lauban's development of the theme, to be sure, is more extensive than that of any of the authors just mentioned; but the prime significance of his text is rather that its author taught the man most closely associated with the pursuit in England several decades later of another and more famous 'instauration': the 'Baconian' intelligencer and universal reformer, Samuel Hartlib. Lauban taught Hartlib elsewhere in Silesia, in Brieg, during the longest and most distinguished posting of an itinerant career, and references to him are scattered throughout Hartlib's correspondence for the rest of the younger man's life. In an undated but obviously early letter to Hartlib from a former classmate in Brieg, Richard Pernham, Lauban is listed alongside Scaliger and Junius as amongst the great humanist scholars of the era.[7] In the autumn of 1632, the year before Lauban's death, Hartlib praised Lauban's services to pedagogy and ecclesiastical reconciliation and sought to engage him in John Dury's recently inaugurated irenical activities.[8] In his earliest letter to Hartlib of 5 June 1646, Cyprian Kinner, Comenius's close collaborator in Elbing and Hartlib's former classmate in Brieg, recalled Lauban as 'noster ille qvondam Præceptor'.[9] And shortly before Hartlib's own death, Lauban was again mentioned in a letter from the Silesian-bred rector of Llandyssil (Wales), Martin Grundmann.[10] Since Lauban's pedagogy in Brieg was consistent with the principles announced in nearby Goldberg, Hartlib presumably encountered the idea of the 'instauratio imaginis Dei in homine' as the purpose of a well-rounded education

6   Martinius, *Idea methodica et brevis encyclopaediae* (Herborn, 1606), dedication, sig. *2^{r-v}.

7   Richard Pernham (Elbing) to Hartlib, 20 June (no year): the letter is addressed to 'Doctissimo Iuvenj Domino Samueli Hartlieb amico suo dilectissimo Bregae': *The Hartlib Papers* (2nd edn, 2 CD-ROMs, Sheffield, 2002), 49/27/1A (hereafter HP).

8   Hartlib (London) to anon., 22 Oct. 1632, in Jan [*alias* Johannes] Kvačala, ed., *Korrespondence Jana Amoso Komenského* (2 vols, Prague, 1898–1902), i, pp. 14, 15; and Johannes Kvačala, ed., *Die pädagogische Reform des Comenius in Deutschland bis zum Ausgange des XVII Jahrhunderts* [Monumenta Germaniae Paedagogica, vols 26, 32] (Berlin, 1903–4), i, pp. 25, 26: 'Laubano, dem wir sämbtlich tausenfältig mit allen möglichen Diensten zum höchsten verpflichtet seyn'.

9   Cyprian Kinner (Elbing) to Hartlib, 5 June 1646 (HP 1/33/5A). The same letter opens with the exclamation, 'Tam mihi scilicet jucunda est scholasticæ qvondam conversationis recordatio: ut nominis tui oblivisci, qvoad vixero, non ausim!'

10 Martin Grundmann (Llandyssil) to Hartlib, 3 Dec. 1660 (HP 10/5/23A). Grundmann, who wrote at least 16 letters to Hartlib beween 1646 and 1661, appears to have been a native of Brieg. In a letter of 7 Jan. 1660 (HP 10/5/13A) he thanked Hartlib for a letter 'out of Silesia from my brother' and asked him to forward a letter 'to my brother in Brig who is a Iuris consultus there'. He also associated his father with Lauban in the letter cited above. It therefore appears that the initials 'B. S'. with which Grundmann signed a letter of 1654 (HP 10/5/6A) refer to 'Brega-Silesius'.

long before he ever heard of the *Instauratio magna* which would lead his English endeavours to be described ever afterwards as 'Baconian'.[11]

The relationship between these two 'instaurations' is extremely important because, presumably in the case of Hartlib and demonstrably in the case of Comenius, it established the intellectual context into which the central European Reformed intellectuals who were to play such central roles in Hartlib's circle inserted the project announced in Bacon's *Instauratio magna*.[12] With the publication of Charles Webster's *Great Instauration*, the specific religious context in which Hartlib's generation read Bacon was made clear.[13] Bacon's first attempt to present his reform of natural philosophy was subtitled *Instauratio magna imperii humani in universum*.[14] What Bacon was proposing to restore was the dominion of mankind over the rest of creation enjoyed by Adam in Paradise and lost in his Fall from grace and expulsion from Eden. In the Genesis account, however, this dominion is repeatedly linked to Adam's own creation in the image and likeness of God.[15] From Patristic commentators onward, Adam's dominion was commonly conceived as an aspect of the image and likeness of the sovereign God, who exercised dominion over creation as a whole. Although it was the aspect most thoroughly elaborated in the Genesis account, dominion over creation was not the feature of the divine image which most appealed to the Church Fathers themselves. Steeped as they were in Platonism, many of the Fathers found the image of God most clearly expressed not in the human body but in the human soul – a single, incorporeal, immortal spirit – and above all in the faculties of intellect, will, and language which set human beings above animals.[16]

11   A briefer and less explicit exposition of the idea has pride of place in the arguments for the necessity of schools included in the oration marking Lauban's return from Danzig to Brieg in 1614: Lauban, *De disciplina scholastica auspicalis oratio* (Brieg, [1614]), pp. 12–14. I am grateful to Dr Noémi Viskolcz (Szeged) for obtaining a copy of this work for me from the university library in Wrocław.

12   For a census of these figures, see Howard Hotson, 'The Thirty Years War and the shape of Hartlib's circle', in Scott Mandelbrote, ed., *The Hartlib Papers: A Universal Correspondency* (Oxford, forthcoming).

13   Webster, *The Great Instauration: Science, Medicine and Reform 1626–1660* (London, 1975), chap. 1.

14   Bacon, *Temporis partus masculus sive instauratio magna imperii humani in universum* (1603), in *Works*, ed. James Spedding, Robert L. Ellis, and Douglas D. Heath (14 vols, London, 1857–74), iii, p. 527; on which see Benjamin Farrington, *The Philosophy of Francis Bacon* (Chicago, 1964), pp. 16–37.

15   Genesis, 1, 26 reads: 'and God said, let us make man in our own image, after our likeness: and let them have dominion over the fish of the sea', etc. Verses 27–8 repeat this coupling in more detail.

16   For a useful survey from a Reformed theological perspective, see David Cairns, *The Image of God in Man* (London, 1953), pp. 73–113. A classic account is Eugenio Garin, 'La "dignitas hominis" e la letteratura patristica', *Humanisme et Renaissance*, 1 (1938), 102–46.

Christian humanism and the *imago Dei*

In emphasizing the restoration of perfection to man's intellect, will, and language rather than his dominion over creation, Lauban was thus operating within a longstanding tradition; and the most recent history of that tradition is clearly suggested by the shape of his intellectual production as a whole. Judging from the curricula in Goldberg and Brieg, Lauban falls neatly into the flourishing early seventeenth-century Silesian tradition of late Renaissance humanism.[17] Prominent amongst his publications are likewise an analysis of Virgil's Aeneid, a work on Greek etymology, and several volumes of neo-Latin poetry which document in detail his relationship with the flourishing humanist circles in Silesia and Heidelberg.[18] Lauban, then, was first and foremost a humanist, and the ideas at the heart of the Goldberg oration were of humanist provenance as well.

Long before Bacon announced the restoration of man's primordial dominion as the collective goal of a reformed natural philosophy, Christian humanists had been pursuing the restoration of the other aspects of the divine image as the ultimate goal of their pedagogical programme. At its core, as Paul Oskar Kristeller famously showed, Renaissance humanism was an educational programme, centred on the *studia humanitatis*.[19] The ultimate goal of the *studia humanitatis*, however, was not the restoration of good letters as an end in itself but the restoration of *humanitas*, that is, the pursuit of human perfection through the cultivation of the three faculties which set humankind above the animal kingdom: speech, reason, and moral freedom. Following Patristic precedent, the central and distinguishing feature of Christian humanism has been described as the 'baptizing' of this

---

17 The Goldberg regulations are printed in Lauban and Feige, *Illustris Scholae Goldbergensis Instauratio*, sigs P1–V1; a valuable and detailed account of Lauban's activities in Brieg is K.F. Schönwälder and J.J. Guttmann, *Geschichte des Königlichen Gymnasiums zu Brieg* (Breslau, 1869). In general, cf. Manfred P. Fleischer, *Späthumanismus in Schlesien* (Munich, 1984); Robert Seidel, *Späthumanismus in Schlesien. Caspar Dornau (1577–1631). Leben und Werk* (Tübingen, 1994).

18 Most extensive and revealing is Lauban's 415-page *Musa lyrica sive poetarum epiphyllidon pars melica* (Danzig, 1607), which documents his contact with leading humanists in Silesia such as Caspar Cunradus, Caspar Dornau, Martin Mylius, and the von Nostitz family; and in Heidelberg such neo-Latinists as Paul Melissus, Jan Gruter, and Abraham Scultetus. Note also the verses to Goclenius on pp. 402–3, and to a 'Martin. Hartliebium' from Lauban's native Sprottau on pp. 181–5, 295–6. Hartlib also mentions an 'Index Ovidianum' in preparation in 1632: Kvačala, ed., *Korrespondence Komenského*, i, p. 15.

19 Kristeller, 'The humanist movement', *The Classics and Renaissance Thought* (Cambridge, Mass., 1955), pp. 3–23; revd version in *Renaissance Thought* (New York, 1961), pp. 3–23 and *Renaissance Thought and its Sources* (New York, 1979), pp. 21–32.

classical ideal 'by subsuming it under the biblical ideal of Man as the *imago Dei*'.[20] 'What else is the philosophy of Christ', as Erasmus asked in the *Paraclesis*, 'than the restoration of human nature originally well formed?'[21]

The absorption of this exalted anthropology, and the educational tradition founded upon it, into an important but neglected strand of Reformed theology was by no means a foregone conclusion. It was after all on the question of the freedom of the will to pursue the good that Erasmus, the prince of the humanists, had clashed with Luther, the first of the great reformers. Luther's conception of the divine image, like everything else in his mature theology, was dictated by his central principle of justification by faith alone. For Luther, the *imago Dei* in Adam was to be found exclusively in his original, righteous relationship to his Creator. Since that righteousness was completely lost to Adam's posterity by his Fall, so too was the image of God; and the only agency which could restore that image was Christ himself.[22] Given this restrictive conception, the project of restoring the image of God through educational or philosophical reform and strenuous human effort could have no place within the strict, 'gnesio-Lutheran' orthodoxy which had been fully consolidated by the time Lauban, Goclenius, and Althusius delivered their orations on the dignity of schools.

Perhaps the most remarkable untold story in the history of late Reformation theology is the account of how this humanist anthropology, so uncompromisingly condemned by Luther himself, re-emerged to become the foundation upon which one of the most ambitious intellectual enterprises of seventeenth-century Protestantism would be built.[23] No full account of this process can be offered here, but it appears to have drawn strength from at least three different sources. One of these, surprisingly, was Calvin himself. Raised more thoroughly than Luther in the humanist traditions of his time, Calvin adopted a perceptibly classical account of

20   See the excellent summary in Brendan Bradshaw, 'Transalpine humanism', in J.H. Burns, ed., *The Cambridge History of Political Thought 1450–1700* (Cambridge, 1991), esp. pp. 101–13: '*Humanitas* and the *imago Dei*'; and the more detailed account in Bradshaw, 'The Christian humanism of Erasmus', *Journal of Theological Studies*, new ser. 33 (1982), 411–47. For general background, see Charles Trinkhaus, *'In Our Image and Likeness': Humanity and Divinity in Italian Renaissance Thought* (2 vols, London, 1970).

21   John C. Olin, ed., *Christian Humanism and the Reformation: Selected Writings of Erasmus* (2nd revd edn, New York, 1975), p. 100. Cf. the very similar quotation from Juan Luis Vives in Comenius, *Didactica magna*, chap. v.1; repr. in *Dilo Jana Amose Komenského* (Prague, 1969–), xv/1, p. 60 (hereafter *DJAK*).

22   Cf. the commentary on Genesis, 1, 26 in Luther, *Werke: Kritische Gesamtausgabe* (58 vols, Weimar, 1883–1948), xxiv, pp. 41, 51; xlii, pp. 41–9; *Luther's Works* (55 vols, St Louis, MO, 1958–86), i, pp. 55–68; and the discussion in Cairns, *Image of God*, chap. 10; and Charles Trinkaus, 'Luther's hexameral theology', *The Scope of Renaissance Humanism* (Ann Arbor, 1983), pp. 404–21.

23   This topic is lacking, for instance, in Erica Rummel's otherwise excellent *The Confessionalization of Humanism in Reformation Germany* (Oxford, 2000).

the perfections which constituted the image of God in prelapsarian man.[24] Another source was probably the emergence of covenant theology from Zurich, Heidelberg, and Herborn, which further reinforced the image of God and its restoration as an important theme within German Reformed theology and pedagogy.[25] No less important may have been the influence of Philip Melanchthon, at once the greatest humanist scholar of Luther's immediate circle and Lutheranism's greatest pedagogue, the celebrated *praeceptor Germaniae*. Melanchthon never broke fully with Erasmus, and mounting frustration with progress in reforming morals eventually led him to re-emphasize human participation in regeneration and sanctification.[26] After Luther's death, a protracted period of Philippist ascendancy within Wittenberg provoked a series of major controversies, which pitted proponents of the co-operation of the human will in justification and the necessity of good works by the justified, against arch-Lutheran opponents. When the gnesio-Lutheran party ultimately triumphed, Philippists were ejected from leading positions throughout the Lutheran world and gravitated to Heidelberg, Marburg, Herborn, Bremen, and other centres of German Reformed learning, with as yet largely unexplored theological and pedagogical consequences.[27]

This mixture of humanism, Philippism, and Reformed theology too is well represented in Lauban's pedigree. He matriculated in Wittenberg in 1588, during the last years of Philippist ascendancy there,[28] before transferring to Heidelberg in

24   Cf. Calvin on Genesis 1, 26: *Opera quae supersunt omnia*, ed. G. Baum, E. Cunitz, and E. Reuss (59 vols, Braunschweig and Berlin, 1853–1900), xxiii, pp. 25–7; *Institutio religionis christianae* (1559), I.xv.3; and the discussion in Cairns, *Image of God*, chap. 11; Mary Potter Engel, *John Calvin's Perspectival Anthropology* (Atlanta, GA, 1988), pp. 37–72; and Susan E. Schreiner, *The Theater of His Glory: Nature and the Natural Order in the Thought of John Calvin* (Grand Rapids, 1991), pp. 55–72.

25   See for instance J. Wienecke, 'Die gesellschaftlichen Lehren der Herborner Hohen Schule zur Studienzeit Comenius', *Studia Comeniana et Historica*, 5 (1973), 37–66, esp. pp. 42, 43, 48. For the theological differences between Lutherans and Calvinists on this point, cf. Richard A. Muller, *Dictionary of Latin and Greek Theological Terms Drawn Principally from Protestant Scholastic Theology* (Carlisle, 1985), pp. 143–6, and Heinrich Heppe, *Reformed Dogmatics*, rev. and ed. by Ernst Bizer, trans. G.T. Thomson (London, 1950), pp. 232–50.

26   Cf. Wilhelm Maurer, *Der junge Melanchthon zwischen Humanismus und Reformation* (Göttingen, 1967–9); Heinz Scheible, 'Melanchthon zwischen Luther und Erasmus', in Scheible, *Melanchthon und die Reformation: Forschungsbeiträge*, ed. Gerhard May and Rolf Decot (Mainz, 1996), pp. 171–96.

27   Cf. Bernhard Lohse and Wilhelm Neuser in *Handbuch der Dogmen- und Theologiegeschichte*, ed. Carl Andresen (3 vols, Göttingen, 1980), ii, pp. 113–17, 121–5, 285–96; Heinz Scheible, ed., *Melanchthon in seinen Schülern* (Wiesbaden, 1997).

28   Karl Eduard Förstemann, Otto Hartwig, and Karl Gerhard, eds, *Album academiae Vitebergensis: Ältere Reihe 1560-1602* (3 vols, 1841–1905; repr. Aalen, 1976), ii, col. 357b, no. 32 (17 June 1588); Thomas Klein, *Der Kampf um die zweite Reformation in Kursachsen 1586-1591* (Cologne, 1962).

1589, where the tradition had been stamped by a series of irenical fellow-Silesians like Zacharias Ursinus and David Pareus.[29] Back in Silesia Lauban pursued a surprisingly conciliatory religious policy: while teaching the sons of Reformed parents from the Heidelberg catechism, he was not averse to using Luther's German catechism and the works of Melanchthon for Lutheran pupils.[30] Hartlib was clearly conscious of his teacher's irenical stance: in forwarding to him Dury's key early treatises in 1632, Hartlib wrote that he was 'well aware that Lauban too has already applied himself very industriously and praiseworthily to these concerns'.[31]

Reformed encyclopaedism and the *imago Dei*

Similar backgrounds and outlooks mark the two figures most responsible for developing the notion of the instauration of the image of God in man into an encyclopaedic pedagogy: Bartholomäus Keckermann and Johann Heinrich Alsted. Keckermann, like Lauban, began his university studies in Wittenberg and Leipzig and moved on to Heidelberg in 1592 after the reimposition of strict Lutheranism on the Saxon universities.[32] Lauban and Keckermann were well acquainted: between January 1605 and 1608 they worked alongside one another in the Danzig gymnasium – the former teaching Greek and Latin, the latter philosophy – and their friendship is recorded in half a dozen epigrams to one another published within their writings.[33] The most detailed discussion of Keckermann to date has noted the centrality of the *imago Dei* to his theology and philosophy, and his

29   G. Toepke, ed., *Die Matrikel der Universität Heidelberg von 1386 bis 1662* (7 vols, Heidelberg, 1884–93), ii, pp. 147 (11 Apr. 1589), 469 (MA 1 May 1591), 552. G. Hecht, 'Schlesisch-kurpfälzische Beziehungen im 16. und 17. Jahrhundert', *Zeitschrift für die Geschichte des Oberrheins*, new ser. 42 (1929), 176–22.

30   Cf. Schönwälder and Guttmann, *Geschichte des Königlichen Gymnasiums zu Brieg*, pp. 107–10; Seidel, *Späthumanismus in Schlesien*, pp. 378–9.

31   Kvačala, ed., *Korrespondence Komenského*, i, pp. 14–15.

32   Förstemann, Hartwig, and Gerhard, *Album academiae Vitebergensis*, ii, col. 373a, no. 19 (4 May 1590); G. Erler, ed., *Die jüngere Matrikel der Universität Leipzig*, I (Leipzig, 1909), p. 216 (1592); Toepke, *Matrikel der Universität Heidelberg*, ii, p. 163, no. 227 (22 Oct. 1592); see also Klein, *Zweite Reformation*, pp. 211–13.

33   Lauban contributed epigrams to Keckermann's *Disputationes philosophicae, physicae praesertim* (Hanau, 1606), sig.):(5ʳ and *Systematis logici plenioris pars altera* (Hanau, 1609), sig.†† 7ᵛ; the latter repr. in Keckermann, *Opera omnia* (2 vols, Geneva, 1614), i, p. 1053. Lauban's *Musa lyrica* includes verses from Keckermann on sig. A7ᵛ and others addressed to him on pp. 195–6, 205–9, 220–1. For Lauban's connections with Danzig, see also his *Postliminium Borusso-Silesiacum, hoc est, ad patronos, maecenates, collegas, fautores, amicos Dantiscos ode valedictoria, cum collegar[um] et amicorum propempticis* ([Danzig], 1614); and Ephraim Praetorius, *Athenae Gedanenses* (Leipzig, 1713), pp. 52–4.

tendency to unite and surpass the most liberal teachings of Melanchthon and Calvin on this topic.[34]

Alsted may also have been in contact with Lauban. His intellectual relations with the circle of Silesian humanists and pedagogues were extremely close in the years around 1610 and generated a frequent exchange of letters, books, and manuscript treatises. Alsted saw several such treatises into print, including an encyclopaedic sketch outlining an 'ad recuperandam Dei imaginem Methodus unica'.[35] A similar epistolary exchange presumably transferred the brief series of musical precepts ascribed to Lauban which Alsted published in 1611 within his earliest encyclopaedic textbook of mathematics.[36] Alsted's greatest debt was to Keckermann, but that to the Philippists and humanists is perhaps nowhere more strikingly evident than in the lengthy excerpts from six authorities included within his most extensive treatment of the philosophical *praecognita* which laid the foundations of his encyclopaedia. Alongside Aristotle, Galen, and Melanchthon himself, these included Niels Hemmingsen, the great Danish Philippist; Viktorin Striegel, the leading 'synergist' translated from Leipzig to Heidelberg; and Franciscus Junius, the Heidelberg humanist and Leiden irenicist.[37]

As Alsted's relations with Silesia eloquently testify, the conditions for developing the *instauratio imaginis Dei* into a fully realized pansophic programme were, at the practical level at least, more favourable in the western than the eastern quarters of the Empire; and it was not in Goldberg, Beuthen, or Brieg but in Heidelberg, Hanau, and above all Herborn that they issued in substantial publications.[38] The fullest explication of this programme is found in the introductory *praecognita* to Alsted's *Cursus philosophici encyclopaedia* of 1620.[39] Following a tradition deriving via Keckermann and Zabarella from Aristotle, Alsted's encyclopaedia divided philosophy objectively into three parts: the theoretical disciplines, which deal

---

34   W.H. Zuylen, *Bartholomäus Keckermann. Sein Leben und Wirken,* Inaugural Dissertation, Tübingen (Leipzig, 1934), esp. pp. 23–6, 86–92.

35   This is the 'Encyclopaediae methodum' (1613) by the physician in Öls/Oleśnica, Heinrich Mylphort, eventually published within Alsted's *Encyclopaedia,* here quoting i, p. 2398. In general, see Howard Hotson, 'Johann Heinrich Alsted's relations with Silesia, Bohemia and Moravia: patronage, piety and pansophia', *Acta Comeniana,* 12 (1997), 13–35, on Mylphort pp. 32–3.

36   Alsted, *Elementale mathematicum* (Frankfurt, 1611), pp. 287–312: 'Elementale musicum': p. 312.

37   Alsted, *Philosophia dignè restituta: praecognitorum philosophicorum complectens* (Herborn, 1612), pp. 16–44.

38   For a more extensive discussion of the development of this idea by Keckermann and Alsted, and a consideration of its orthodoxy, see Hotson, *Johann Heinrich Alsted 1588–1638: Between Renaissance, Reformation, and Universal Reform* (Oxford, 2000), pp. 66–78.

39   A key text is Alsted, *Cursus philosophici encyclopaedia* (2 vols, Herborn, 1620), i, cols 78, 80. Cf. Alsted, *Consiliarius academicus* (Strasbourg, 1610), p. 10; *Philosophia restituta,* pp. 101–10; *Compendium philosophicum* (Herborn, 1626), p. 11; *Encyclopaedia septem tomis distincta* (2 vols, Herborn, 1630), i, p. 66.

with necessary things; the practical disciplines, which deal with contingent things; and the instrumental disciplines, which deal with secondary notions. His key move was to emphasize that these three main divisions corresponded to the faculties of the human subject which respectively study them (see Table 1).[40] The subject of theoretical

Table 1   The instauration of the divine image as the objective of
**   *encyclopaedia, pansophia* and universal reform**

Alsted, *Encyclopaedia*

divisions of philosophy:	theoretical	practical	instrumental
human faculties:	contemplative (= intellect)	practical (= will)	poetical or factive (= operation)
kinds of imperfection:	ignorance	vice	ineptitude

Comenius, *Consultatio catholica*

Trinitarian properties:	*nosse*	*velle*	*posse*
human faculties:	intellect	will	operation
principles of these faculties:	ideas	instincts	faculties
universal disciplines built on these principles:	philosophy/ learning	religion/ ethics	politics/ technology
objectives of disciplines:	wisdom in the mind	piety in the heart	tranquillity in life
objects of study:	man (around us)	God (above us)	world (below us)
sources of intellectual light:	reason	faith	sense
methods employed:	synthetic	syncritic	analytical
co-ordinating institutions:	College of Light	Ecumenical Consistory	Court of Peace

philosophy is the intellect – that is, the theoretical or contemplative faculty through which man is disposed to the contemplation of things. The subject of practical philosophy is the will – that is, the practical or operative faculty through which he is disposed to pursue virtue and to flee vice. The subject of the factive or instrumental disciplines is that faculty by which man is inclined towards and well-adjusted to artificial works.[41] Since each of these three faculties was to a greater or lesser extent damaged by the Fall, they also correspond to 'the chief kinds of human imperfection', namely ignorance in contemplation, vice in action and ineptitude (*inertia*) in art. The three main kinds of disciplines thus provide three general remedies for the defects of the three main faculties of the human mind, 'which philosophy ought to cure, for which reason

40   Alsted, *Cursus philosophici encyclopaedia*, i, cols 378–91; *Encyclopaedia*, i, pp. 662–6.

41   These distinctions are explained best in Keckermann, *Opera*, i, pp. 27G–28B. Cf. also the distinction between *intellectus, voluntas*, and *agendi potentia* in Martinius, *Idea encyclopaediae*, p. 13.

it is called by Platonists the medicine for curing the diseases of the soul. For theoretical philosophy removes the darkness of ignorance, practical philosophy the vice of the will, and poetical philosophy the ineptitude in the poetic intellect'.[42]

Finally, as this passage continues, 'individual disciplines remove individual diseases': 'for any discipline whatsoever is concerned with its own peculiar perfection opposed to a definite and determined defect of nature, and treats its own peculiar means for attaining [that perfection] which are not taught in any other discipline'.[43] The same doctrine is elsewhere rephrased in theological language: since the image of God is chiefly located in wisdom and justice, that is, in the soundness of the intellect and the sanctity of the will, and since the purpose of all the disciplines is to instil in the student one or the other of these, all disciplines, each in its own way, restore the ruined image of God in us.[44] Every component of the *encyclopaedia* is thus subordinate to one all-encompassing aim; each discipline is dedicated to repairing a particular defect of human nature caused by the Fall; and the cycle of these disciplines as a whole is intended to create a new man, to restore the individual *as a whole* to his original state, to recreate within him the image of divine perfection. As Alsted explained at the very outset of the *Encyclopaedia*, 'Although God alone is all-wise and all-knowing [πάνσοφια κι πανεπιςήμων], nevertheless he impresses the image of his perfection on men who desire to learn, as is seen especially in those who by vehement force of mind embrace the whole orb of the disciplines', that is to say, 'what is commonly called the *encyclopaedia*'.[45] Those who master the entire *encyclopaedia*, therefore, most clearly manifest the restored image of God in themselves.

Comenian pansophia and the *imago Dei*

Alsted was, by all accounts, the most influential teacher of the young Comenius;[46] and the pupil picked up this tradition at the point at which his teacher had left it and carried it forward with striking but as yet little recognized results. In the preface to his very first pansophic work, for instance – the *Pansophiae praeludium* published by Hartlib in 1637 – Comenius likewise announced that universal learning was to be pursued 'in order that man's mind may indeed become what it ought to be:

42   Alsted, *Cursus philosophici encyclopaedia*, i, col. 80.
43   Alsted, *Philosophia restituta*, p. 412.
44   Alsted, *Encyclopaedia*, i, p. 74.
45   *Ibid.*, i, p. 27.
46   On Comenius's studies under Alsted, see Franz Hofmann, 'Der enzyklopädische Impuls J.H. Alsteds und sein Gestaltwandel im Werke des J.A. Komenský', in Hans Schaller, ed., *Comenius. Erkennen – lauben – Handeln* (Sankt Augustin, 1985), pp. 22–9; Gerhard Menk, 'Johann Amos Comenius und die Hohe Schule Herborn', *Acta Comeniana*, 8 (1989), 41–59.

pansophi Dei imago, an image of the all-wise God'.[47] There can be little doubt that Comenius was familiar with Alsted's writings on this subject. It was in the early writings published before and during their extended encounter in Herborn – the *Panacea philosophica* (1610), the *Theatrum scholasticum* (1611), and especially the *Philosophia digne restituta* (1612) – that Alsted developed Keckermann's suggestions into a fully encyclopaedic approach to the *instauratio imaginis Dei in homine*.[48] By the time he began roughing out his own pansophic project in the late 1630s, Comenius was also thoroughly familiar with Alsted's mature encyclopaedic works, above all with the preliminary *praecognita* in which these ideas are worked out most fully.[49] In subsequent years, Comenius inserted the project of the restoration of the image of God more fully into his pansophic programme, elaborated it still more systematically, and above all developed it more boldly than any of his predecessors had dared to do.[50]

Alsted, as we have just seen, conceived the three main divisions of the encyclopaedia as a means for restoring the image of divine perfection to the three faculties of Aristotelian psychology: theoretical, practical, and operative. The central move of Comenian pansophia was to ground this whole project more thoroughly in Trinitarian theology. A classic account of the Trinity, stemming ultimately from Augustine, associates the three persons of the Godhead with *posse*, *nosse*, and *velle* – the properties of power, knowledge, and will. As Comenius

47   Comenius, *Pansophiae praeludium* (1637), preface (*DJAK*, xv/2, p. 15). Cf. Comenius, *Didactica magna*, chap. iv (*DJAK*, xv/1, pp. 58–60); *Scholae pansophicae delineatio* (1651), paragraph 7 (*DJAK*, xv/3, pp. 195–6); *De rerum humanarum emendatione consultatio catholica* (2 vols, Prague, 1966), ii, cols 5, 25, 31, 85–6 (hereafter *Consultatio*); *Pampaedia*, trans. A.M.O. Dobbie (Dover, 1986), chaps i.8; iii.14, 31; vii.7.

48   Comenius also encountered the idea in the *Physica et ethica mosaica* (Hanau, 1613) by the Norwegian Philippist in Herborn, Kort Aslakssøn: see Milada Blekastad, *Comenius: Versuch eines Umrisses von Leben, Werk und Schicksal Jan Amos Komenský* (Oslo and Prague, 1969), p. 31.

49   Comenius, *Conatuum pansophicorum dilucidatio* (1639), no. 10 (*DJAK*, xv/2, p. 66); Dagmar Čapková, 'A "working diary" of J.A. Comenius', *Acta Comeniana*, 4 (1979), 367–87, esp. pp. 374–6.

50   Comenius's earlier works experiment with a number of trinitarian formulae: for instance, the *Pansophiae praeludium*, no. 107 and *Didactica magna*, x. 7 (*DJAK*, xv/1, p. 78; xv/2, p. 47) employ the triad of intellect, will, and memory; the *Novissima linguarum methodus*, chap. i uses *ratio*, *oratio*, and *operatio*; chap. xxv of the same work prefers *sapere*, *agere*, and *loqui* (*DJAK*, xv/2, pp. 108–11, 306). The first of these triads derived from Augustine, the second from Cardano, while the third (producing the acronym 'sal') is used in Martinius, *Idea encyclopaediae*, preface, sig. α2^{r-v}: cf. also Alsted, *Cursus philosophici encyclopaedia*, ii, col. 799; Comenius, *Pampaedia*, chap. iii.9; *Consultatio*, ii, col. 23; *The Analytical Didactic of Comenius*, trans. Vladimir Jelinek (Chicago, 1953), pp. 80–1. Despite this variation, the basic structure of the scheme outlined from the *Consultatio catholica* was worked out as early as the *Pansophiae seminarium* of 1634–5 (*DJAK*, xiv, pp. 13–47).

writes near the outset of the *Panegersia* (the first of the seven books of his unfinished masterpiece, the *Consultatio catholica*), 'all the world knows that God's outstanding virtues are *power* (with which he created and preserved the world), *wisdom* (which has enabled him to know, see, maintain, and govern it), and *goodness* (wherewith he is sanctified and dispenses justice and mercy towards all his Creation)'.[51] These same 'three divine characters – namely, the wish to know, the wish to dominate, and the wish to enjoy eternal blessedness – are indelibly stamped upon our nature'.[52] It is above all these three faculties which, for Comenius, represent 'the living image of the living God' in man.[53] The purpose of Comenian pansophia, as of Alstedian encyclopaedism, was to restore the image of the triune God to this triad of human faculties.

This task of instauration must begin, as Lauban already recognized, by re-assembling the fragments of the broken image of God still remaining in fallen man. Keckermann had begun this process in his pioneering treatment of the philosophical *praecognita*. Alsted had carried it further, devoting the first book of his original encyclopaedia, the 'Archeologia', to collecting and co-ordinating these principles.[54] Here too Comenius used his more explicitly Trinitarian structure to produce a more systematic, complete, and optimistic foundation for the *instauratio imaginis Dei*.[55] Alsted had divided the principles upon which the encyclopaedia was founded into two main groups: the *principia cognitionis*, which included the true, necessary, and fundamental first principles from which philosophical conclusions were deduced; and the *principia essendi philosophiae*, which included universal innate instincts or desires which prompted the pursuit of knowledge in the first place.[56] Comenius generalized this second set of principles and added a third component to them to complement the operative dimension of his tripartite scheme: in Comenius's mature scheme, universal, innate *ideas* equip the intellect for distinguishing truth from falsity; universal, innate *instincts* incline the will toward good and away from evil; and universal, innate *faculties* form the basis of man's successful intervention in the world around him. 'These three factors', he concludes, 'are the foundations of all true reasoning, all goodwill, and all effective action' and also of 'universal agreement and concord', since they are common to

51   *Panegersia*, trans. A.M.O. Dobbie (Shipton-on-Stour, 1990), chap. iv.14 (= *Consultatio*, i, col. 31); cf. *Pansophiae praeludium* (1637), no. 64 (*DJAK*, xv/2, p. 36).

52   *Panegersia*, chap. iv.18; cf. chap. ix.14 (= *Consultatio*, i, cols 32, 85).

53   *Panegersia*, chap. iv.7 (= *Consultatio*, i, col. 29).

54   Keckermann, *Praecognitorum philosophicorum libri duo* (Hanau, 1607); in Keckermann, *Opera*, i, pp. 1–74; Alsted, *Philosophia restituta*, pp. 48–250; *Cursus philosophici encyclopaedia*, i, pp. 1–58; *Encyclopaedia*, i, pp. 73–88; and Hotson, *Alsted*, pp. 78–81.

55   Cf. *Didactica magna*, chap. v (*DJAK*, xv/1, pp. 60–7).

56   Many of these distinctions were already sketched out in Martinius, *Idea encyclopaediae*, pp. 1–3, 13–26.

all humankind.[57] 'All our corruption is rooted in the deterioration of our instincts, our ideas, and our faculties, and our hope of salvation [*tota salutis spes*] depends entirely upon our ability to rectify these on the same principle as diseases of the human body'.[58] The starting point for the Comenian *emendatio rerum humanarum* was therefore to collect, co-ordinate, and harmonize these universal principles, something which Comenius (forgetting the efforts of Keckermann, Alsted and his other predecessors) claimed had never been attempted before.[59]

Just as Alsted sought to use the theoretical, practical, and operative disciplines of the encyclopaedia to restore the image of divine perfection to each of the human faculties, Comenius sought to use three master disciplines to restore those three faculties to an image of God's knowledge, will, and power: philosophy, religion, and politics. Generalizing (like his predecessors) on Aristotle's famous maxim at the outset of the Metaphysics, Comenius held that 'every man without exception naturally desires to know'; and this 'hunger for the truth produces philosophy or the study of wisdom'. In a similar manner, 'every man desires his own welfare', and this 'desire for the good creates religion or the cultivation and enjoyment of the highest good'. Finally, 'it is the insatiable desire of human nature to control its present environment and to fashion and refashion a new one, or in a word, to be the complete master of its affairs'; and this 'eagerness to manage affairs effectively in freedom leads in the end to a political system which restores good order to men'.[60] Comenius therefore defines 'human affairs as consisting of *wisdom* in the mind, *piety* in the heart, and *tranquillity* in life, in association with the philosophy, the religion, and the politics which seek these elements and maintain and increase them'.[61]

This set of three triads – the three faculties of intellect, will, and operation; the three universal principles (ideas, instincts, and faculties) on which they are based; and the three disciplines of philosophy or learning, religion or ethics, politics or technology which cultivate the principles to restore the faculties to health – structure the *Consultatio* at every level. As Comenius writes in the same chapter of the *Panegersia*, 'These three (philosophy, religion, and politics) are the most important

---

57   *Panegersia*, chap. ix.15–16; *Panorthosia*, chap. x.4 (= *Consultatio*, i, col. 86; ii, cols 478–9). Awkwardly, Comenius uses the term 'facultates' here to refer to both (a) the three basic powers of the soul (the *facultas intellectiva* or *mens*, the *facultas volitiva* or *volutas*, and the *facultas potestativa* or *vis exsequutiva*) and (b) the universal principles or instruments peculiar to the third of these powers ('Habet...Vis exsequutiva sua Organa,...Et haec...Communes Facultates dici merentur').

58   *Panegersia*, chap. ix.33 (= *Consultatio*, i, col. 96).

59   Cf. *Panegersia*, chap. ix.23; *Panaugia*, chap. vi.23–5, trans. A.M.O. Dobbie (Shipton-on-Stour, 1987); *Panorthosia*, chap. xi.10, trans. A.M.O. Dobbie (2 vols, Sheffield, 1995), ii, col. 178 (= *Consultatio*, i, cols 90, 151–2; ii, col. 502, resp.).

60   Quoting *Panegersia*, chap. iv.8–12 (= *Consultatio*, i, cols 29–30).

61   *Panegersia*, chap. iv.26 (= *Consultatio*, i, col. pp. 34).

features of human society, and everything else is secondary'.[62] 'Therefore in my account of human affairs, education, religion, and politics undoubtedly ought to be emphasized and presented as the main topics of this *Consultation*'.[63] 'The objective environment in which the human race must live', first of all, 'is also threefold, consisting of the *world* full of things, the *people* who inhabit it, and *God* who presides over both'.[64] These three domains constitute, secondly, the three objects of study and the three sources of intellectual light: the image of God as imprinted on his creatures (the natural world below us), on the human mind (the world within and around us), and on the Word of God itself (scripture).[65] To these correspond, thirdly, three ways of apprehending the intellectual light radiating from these three worlds: '*[S]ense* governs our relationship especially with objects, *reason* governs that with men, and *faith* governs that with God'.[66] To these three domains apply, fourthly, three basic intellectual methods: the *analytical method* for resolving the objects exposed to our senses into their components; the *synthetic method* for looking into our minds with their inborn ideas, instincts, and faculties; and the *syncritic method* for contemplating divine matters, which can only be understood through comparison with other things.[67] Universal light will result from scrutinizing the three sources of 'light' (the world, mankind, and God) with these three 'eyes' (of sense, reason, and faith) with the assistance of the three kinds of method (analysis, synthesis, and syncrisis). Universal harmony will result from bringing these three into concord with one another.[68] Finally, the universal institutions prescribed in the penultimate section of the *Consultatio*, the 'Panorthosia', for restoring these three domains to perfection are likewise based on the same triad: the universal bond of learning will be established by a College of Light, the universal bond of politics by a Court of Peace, and the universal bond of religion by an Ecumenical Consistory.[69] From the intimate details of his pedagogy to the grandiose plans for a new world order, everything in Comenius's *Consultatio*

---

62 *Panegersia*, chap. iv.13; *Panorthosia*, chaps xi–xiii (= *Consultatio*, i, col. 30; ii, cols 499–526).

63 *Panegersia*, chap. iv.25 (= *Consultatio*, i, col. 34).

64 *Panaugia*, chap. viii.8; cf. *Pampaedia*, chap. iii.10; *Panorthosia*, chap. x.51–2 (= *Consultatio*, i, cols 166–70; ii, cols 23, 497); *Didactica magna*, chap. x.5 (*DJAK*, xv/1, p. 78).

65 See *Panaugia*, chaps v, vi, vii resp. (= *Consultatio*, i, cols 138–66).

66 *Panaugia*, chap. viii.8 (= *Consultatio*, i, col. 169).

67 Paraphrasing *Panaugia*, chap. ix.12; cf. *Pampaedia*, chap. vii.16 (= *Consultatio*, i, cols 170–6; ii, cols 89–90); *Analytical Didactic*, pp. 134–7 (*DJAK*, xv/2, pp. 192–3). The Greek noun 'syncrisis' (from *syn*, together, and *krisis*, a choosing, from *krinein*, to decide, judge) means 'a comparison'. In Comenius's scheme, analysis reduces composite wholes to their simplest parts, synthesis recombines these parts to understand complex entities, and syncrisis compares complex entities and their parts with one another.

68 *Panaugia*, chap. x; *Panorthosia*, chap. xiii.12 (= *Consultatio*, i, cols 177–85; ii, cols. 522–5).

69 *Panorthosia*, chaps xv–xviii (= *Consultatio*, ii, cols 533–59).

catholica is therefore designed to bring about the instauration of the image of God in man. The universal reform of human affairs, in other words, was grounded in a conception of human nature. The 'instauratio imaginis Dei in homine' provided the blueprint for the 'rerum humanarum emendatio'.

Universal reform and Reformed orthodoxy

Having grasped the purpose of Comenian universal reform as an *instauratio imaginis Dei in homine*, it is now possible to describe concisely its relationship to the purpose of Baconian reform as an *instauratio magna imperii humani in universum*. In essence, the Baconian programme provided the operative element least well developed in the encyclopaedic tradition of Heidelberg, Danzig, and Herborn. A strong practical orientation, to be sure, was fundamental to this tradition from the beginning. The Calvinizing wave of further reform from which this encyclopaedic project emerged was ultimately devoted to the reformation of a broad range of practical affairs. The Ramist tradition institutionalized as a key agent of that reform, with its emphasis on *praxis* and *usus*, reinforced this practical aspect of Herborn pedagogy from the start.[70] Alsted included the reform of the operative or poetic faculty in his encyclopaedic plans, added to the second and definitive edition of the *Encyclopaedia* an unprecedented systematic treatment of the mechanical arts (to complement the previous attention to the liberal arts), and also reprinted a list of desired natural histories taken directly from Bacon's *Novum Organum*.[71] But the academic setting dictated that this practical emphasis would be secondary, and the Herborn encyclopaedic tradition had reached its final shape before Bacon's programme was announced in print. It was therefore left to Comenius to insert the Baconian instauration into the Alstedian one. The Baconian restoration of man's dominion over nature added precisely the operative dimension least well developed in the Herborn encyclopaedic tradition. Simply formulated, the broad contours of the Comenian 'emendation of human affairs' resulted from slotting the Baconian restoration of man's dominion over creation into the central European Reformed encyclopaedic project of restoring the image of God as a whole, of which dominion over creation was one part.

The theological boldness with which Comenius developed this idea, disregarding the constraints of Reformed theology, would have surprised even his most liberal predecessors. In the cases of Keckermann and Alsted, it is difficult to determine precisely at which point, if at all, they slip outside the theological mainstream of the Reformed tradition.[72] Comenius, raised as he was outside the

---

70   Gerhard Menk, *Die Hohe Schule Herborn in ihrer Frühzeit* (Wiesbaden, 1981), pp. 203–17; Hotson, *Alsted*, pp. 15–24.

71   Alsted, *Encyclopaedia*, ii, pp. 1859–1956. Cf. *ibid.*, ii, p. 2021 with Bacon, *Works*, i, pp. 406–10.

72   Hotson, *Alsted*, pp. 73–8.

heartland of the Reformed tradition, strained the limits of Reformed orthodoxy from the outset and became still bolder as his plans developed. Erasmus had sought to preserve a tiny contribution of human activity in the process of redemption; in the face of Luther's condemnation, Comenius boldly affirmed it.[73] The Philippist Georg Major provoked furious debate by reasserting 'the necessity of good works by the justified for salvation'; Comenius boldly broke with the fundamental doctrine of *sola fide* in emphasizing that it is faith and works together which justify.[74] The Philippist Viktorin Striegel touched off the 'synergist' controversy by insisting that man must work with God in the process of justification and sanctification; Comenius confidently affirmed that God wants man's co-operation in all things.[75] Calvin retained the humanist conception of the image of God as the perfection of man's original faculties, but strongly emphasized that the Fall had damaged, distorted, twisted, and vitiated this original perfection, completely so in regard to man's eternal salvation. Comenius argued in contrast that 'we possess the true originals of God's works fundamentally uncorrupted (meaning the same world which Adam beheld when it was newly created, the same instincts, ideas, and faculties which Adam received from God in the beginning, and the same holy word which flowed from the lips and pens of the saintly prophets and apostles)'.[76] Man's originally sound ideas, desires, and instincts, he insisted, 'do not need to be restored or re-created', but merely, with God's help, 'brought into harmony and controlled'.[77] And he therefore criticized those who 'continually complain of our corrupt state, but make no effort to reform it'.[78] Indeed, what had seemed impossible to the first generation of reformers Comenius proclaimed to be easy: 'it is more natural, and, through the grace of the Holy Spirit, easier for man to become wise, honest, and holy [*sanctum*], than for his progress to become hindered by incidental depravity. For everything returns easily to its own nature'.[79] In short, as the attention of scholars has turned during the past decade for the first time to

73 Cf. for instance *Panegersia*, chap. viii.26; *Panorthosia*, chap. iii.1–15 (= *Consultatio*, i, cols 78–9; ii, cols 399–407).

74 Josef Smolík, 'Comenius on justification and sanctification', *Communio viatorum*, 4 (1998), 137–44; repr. in *Justification and Sanctification in the Traditions of the Reformation*, ed. Milan Opocenský and Páraic Réamonn (Geneva, 1999), pp. 123–8.

75 *Panegersia*, chap. viii.24–6; *Panorthosia*, chap. iii.5–15 (= *Consultatio*, i, col. 77–8; ii, cols 402–7). Otokar A. Funda, 'Der Gedanke des Synergismus in der Theologie von Johann Amos Comenius', and Stanislav Sousedík, 'Comenius' chiliastische Rechtfertigungslehre', in Vladimír J. Dvořák and Jan B. Lášek, eds, *Comenius als Theologe* (Prague, 1998), pp. 155–9, 174–83 resp.

76 *Panaugia*, chap. xv.11 (= *Consultatio*, i, col. 231).

77 *Panegersia*, chap. viii.2 (= *Consultatio*, i, col. 68). Cf. *Didactica magna*, chap.v.13–17 (*DJAK*, xv/1, pp. 64–5); *Panegersia*, chap. viii.14 (= *Consultatio*, i, col. 72).

78 *Didactica magna*, chaps v.21–5, xii.14 (*DJAK* xv/1, pp. 65–7, 85–6).

79 *Didactica magna*, chap. v. 25 (*DJAK*, xv/1, pp. 66–7); cf. *Analytical Didactic*, p. 111 (*DJAK*, xv/2, p. 180); *Pampaedia*, chaps ii.21–2, iv.16, vii.17; *Panorthosia*, chap. iii.16–18 (= *Consultatio*, ii, cols 21–2, 52, 91, 407–9).

Comenius's theology, the proximity of his soteriology to humanist teaching has become increasingly apparent.

Given these innovations, it is scarcely surprising that Comenius was repeatedly charged with Pelagianism, that is, with implying that the human will plays an active part in the process of salvation and sanctification. The very first publication of a sketch of his pansophic project, the *Pansophiae praeludium*, provoked such charges both within and outside his own confession. When Joachim Hübner, acting on Hartlib's behalf, sought to obtain permission to print the work in Oxford in 1637, the vice-chancellor of the university, acting as censor, objected that Comenius 'Pelagianizes in various places'. Fortunately, a Moravian theologian was in Oxford at the time and managed to convince the censor 'that he, Mr. Comenius, was indeed orthodox, and stands neither with Pelagians nor Socinians, and what he says *de excellentia Naturae humanae*, refers only *ad Philosophiam* and by no means *ad Theologiam*' – precisely the arguments which Keckermann and Alsted had used to deflect theological criticism from their encyclopaedic efforts to repair man's fallen faculties.[80] Far more strenuous, detailed, and damaging was the assault against the work by a leading lay member of Comenius's own confession: the Senior of the Polish Unity of Brethren, Hieronim Broniewski. Broniewski catalogued fifty theological objections to the mere fifty-two pages of the *Praeludium*, accusing Comenius of a host of errors: of mixing heaven and earth, the light of revelation and human reason, the saving work of Christ and the depraved human will, the *status integritatis, corruptionis, et gratiae*; of failing to acknowledge the burden of original sin; and of attempting to restore the ruined divine image not through the central dogmas of faith but by means of a rational, pedagogical discipline.[81] Whether judged by the prevailing standards of Reformed orthodoxy or by the particular rules of the Unity of Brethren, Comenian pansophia transgressed the boundaries of orthodoxy from the very outset. Similar criticisms would dog Comenius throughout his long career.[82]

80   Hübner (Oxford) to Hartlib, 12 June 1637; in Kvačala, ed., *Korrespondence Komenského*, i, p. 28; and Kvačala, ed., *Reform*, i, p. 91; cf. Blekastad, *Comenius*, p. 253; Hotson, *Alsted*, p. 74.

81   Broniewski, 'Annotatiuncula quædam in præludia Comeniana ad Portam Sapientiæ' (HP 7/62/1A–4B); Broniewski (Skoki) to Orminius. 5 Jan. 1639 (HP 7/62/4B–6A); both printed in G.H. Turnbull, *Hartlib, Dury and Comenius: Gleanings from Hartlib's Papers* (London, 1947), pp. 452–7. For context, cf. *ibid.*, p. 348; Blekastad, *Comenius*, pp. 257–60.

82   Equally critical is the anonymous manuscript 'In pansophiae librum annotationes' (HP 18/22/1A–6B), on which see Dagmar Čapková, 'The reception given to the *Prodromus pansophiae* and the methodology of Comenius', *Acta Comeniana*, 7 (1987), 37–59. Maresius also apparently accused Comenius of being a synergist and condemned his views on justification: cf. Smolík, 'Comenius on justification', p. 137; Wilhelmus Rood, *Comenius and the Low Countries* (Amsterdam, Prague, and New York, 1970), p. 202.

Boldly reasserting synergism and justification by works, however, did not exhaust Comenius's novelty on this crucial point. Beyond passive justification by faith and active justification by works, Comenius glimpsed a still higher prospect: the everlasting justification by the essential righteousness of God, participation in the very being of God, in a word 'deification'. Alien as such a doctrine may seem to mainstream Protestant theology, it represents a straightforward extension – one might say an apotheosis – of this tradition of the instauration of the image of God in man.

For Keckermann and Alsted, the motivations driving the attempt to repair the divine image were certain principles of action, intrinsic to human nature and damaged but not destroyed by the Fall, such as that enunciated at the outset of Aristotle's metaphysics: 'All men by nature desire to know'.[83] Knowledge, however, is one of the three key components of the image of God in man; and since God's knowledge is infinite, Comenius argued that human beings, made in God's image, likewise desire not only to know but to know all things. The same applies to the volitional and active faculties as well: 'The three faculties are of infinite extent, since as a rule the mind can think infinite thoughts, the will can wish infinite wishes, and the active faculty can contrive one action after another unto infinity. Clearly God has stamped the human soul with his own infinite powers of omniscience, omnivolence, and omnipotence'.[84] In a word, 'human nature positively seeks perfection'.[85] Pushing the Aristotelian dictum to its greatest possible level of generality, Comenius ultimately grounded the entire pansophic undertaking in the observation that 'man by nature desires to be deified'. In fact, 'every being desires to be perfected and elevated'; and since 'man regards nothing as more elevated than God, he therefore desires to become like God'.[86] It was, Comenius acknowledged, by this very desire that man was caught and deceived by Satan at the beginning; but Comenius, at the very end of his long life, had clearly concluded that this same desire, like the other innate appetites which motivated the entire pansophic striving, was put in place by the Creator, preserved from the Fall, and would ultimately be fulfilled by the highest form of justification, the 'justification by the essential righteousness of God'.[87]

---

83   Aristotle, *Metaphysics*, book I (A) 1.

84   *Panegersia*, chap. ix.14 (= *Consultatio*, i, col. 149). Cf. *Didactica Magna*, chap. v.4 (*DJAK*, xv/1, p. 61); *Panegersia*, chap. ix.17, 37; *Panaugia*, chap. vi.17, 25; *Panorthosia*, chap. ii.15 (= *Consultatio*, i, cols 87, 97–8, 149, 151–2; ii, col. 377 resp.)

85   *Panegersia*, chap. viii.3, 9 (= *Consultatio*, i, cols 68–9, 70).

86   Comenius, *Unum necessarium* (Amsterdam 1668), chap. viii.4 (*DJAK*, xviii, p. 115): 'Si sublimiùs vellemus loqui, *Christianus homo Christo conformis perque conformitatem illam Deificandus*. Nam homo per naturam Deificari appetit: quia cùm omne ens perfici ac sublimari appetat, homo autem nihil se sublimius habeat praeter Deum, appetit ergò fieri sicut Deus'.

87   See *Panorthosia*, chap. viii.49–53 (= *Consultatio*, ii, cols 459–63), esp. chap. viii.52, where Comenius distinguished between three kinds of justification: 'justificari fide', 'justificari operibus', and 'justificari essentiali justitiâ Dei, quae et ipsa jam nobis

Josef Smolík, commenting recently on several of these passages, has described this emphasis on 'deification' as 'an absolutely new element in Comenius' concept of justification' and one 'wholly alien to Reformation teaching on justification and sanctification'.[88] The doctrine of *theosis* has in fact a pedigree which is both long and unorthodox: it can be traced back through Anabaptists, mystics, and gnostics to Patristic Neoplatonists such as Origen, whom Comenius cited in this regard in the *Unum necessarium*.[89] It was not, moreover, entirely unknown to Comenius's immediate teachers: within his *Encyclopaedia*, Alsted discusses 'deification' both in the peroration of his treatment of theology and, more strikingly still, as the summit of the ten grades of cabbalistic knowledge. Moreover, the key passage on cabbalistic knowledge in the *Encyclopaedia* of 1630 is reproduced almost without alteration from Alsted's first encyclopaedic work, the *Systema mnemonicum maius* of 1609/10, which antedates Comenius's studies with him in Herborn.[90]

Tracing the most radical expression of Comenius's pansophic aspirations not only to Reformed, Philippist, and humanist theology and pedagogy but to the Cabbala concludes this brief excavation with an unexpected but suggestive finding. Closely intertwined with the roots of this tradition of encyclopaedic pedagogy in Reformed theology and Christian humanism were other roots – often more subtle, but perhaps also more profound – in still less orthodox intellectual traditions. The Neoplatonic themes and humanist anthropology, first enunciated by the church Fathers, revived during the Renaissance by Christian humanists, preserved in various modified forms by Calvin, Melanchthon, and the Philippist 'crypto-Calvinists', and developed by Keckermann and Alsted as the foundations for that community's great encyclopaedic enterprise, were also being developed simultaneously in more radical ways by representatives of other intellectual traditions overlapping in still poorly understood ways with the Reformed: Paracelsians, alchemists, Hermeticists, Lullists, mystics, would-be Rosicrucians, spiritualists, Arminians, and Socinians to name a few of the most important. While Althusius, Martinius, and Keckermann shunned such traditions, Alsted was clearly fascinated

---

communicatur per Christum Deum-hominem': 'Denum in ipsam usque Christi divinitatem penetrandum...: quatenus Filius Dei particeps factus humanae naturae, nos rursum participes fecit divinae naturae (2 Pet. 1. 4.)'.

88   Smolík, 'Comenius on justification', pp. 139–40; reprinted with improved translation in Opocenský and Réamonn, *Justification and Sanctification*, pp. 125, 126.

89   For the history of the term, cf. Cairns, *Image of God*, pp. 102–9; Jaroslav Pelikan, *The Christian Tradition* (5 vols, Chicago, 1971–89), i, pp. 344–6; ii, pp. 10–16; iv, pp. 66–8, 319, 359; Ben Drewery, 'Deification', in Peter Brook, ed., *Christian Spirituality: Essays in Honour of Gordon Rupp* (London, 1975), pp. 33–62; Martin Schmidt, *Wiedergeburt und Neuer Mensch. Gesammelte Studien zur Geschichte des Pietismus* (Witten, 1969), pp. 238–98.

90   Cf. Alsted, *Systema mnemonicum duplex, I. minus...II. maius...*(2 parts, Frankfurt am Main, 1610), part i (= *Artium liberalium systema mnemonicum*, 2 vols), i, pp. 374–6 with *Encyclopaedia*, ii, pp. 1690.b, 2271.a.2. For discussion see Hotson, *Alsted*, pp. 158–60.

by many of them from his youth onward and passed on his fascination to favoured students such as Josua von der Tann, Johann Heinrich Bisterfeld, and Jan Amos Comenius.[91] Within these traditions, ostensibly orthodox writers like Alsted found many of the leading ideas and aspirations expressed and developed with a boldness which both inspired them and prevented them from citing these works as defensible authorities. The necessary brevity of the present essay provides a convenient pretext for declining to trace the still deeper but even more elusive roots of the 'instauratio imaginis Dei' through these tangled traditions. More plausible still is the closing disclaimer that, if any living scholar is equipped to undertake this daunting task, it is the person to whom this volume is dedicated: Charles Webster.

---

91   On von der Tann see Hotson, *Alsted*, pp. 144–53; on Alsted's encouragement of Bisterfeld's interests in these traditions, cf. *ibid.*, pp. 160, 180, 173, 231; Maria Rosa Antognazza, 'Bisterfeld and *immeatio*: origins of a key concept in the early modern doctrine of universal harmony', in Martin Mulsow, ed., *Spätrenaissance-Philosophie in Deutschland, 1570–1650* (Wiesbaden, forthcoming).

Chapter 2

Harmony, Health, and Healing: Music's Role in Early Modern Paracelsian Thought

Penelope Gouk

Probably the first of the great European physicians to exhibit a love for music was Paracelsus (1493–1541), who achieved fame as the precursor of chemical pharmacology and therapeutics. He is known as the most original medical thinker of the sixteenth century. Music played an important part in his fascinating life. As a boy Paracelsus worked for Orgelmeister Konrad Parimaun of Nuernberg. In 1480 [sic] he was taken by Prince Sigismund to Innsbruck where he became the palace organist. Later, he was palace organist for King Maximilian, who knighted him in 1525. After the king's death Paracelsus became church organist in Salzburg. He was famous throughout all Germany as an organist, composer, and instrument builder as well. Among his published musical compositions were 'Marienlieder', 'Ach Lieb mit Leid' and some twenty others.[1]

Or so claimed Willard Marmelszadt in *Musical Sons of Aesculapius*, a work the author saw into print in 1946 despite being on active duty with the Medical Corps of the United States Navy. In reality, Paracelsus was neither composer nor organist, and to the best of my knowledge, music played no significant part in his life or thought. The reason why no other scholar has ever noticed Paracelsus's extraordinary musical skills is that Marmelszadt seems to have confused him with another (yet to be identified) historical figure altogether.

I encountered this ridiculous statement shortly after deciding to write on the subject of music and Paracelsianism for my contribution to this volume, which seemed especially appropriate since I first wrote about Paracelsus as an undergraduate taking Charles Webster's Special Subject in the Scientific Revolution, and it was at his suggestion that I went on to study the role of music in early modern scientific thought at the Warburg Institute.[2] My choice of topic was prompted by the realization that although several well-known Paracelsian physicians – notably

---

1 Willard Marmelszadt, *Musical Sons of Aesculapius* (New York, 1946), pp. 24–5.
2 Penelope Gouk, 'Music in the natural philosophy of the early Royal Society', unpublished London University Ph.D. thesis (1982).

Heinrich Khunrath (1560–1605), Robert Fludd (1574–1637), and Michael Maier (1568–1622) – figure prominently in my latest research project, which is exploring how medical theories about music's effects changed during the early modern period, I had not yet addressed the relationship between the explicitly 'Paracelsian' interests of these doctors and their musical interests.

The existence of such a relationship is not in doubt. Maier, for example, composed his own music for the *Atalanta Fugiens* (1618) which was published by Johann Theodore de Bry at Oppenheim. This is a book of fifty alchemical emblems which have a musical, as well as pictorial, mode of expression. Each emblem comprises an image (engraved by Matthieu Merian, De Bry's son-in-law), a motto and epigram drawn from well-known Latin and Arabic alchemical sources, and a three-part musical setting of the epigram, where each voice represents one of the three Paracelsian principles of salt, sulphur, and mercury.[3] A comparable linkage between alchemical and musical principles is made in Fludd's striking image of 'man the microcosm' found in his *Utriusque cosmi...historia*, a work which not coincidentally was also published in Oppenheim by De Bry between 1617 and 1619. Here the harmony between body and soul, a connection which physicians understood to be mediated through the animal spirits, is represented metaphorically as a musical string, the basic premise being that the human body is the instrument of the soul, and therefore its response to being 'played on' can be understood as analogous to the sympathetic response of a musical instrument to the performer's hand. Fludd's well-known picture of the 'divine monochord' located in an earlier section of his book shows how the relationship between God and his creation is also mediated by both spirit and musical ratios.[4]

By the early eighteenth century, the idea that human bodies were governed by the same mathematical laws as planetary bodies was a medical commonplace. The Leiden medical educator Hermann Boerhaave (1668–1738), for example, notably used Newtonian dynamics to underpin his model of the body as a system reduced

---

3   For a modern translation and edition of this work see Joscelyn Godwin, *Michael Maier's Atalanta Fugiens – An Edition of the Emblems, Fugues, and Epigrams*, with a commentary by Hildemarie Streich (Grand Rapids, 1989). For the broader intellectual and political context of Maier's alchemy see Bruce T. Moran, *The Alchemical World of the German Court: Occult Philosophy and Chemical Medicine in the Circle of Moritz of Hessen (1572–1632)* (Stuttgart, 1991), pp. 102–14.

4   Penelope Gouk, *Music, Science and Natural Magic in Seventeenth-Century England* (New Haven and London, 1999), especially pp. 146–7, 95–101; Gouk, 'Music, melancholy and medical spirits in early modern thought', in P. Horden, ed., *Music as Medicine: The History of Music Therapy since Antiquity* (Aldershot, 2000), pp. 173–94; also Joscelyn Godwin, *Robert Fludd: Hermetic Philosopher and Surveyor of Two Worlds* (London, 1979). On the links between Fludd and Maier see Moran, *Alchemical World*, pp. 107–11, and Frances A. Yates, *The Rosicrucian Enlightenment* (London, 1972), chap. 6.

to the motion of fluids (humours) and solids (fibres).[5] However, it is Fludd who seems to have been the first physician actually to 'picture' the occult mechanisms of the body in terms of vibrating strings and subtle fluids. Long before Newton provided the mathematics to legitimate this kind of physiological model, Fludd asserted that the same invisible mechanisms were governing cosmic and human bodies, as well as the relationships between these realms.[6] Such a belief was hardly unique to Fludd, of course; the harmony between macrocosm and microcosm was something every early modern Paracelsian, and indeed most intellectuals at the time, apparently took for granted.

The search for harmony and the 'patronage of despair'

One of the best pieces of evidence to support this statement is the image of Heinrich Khunrath's alchemical laboratory, an engraving which Allen Debus in particular has used to characterize the most distinctive features of Paracelsian natural magic and chemical philosophy (Figure 1). Taken from Khunrath's *Amphitheatrum sapientiae aeternae* (1st edn 1595, 2nd edn 1609), this picture is the earliest known representation of a 'laboratory', or rather laboratory-cum-oratory, a private inner sanctum where Khunrath, presenting himself as a pious Christian magus, is depicted at prayer and experimental work. Over the last few decades this image has served historians well, not only as a means of demonstrating the connection between Paracelsianism as an experimentally-grounded practice and the emergence of modern science, but also for exploring the linkage between Paracelsianism as a system of reformed medicine and the Reformation itself.[7]

Of course, the emerging new science was hardly a Protestant monopoly, but recent work by Heller, Grell, and Cunningham certainly confirms the intimate

---

5   See, for example, Andrew Cunningham, 'Medicine to calm the mind: Boerhaave's medical system, and why it was adopted in Edinburgh', in A. Cunningham and R. French, eds, *The Medical Enlightenment of the Eighteenth Century* (Cambridge, 1990), pp. 40–66.

6   Penelope Gouk, 'Musical models in natural philosophy in the time of Thomas Harriot', *Durham Thomas Harriot Seminar Occasional Papers*, 29 (1999), 1–32; also Gouk, 'The role of harmonics in the Scientific Revolution', in *The Cambridge History of Western Music Theory*, ed. Thomas Christensen (Cambridge, 2002), pp. 223–45.

7   Allen G. Debus, 'The medico-chemical world of the Paracelsians', in *Changing Perspectives in the History of Science: Essays in Honour of Joseph Needham*, ed. M. Teich and R.M. Young (London, 1973), pp. 85–99. The same image is used in Urszula Szulakowska, 'Geometry and optics in Renaissance alchemical illustration: John Dee, Robert Fludd and Michael Maier', *Studies in Hermeticism*, 14 (1995), 1–12, and Szulakowska, *The Alchemy of Light. Geometry and Optics in Late Renaissance Alchemical Illustration* (Leiden, Boston and Koeln, 2000).

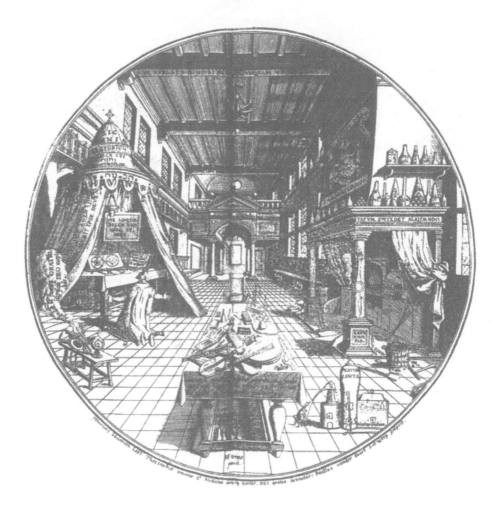

Figure 1   Alchemical laboratory from Heinrich Khunrath, *Amphitheatrum sapientiae aeternae* **(1609)**

association that Webster first argued for in the *Great Instauration* between new, experimentally-based methods of advancing knowledge, and the anticipation of Christ's second coming among those who considered themselves as God's elect.[8] And while it may be simplistic to treat this picture as representative of Paracelsianism as a whole, it is certainly an apt portrayal of the 'cosmotheological Paracelsianism' that Khunrath, Fludd and Maier were promoting in (mostly Protestant) courts across Europe during the first decades of the seventeenth century.[9] In particular they looked to support from the Landgraf Moritz of Hessen (1572–1632), whose court at Kassel outflanked even that of the Holy Roman Emperor as the centre of occult patronage prior to the outbreak of the Thirty Years' War.[10]

The zeal with which the Landgraf promoted his universalist vision arose from the fragmentation he saw around him. While his political authority deteriorated, Moritz increasingly focused on integrating the occult arts with the traditional theology, medicine and philosophy taught at the university of Marburg. At the same time his Kassel court acted as a magnet for a wide spectrum of alchemists, Paracelsians, and other mystical philosophers whose universalist doctrines offered an 'intellectual balsam' for religious and political confusion.[11] As Bruce Moran has persuasively argued, this official court ideology 'became a surrogate reality, and it is in this sense that its patronage, as much at Hessen-Kassel as at other German courts, became finally a patronage of despair'.[12] Moran sees Moritz gradually turning inwards, finding 'psychological refuge' in a magical and experimentally-

---

8   Henry Heller, *Labour, Science and Technology in France 1500-1620* (Cambridge, 1996); Ole Peter Grell, ed., *Paracelsus: The Man and his Reputation, his Ideas and their Transformations* (Leiden and Boston, 1998); also Ole Peter Grell and Andrew Cunningham, eds, *Medicine and the Reformation* (Cambridge, 1993).

9   I borrow the term 'cosmotheological' from Stephen Pumfrey, 'The spagyric art: or, the impossible work of separating pure from impure Paracelsianism: a historiographical analysis', in *Paracelsus*, ed. Grell, pp. 21–51 (especially p. 51). For more details on the place of music in the cultural lives of Khunrath, Fludd and Maier, see my article 'Doctors and practitioners: music and medicine as paradigms of the arts-science divide in early modern Europe', in *Scientiae et artes. Die Vermittlung alten und neuen Wissens in Literatur, Kunst und Musik*, ed. Barbara Mahlmann-Bauer (Wiesbaden, 2004), pp. 161–88.

10   Moran, *Alchemical World*, p. 8.

11   *Ibid.*, p. 25. The relationship between Paracelsianism (and other occult disciplines) and specific confessional and political loyalties is a vexed one. As Howard Hotson aptly puts it, 'we lack an adequate map of the confessional options in learned Germany in this period and how they relate to one another' (personal communication with the author). For the purposes of this chapter, what seems to be significant about the 'cosmotheological' or 'courtly' Paracelsianism I am describing here is its elusive and transformative nature; i.e. it is not tied to a specific creed or dogma, but is rather a mode of being or 'form of life' guided by mystical revelation and the inner light of Christ.

12   Moran, *Alchemical World*, p. 25.

based philosophy that would not only provide effective medicines for individuals, but would also restore health to the social body through enlightened religious reform. According to Robert Evans, spiritual contemplation and experimental practice were equally central to the occult philosophy cultivated at Prague: just like Moritz, who also abdicated in despair, Rudolf became ever more devoted to the pursuit of arcane knowledge and secret power as his temporal power ebbed away.[13]

This convergence between failing political aspirations, occult philosophy and Paracelsian medicine is already familiar to historians, even if not entirely understood. Moritz and Rudolf were not alone in finding the extravagant claims of learned Paracelsian physicians like Khunrath deeply attractive. Their occult philosophy promised the salvation of mankind through the intuitions of an intellectual elite, extraordinary individuals who alone among men were equipped to take on this arduous task. Thus, for example, although the alchemical laboratory depicted in the *Amphitheatrum sapientiae aeternae* is meant to be Khunrath's place of work and prayer, the image is also meant to embody the lofty ideals and pious practices of Europe's most noble living alchemists. There is, however, a paradox at the heart of Khunrath's picture which has been explored neither in relation to early modern Paracelsian thought, nor even in relation to Paracelsus himself.

One of the most prominent features of Khunrath's Paracelsian laboratory is the group of musical instruments and music books lying on the table at the very front of the picture, the tablecloth itself being decorated with an inscription that may be translated as 'Sacred music is the escape from sadness and evil spirits because the spirit (SPIRITUS) rejoices cheerfully in a heart filled with pious joy' – a sentiment whose significance we shall return to shortly below. However, despite evidently being central to Khunrath's vision, music's relevance to his laboratory, and the functions it serves in this private sanctum, have not been adequately investigated by historians. Debus, for example, explains the presence of these instruments simply in terms of music being a metaphor for the harmony between macrocosm and microcosm, which is a central principle of Paracelsian magical doctrine. However, he says nothing about the musical instruments themselves, nor does he speculate how they might be relevant to either alchemy or prayer beyond a general appeal to Neoplatonic principles.

This neglect by Debus is hardly surprising, given Paracelsus's own apparent neglect of music. Despite Marmelszadt's wishful portrayal of the reformer as composer and organist, Paracelsus was clearly not a musician, and although he used the concept of 'harmony' in his writing, he never explored the musical significance of this harmony. Indeed – with what seems to be a single exception to prove the rule – he never wrote on music at all. Paracelsus's own reticence on the subject

13   Robert Evans, *Rudolf II and His World: A Study in Intellectual History 1576–1612* (Oxford, 1973, paperback edition 1984), especially pp. 196–42.

is surely the most likely reason why historians have overlooked music in their exploration of his ideas as well as their later transmission and reception.[14]

The brief remarks that Paracelsus did make about music are found in his early treatise, *De religione perpetua* [On the perennial religion], a text that was widely copied in manuscript form, and therefore may conceivably have been known to Khunrath and other later Paracelsians.[15] The context is a discussion of the benefits that come to the pious doctor from following the 'religion of medicine'. These include an intuitive grasp of appropriate remedies for particular ailments, empirical knowledge that is based on the localized, every-day experience of practitioners, and the magical 'doctrine of signatures' rather than elite university learning. Crucially for my analysis of Khunrath's image in the following section, Paracelsus identifies '*Musica*' (the word harmony is not used here) as a cure for melancholy and morbid imagination [*Fantasey*], notably its capacity to take away the melancholy of those 'who belong to the Baptists and similar sects', being a remedy which also drives away 'the spirits used by witches, by the malevolent, and in sorcery' to inflict suffering on people. Paracelsus likens music to a garden, in that just as there are appropriate plants for curing particular illnesses, so appropriate music can be used to cure disorders of the brain and mind.[16] Here, in a nutshell, is everything that mattered about music to those early modern doctors who, like Paracelsus, sought to heal souls as well as bodies: that is, its power to counteract melancholy, and its natural affinity with spirits that can be used to affect the human imagination. Although the *De religione perpetua* does not state it explicitly, Paracelsus evidently regarded music (or certain types of music) as a kind of natural magic. That is to say, its power to inflame or moderate the passions of the soul (and thereby to either cause or cure disease), arose from an individual's ability to manipulate spirit at a distance, by purely natural means, rather than by the employment of intelligences or miraculous powers.[17]

Paracelsus has nothing further to say about the place of music in this complex of ideas on the 'religion of medicine'. Indeed, given that his own religious

---

14   See, for example, the essays in Grell, ed., *Paracelsus*. Christoph Meinel earlier argued for a lack of any 'real' connection between these arts in his 'Alchemie und Musik' in Christoph Meinel, ed., *Die Alchemie in der europäischen Kultur- und Wissenschaft Geschichte* (Wiesbaden, 1986), pp. 201–27.

15   Charles Webster, 'Paracelsus, Paracelsianism, and the secularization of the worldview', *Science in Context*, 15 (2002), 9–27, at p. 21.

16   Extract from Karl Sudhoff, *Versuch einer Kritik der Echtheit der Paracelsischen Schriften*, II, pt 1 (Berlin, 1898), p. 419, partly translated in Horden, *Music as Medicine*, p. 152.

17   On natural magic see Charles Webster, *From Paracelsus to Newton: Magic and the Making of Modern Science* (Cambridge, 1982), especially pp. 57–62; also Walker, 'General theory of natural magic', in his *Spiritual and Demonic Magic from Ficino to Campanella* (London, 1958), pp. 75–84; and Penelope Gouk, 'Natural philosophy and natural magic', in E. Fuciková, ed., *Rudolf II and Prague: The Court and the City* (London, 1997), pp. 231–8.

radicalism 'made him generally hostile to liturgy and ritual incantation' (to use Peregrine Horden's words), these fleeting remarks on the curative virtue of music seem even more puzzling.[18] Yet although Paracelsus's own ideas may never be recovered, we can, I believe, begin to establish why music mattered so much to a Paracelsian like Khunrath (or Maier, or Fludd), in particular why it should occupy centre stage, as it were, in the representation of his alchemical laboratory. This image has already revealed a great deal to historians about the experimental form of life that occult and courtly Paracelsians were representing to their audiences.[19] My suggestion is that we should also enter imaginatively into the aural, as well as visual, space occupied by Khunrath's laboratory design.[20] This is because in keeping with the magical worldview shared by these Paracelsians, simply 'reading' an image such as this is not sufficient; its inner meaning must also be grasped through 'listening' to the sounds that are tacitly embodied here.[21] We can then begin to investigate why music – as articulated sound, as a body of instrumental practices – was so important to their experimental agenda; and also where they got this idea from, if not from Paracelsus himself.

Experimental identities: the Christian magus

The image of Khunrath as a Christian magus was designed by Hans Vredeman de Vries, a Huguenot exile from Antwerp who was in Hamburg around 1595 (when Khunrath was there), and engraved by Paul van der Doort, another Huguenot who was at that time superintendent of the Dutch poor in Hamburg. Through a skilful use of perspective the reader is invited to enter the alchemist's laboratory where he is engaged in his private labours and devotions. In fact the picture itself (as its mandala form signifies) is intended to serve as a meditative vehicle for lifting the viewer's soul up towards the divine, in sympathy, as it were, with Khunrath's own spiritual exercises. In terms of iconography the picture belongs to an emblematic tradition of 'Melancholia', a visual convention that began with Albrecht Dürer's famous engraving *Melencholia I* of 1514, but which had its theoretical origins in Marsilio Ficino's *De triplici vita*, or *Three Books on Life* (1489) and was further

18   Horden, *Music as Medicine*, p. 152.
19   See for example Szulakowska, *Alchemy of Light*, pp. 129–37. For other relevant examples of early modern laboratory design and experimental identity, see Owen Hannaway, 'Laboratory design and the aim of science', *Isis*, 77 (1986), 585–610, and Steven Shapin, '"A scholar and a gentleman": the problematic identity of the scientific practitioner in early modern England', *History of Science*, 29 (1991), 279–327.
20   I am grateful to Peter Forshaw for allowing me to read sections of his forthcoming University of London Ph.D. thesis on '*Ora et labora*: alchemy, magic, and Cabala in Heinrich Khunrath's *Amphitheatrum sapientiae aeternae* (1609)'.
21   For an introduction to how this might be done, see Bruce R. Smith, *The Acoustic World of Early Modern England: Attending to the O-Factor* (Chicago and London, 1999).

popularized in Heinrich Cornelius Agrippa's *De occulta philosophia* (published 1533, circulated in manuscript already around 1510).[22]

In brief, this tradition assumes that the philosopher engaged in pursuit of the higher, contemplative sciences which are under the influence of Saturn is likely to suffer melancholy, a condition normally ascribed to an excess of black bile (choler) which was concocted in the spleen and tended to gather around the heart. This state was thought to be exacerbated by depletion of the animal spirits, which early modern physicians understood to be a vital, vaporous substance generated out of the blood and stored in the brain, and which served as the first instrument of the soul. Loss of spirit allowed choler to accumulate in the blood and caused it to be sluggish, a condition which in turn led to a whole array of symptoms, from torpor to flatulence. Although the condition of melancholy was familiar to western physicians through their knowledge of Galen, it was Ficino who first observed that introspective philosophers are liable to become melancholic because they 'seem wholly to neglect that instrument with which they are able in a way to measure and grasp the whole world', and therefore to maintain health, need constantly to replenish and nourish these spirits.[23]

Around 1600, just as in Ficino's time, most types of melancholy were thought to be unpleasant states of disease, in which balance of mind was temporarily upset due to a range of psychological and/or physical factors triggered by too much choler. The kind of melancholy Khunrath presents here (and which Ficino had been most interested in), was an altogether more attractive and rare condition, possessed by those who are constitutionally melancholic rather than suffering a temporary imbalance of humours. The natural melancholic has a special sensibility which makes him permanently different from other men, a condition limited to those 'most fit to undertake matters of weightie charge and high attempt', according to Andreas Laurentius, Huguenot physician-in-ordinary to Henri IV and author of the

22   These texts were also key sources for the aural/musical dimension of this tradition, first explored in Walker, *Spiritual and Demonic Magic*. See also Raymond Klibansky, Ernst Panofsky and Fritz Saxl, *Saturn and Melancholy: Studies in the History of Natural Philosophy, Religion and Art* (Cambridge, 1964).

23   The linkage which Ficino makes between the medical notion of melancholy and Platonic frenzy, or enthusiasm, was first made in the pseudo-Aristotelian *Problems* XXX and later taken up by Rufus of Ephesus. The latter's treatise *On melancholy* (first half of second century AD) made activity of the mind the direct cause of melancholy illness; see Klibansky et al., *Saturn and Melancholy*, pp. 17, 49; also Carol V. Kaske and John R. Clark, eds, *Marsilio Ficino: Three Books on Life. A Critical Edition and Translation with Introduction and Notes* (Binghampton, NY, 1989), quotation p. 111. Compare Agrippa's explanation in Book I, cap. 60 of Henry Cornelius Agrippa, *Three Books of Occult Philosophy Translated by J.F.* (London, 1651). For later theories of spirits, see D.P. Walker, 'Medical spirits in philosophy and theology from Ficino to Newton', in *Arts du spectacle et histoire des idées* (Tours, 1984), pp. 287–300, reprinted in D.P. Walker, *Music, Spirit and Language in the Renaissance*, ed. P. Gouk (London, 1985). See also Gouk, 'Music, melancholy and medical spirits'.

internationally best-selling treatise *On Melancholike Diseases* (first published in French 1594, English edn 1599). These extraordinary and noble individuals had extremely pure spirits, which on being heated up occasioned 'divine ravishment, commonly called *Enthousiasma*, which stirreth men up to plaie the Philosophers, Poets, and also to prophesie much'.[24] Although enthusiasm was to become totally discredited by the end of the seventeenth century, in Khunrath's ideal world, a world inhabited by melancholic patrons like Rudolf and Moritz, it was a state to be aspired to by the pious Christian 'Theosopher' – the lover of divine wisdom and enlightened doctor of medicine he was being portrayed as here.

The altar on the left and the alchemical apparatus on the right together represent the dual means by which divine knowledge is to be achieved, that is through revelation and empirical investigation. Leaving aside the complexities of Khunrath's cabbalistical theology for the moment, we may simply note that this twofold approach is identical to that articulated by another courtly Protestant Paracelsian, Oswald Croll (c.1560–1609), whose *Basilica Chemica* of 1609 'firmly established Paracelsus in the iconography of wisdom in science and medicine'.[25] For Croll, the physician's vocation was nothing less than to be a true follower of Christ; a reformer of medicine who is illuminated by the light of grace and guided by the Book of Scripture on the one hand, and by the light of nature and its corresponding 'Book' on the other. As suggested in Khunrath's image, adherence to these twin Paracelsian goals of higher knowledge and improvement involves a balance between the search for medicines to heal bodily ills (material alchemy), and the search for medicines to heal and purify the soul, the ultimate purpose of which is to achieve mystical union with the divine (spiritual alchemy).[26] In Khunrath's own case the balance was tipped entirely towards the latter goal, but

24   Andreas Laurentius, *Of Melancholike Diseases; or Rheumes, and of Old Age. Composed by M. Andreas Laurentius, Ordinarie Phisition to the King...Translated out of French into English, According to the Last Edition by Richard Surphlet, Practitioner in Phisicke* (London, 1599), chap. 3, pp. 84–6. The original French version was first published in 1594. On the Platonic theory of the four kinds of enthusiasm (poetic, religious, prophetic, erotic) and its transmission in French literature via Pontus de Tyard's *Solitaire premier* (Lyons, 1552), see Frances A. Yates, *The French Academies of the Sixteenth Century* (London, 1947), pp. 77–87. On the musical representation of melancholy see Richard Freedman, 'Listening to melancholy: Lasso's "Un triste coeur" and the French medical tradition', unpublished paper presented at conference on 'Music and Melancholy, 1400–1800', Music Department, Princeton University, October 2002.

25   Webster, *Paracelsus to Newton*, p. 6. For a masterly exposition of Croll's Paracelsian ideas, and how they differed from those of Paracelsus himself, see Owen Hannaway, *The Chemists and the Word: The Didactic Origins of Chemistry* (Baltimore and London, 1975), esp. chaps 1–3.

26   For further discussion see Karen-Claire Voss, 'Spiritual alchemy: interpreting representative texts and images', in *Gnosis and Hermeticism from Antiquity to Modern Times*, ed. R. van den Broek and Wouter J. Hanegraaff (New York, 1998), accessed on http://www.istanbul-yes-istanbul.co.uk/alchemy/index.htm 8/11/2002.

even in this most rarefied practice there is still the emphasis on instrumental techniques which are used to bring about desirable results through manipulating hidden forces, a context in which music has particular relevance because of its extraordinary power over the imagination and human spirit.

The essential link between prayer and alchemy, of course, is *spiritus*, the vital medium which links the earth to the heavens, dwells within all living things (including metals and stones), connects body and soul, and serves as the vehicle through which the adept's prayers communicate with the divine. In Khunrath's laboratory, however, musical instruments are not just a metaphor for this linkage, but are identified as a third means of facilitating it experimentally. Laid out on the table in the foreground is a group of stringed instruments, together with a set of three part-books, of which one is lying open showing musical staves. On the left are a harp and a bowed stringed instrument (possibly a viol, or a *lira da braccio*; its identity is uncertain), on the right are a lute and a cittern. As I have noted earlier, the inscription on the tablecloth translates as 'Sacred music is the escape from sadness and evil spirits because the spirit (SPIRITUS) rejoices cheerfully in a heart filled with pious joy'. Here is the essence of Khunrath's message: practised in the right way, music may serve as a spiritual discipline which, along with alchemy and prayer, empowers the pious Paracelsian doctor to achieve harmony and well-being – a state desirable not just for his own health, but for that of society more generally. However, not just any music will serve; it is specifically *sacred* music. Again using Agrippa's words, 'there is nothing more efficacious to drive away evil spirits then [sic] Musicall Harmony (for any true consent, as being an enemy to them, but fly from it) as David by his Harp appeased Saul, being troubled with an evil spirit. Hence by the ancient Prophets and Fathers, who knew these Harmonicall mysteries, singing and Musical sounds were brought into sacred services'.[27]

Khunrath's kneeling magus is indeed immediately identifiable with King David, the charismatic leader of the Israelites who was inspired by the Holy Spirit to sing God's praises through voice and harp. David's hymns and incantations evidently served as a direct channel of communication between God and his chosen people. The authority of the Bible made it clear that David's singing or chanting of these words, coupled with the tones of the harp itself, provided a vehicle through which divine mercy and relief from suffering were asked for, and received. Furthermore, as Laurentius points out in his *Of Melancholike Diseases*, it was also via psalmody that David possessed the gift of prophecy, and the power to cure Saul's melancholy – a condition which the French physician ascribed to a physiological disorder in the brain rather than the inspired form of melancholy experienced by the healer himself (i.e. David).[28]

Given this unmistakable reference to the miraculous power of ancient Jewish ceremonies, it is all the more important to realize that the sounds most immediately

27   Agrippa, *Occult Philosophy*, Book II, chap. 28.
28   '*David* also when the evil spirit came upon Saul, made him merrie with his harpe, and
        he found ease thereby': Laurentius, *Of Melancholike Diseases*, p. 107.

evoked in the minds of seventeenth-century readers by this picture would have been modern and popular, rather than ancient and esoteric. The combination of these particular stringed instruments, together with the part-books, strongly suggests a four-part (i.e. polyphonic) motet-like setting of one of the Psalms of David. These were sounds unequivocally associated with a Protestant way of life. The historical reason for this association was that Calvin regarded the psalms as the ideal instrument for restoring to Christianity the authentic and unadulterated worship of the ancient church.[29] While Lutherans certainly included them in their congregational hymns, Calvin believed psalms were the only kind of song that should be used in public worship, since they had been sung by Christ's apostles as well as the Jews. In 1539 Calvin published his first psalter and went on to support an initiative to produce a complete edition of the 150 psalms set to simple melodies, that was first published at Geneva in 1562. Such was the popularity of the Genevan Metrical Psalter that thousands of copies were soon being issued by every major centre of the Protestant book trade. The importance of psalm-singing for the spread of Calvinism across western Europe cannot be overstated; already by the 1540s it had become one of the principal means through which Huguenots maintained their religious identity, sustained themselves in the face of persecution, and attracted new converts to the Protestant cause.[30]

In the wake of this phenomenal success, composers began to use the Genevan Psalter as a basis for more elaborate polyphonic settings (usually in four parts that could be performed with voices and/or instruments including those depicted by Khunrath). These works were initially targeted at Calvinists for their private devotional use, though they became equally popular among other Protestants, and even Catholics. This was because although Calvin explicitly forbad godly citizens to use elaborate polyphony in church, and regarded virtually all secular music as corrupting, he nevertheless held the (Platonic) belief that the *right* kind of harmony, performed under properly controlled conditions, is conducive to a virtuous society, and serves as an indicator of spiritual harmony.[31] Devotional polyphony based on the psalms clearly met these rigorous criteria, and by the time Khunrath's

29   Charles Garside, 'The origins of Calvin's theology of music: 1536–1543', *Transactions of the American Philosophical Society*, 69 (1979), 1–36. See also the extensive entry on 'Psalms, metrical' in Stanley Sadie, ed., *The New Grove Dictionary of Music and Musicians, Second Edition* (29 vols, London, 2001), xx, pp. 483–518.

30   Barbara B. Diefendorf, 'The Huguenot psalter and the faith of French Protestants in the sixteenth century', in *Culture and Identity in Early Modern Europe (1500–1800): Essays in Honor of Natalie Zemon Davis*, ed. Barbara B. Diefendorf and Carla Hesse (Ann Arbor, MI, 1993), pp. 41–63. See also Richard Freedman, *The Chansons of Orlando di Lasso and their Protestant Listeners: Music, Piety and Print in Sixteenth-Century France* (Rochester, NY, 2000) and Rebecca Wagner Oettinger, *Music as Propaganda in the German Reformation* (Aldershot, 2001).

31   See, for example, Plato, *Republic*, 397–401b, 410a–412b, 423d–425a, translated in Andrew Barker, *Greek Musical Writings Volume I: The Musician and his Art* (Cambridge, 1984).

image first appeared in print (1595), more than three thousand works of this kind had been published in France and Switzerland alone, leaving aside the extensive repertory which also appeared in the Low Countries, Germany and England over the same period.

With this necessarily brief digression into the musical politics of religious reform, we are now in a better position to understand why courtly Paracelsians would have taken for granted that psalms were the most effective form of soul medicine, and why they would have seen the instruments and music lying on the table as essential to their form of experimental life. For quite apart from the occult practices which it is clearly meant to evoke (and to which we shall shortly return), Khunrath's emblem taps into a powerful form of 'music therapy' that godly citizens around 1600 were using to heal and uplift their souls on an every-day basis: the communal activity of singing or playing psalms together, a practice which took for granted that all disease and sickness were visited by God on human-kind as punishment for sin, and therefore the best medicine was to worship Him, to ask for mercy and release from suffering.

In sum, it is clear that sacred music, especially psalmody, was a recognized vehicle for healing and restoring the soul among all Protestants (especially Calvin-ists) around 1600, and was certainly not an esoteric practice limited to a handful of occult philosophers. Most Protestants of the time would have vehemently rejected any suggestion that they were engaging in magic when they sang psalms. Yet there is definitely something more to Khunrath's soul medicine than every-day psalm-singing, because he makes clear that the magus is an extraordinary individual whose melancholic disposition signals a rare capacity to discern hidden powers and influences, and to harness them for extraordinary ends. Since it has been established that Paracelsus himself saw no obvious relationship between music and astrological medicine, we need to consider where and when this connection originated, and why it became identified with Paracelsianism at all.

Experimental hymns to the stars

The most obvious place to find music being used as a form of spiritual medicine is Ficino's *De vita* (1489), the original source for Khunrath's image of the divinely inspired Christian magus, and the first Renaissance text to treat melancholy as a positive affliction to which philosophers were particularly prone. Significantly, the *De vita* was also the first Western work to suggest how music might be used as a means of allieviating this condition. However, Ficino's remedy was not based on the intrinsic properties of musical sound alone, even though he offered an early ex-planation of how musicians could alter people's mood through their ability to move the passions. Instead, what Ficino recommended was a magical technique for drawing down celestial influences into one's own spirit via music, one of a variety of techniques for harnessing astral forces via the quintessence that would-be modern magi could legitimately use to improve their health and longevity, even though these were secrets best kept hidden from the vulgar.

It is in the third part of the *De vita*, 'on obtaining life from the heavens' (or 'on fitting one's life to the heavens') that Ficino sets down guidelines for capturing the particular qualities of each planet by means of songs designed to draw down their influences, especially those of the sun (Apollo), which can be used to offset the melancholic influence of Saturn.[32] There is no way of knowing what Ficino's solarian hymns actually sounded like, although the suggestion is that he declaimed verses taken from his own edition of the *Orphic Hymns* (1462) and the 18th psalm to his own accompaniment on the lute or *lyra da braccio*, in the manner of the *'improvvisatori'* who were especially popular in fifteenth-century Italian courts.[33] What matters in this context is that his aim was nothing less than to recreate the healing and purifying effects that the ancient magi – especially Orpheus, Pythagoras, and, above all, David – achieved by means of hymns sung to their respective deities.[34] He was particularly keen to emulate their ability to cure diseases of the soul, to expel evil passions (as, most famously, in the case of David curing Saul), and to bring the soul into a state of virtuous harmony.[35] Put another way, the *De vita* is witness to experiments which may arguably be counted among the earliest examples of 'scientific' medical research, in that they embody a series

32   Apart from Walker's groundbreaking discussion in *Spiritual and Demonic Magic*, see also Gary Tomlinson, *Music in Renaissance Magic: Toward a Historiography of Others* (Chicago and London, 1993), especially chap. 4, and Angela Voss, 'Marsilio Ficino, the second Orpheus', in *Music as Medicine*, ed. Horden, pp. 154–72; Voss, 'The musical magic of Marsilio Ficino', in Michael J.B. Allen and Valery Rees, eds, *Marsilio Ficino: His Theology, His Philosophy, His Legacy* (Leiden, Boston and Koeln, 2002), pp. 227–42. On al-Kindi as a source for Ficino's astrological medicine, see these articles by Voss and also Charles Burnett, '"Spiritual medicine": music and healing in Islam and its influence in western medicine', in P. Gouk, ed., *Musical Healing in Cultural Contexts* (Ashgate, 2000), pp. 85–91.

33   Walker, *Spiritual and Demonic Magic*, pp. 19–24; also Voss, 'Marsilio Ficino', pp. 161–9. Voss suggests that Ficino may have used a harp, or a lute, or a *lira* to accompany his hymns; certainly all three types of instrument are depicted in Khunrath's laboratory.

34   Note the parallels between Ficino's enterprise and the efforts of later medical humanists to recover the lost techniques of ancient anatomy as part of a broader programme of medical improvement: see Andrew Cunningham, *The Anatomical Renaissance: The Resurrection of the Anatomical Projects of the Ancients* (Aldershot, 1997). On David as a model for modern rulers, see Esan Ahmed, *The Law and the Song: Hebraic, Christian and Pagan Revivals in Sixteenth-Century France* (Birmingham, Alabama, 1997). For equivalent interests among the so-called 'musical humanists' see D.P. Walker, 'Musical humanism in the sixteenth and early seventeenth centuries', reprinted in Walker, *Music, Spirit and Language in the Renaissance*.

35   D.P. Walker, *The Ancient Theology: Studies in Christian Platonism from the Fifteenth to the Eighteenth Century* (London, 1972), especially chaps 1 and 3.

of mathematically based, but essentially empirical, operations designed to improve mental health and heighten cognitive awareness by altering body chemistry.

Of course, Ficino was not trying to be an experimental scientist, but regarded his songs as powerful examples of the kind of natural magic that he was advocating in the *De vita*, a work which by 1600 was already recognized as one of the key texts of Renaissance magic.[36] Although having had no discernible impact on mainstream medical theory for most of the sixteenth century, the *De vita*'s influence is clearly evident in the portrayal of Khunrath's laboratory, a space in which performing sacred, magical music in the manner of King David is presented as a desirable part of the Paracelsian physician's experimental form of life. Inconveniently for this claim, however, Khunrath nowhere mentions Ficino or the *De vita* in his *Amphitheatrum*.[37] We therefore have to look elsewhere to establish a definite connection between Ficino's planetary songs and courtly Paracelsian medicine. In fact, since Ficino himself does not mention alchemy in the *De vita*, and derides both alchemy and transmutation elsewhere in his writings, it is all the more necessary to discover under what circumstances Ficino's songs for learned melancholics and Paracelsus's radical agenda for moral and medical reform could ever have come together in the first place.

Jacques Gohory and French Paracelsianism

The crucial linkage between Paracelsian alchemy and Ficino's astrological music seems to have been made by Jacques Gohory (1520–1576), writing under the name of Leo Suavius.[38] Gohory, a Catholic, was one of the first generation of authors to introduce Paracelsian thought into France, a period before Paracelsianism had become 'an ill-defined Protestant heresy' and before Paracelsus's works had been placed on the Index (1599).[39] His *Theophrasti Paracelsi philosophiae et medicinae utriusque universae, compendium* was first published at Paris in 1567, reprinted there and published at Basel and Frankfurt in 1568, thereby achieving a Europe-wide circulation. The Paracelsus who emerges from the *Compendium*, however, was quite different from the figure presented in other Paracelsian texts circulating

36   Brian Copenhaver, 'Astrology and magic', in *The Cambridge History of Renaissance Philosophy*, ed. Charles B. Schmitt et al. (Cambridge, 1988), pp. 264–300, esp. pp. 274–85.

37   Peter Forshaw, personal communication. On Agrippa's dangerous interpretation of Ficino's music-spirit theory, see Walker, *Spiritual and Demonic Magic*, pp. 90–6.

38   Didier Kahn, 'Le paracelsisme de Jacques Gohory', *Aries*, 19 (1995), 81–130, offers a useful complement to earlier discussions of Gohory in Allen G. Debus, *The French Paracelsians. The Chemical Challenge to Medical and Scientific Tradition in Early Modern France* (Cambridge, 1991), pp. 26–31, and Walker, *Spiritual and Demonic Magic*, pp. 96–106.

39   Hugh Trevor-Roper, 'Paracelsianism made political, 1600–1650', in Grell, ed., *Paracelsus*, pp. 119–34 (quotation at p. 121).

at the time, and Gohory certainly does not fall into the mainstream of Paracelsian thought. This is because his main concern was to appropriate Paracelsus for his own philosophical agenda, rather than establishing Paracelsianism as a distinctively new movement. In brief, Gohory transformed Paracelsus into his own ideal of a Renaissance magus, a manoeuvre which not only allowed him to integrate what he regarded as the most useful aspects of Paracelsian alchemy into his own occult system of knowledge, but also integrated Paracelsus into the framework of French literary humanism, a republic of letters in which Neoplatonic philosophy predominated.[40]

The way Gohory avoided Paracelsus's appearing iconoclastic was by claiming that Paracelsus's *De vita longa* (the text of which he edited and attached to the *Compendium*) was modelled on Ficino's *De vita*. In so doing, he identified Paracelsus as a learned magus who was following the tradition of the *prisca theologia* or ancient theology, a body of secret pagan and Jewish wisdom that providentially harmonized with Christianity. Ficino was among the first scholars to develop this esoteric tradition of perennial philosophy, one which legitimated his interest in ancient magic and underpinned his learned editions of the works of 'Hermes' (1463), Plato (1484) and the Neoplatonists (1492) as well as the *De vita* itself. As we have already seen from the last work, this tradition assumed that the ancient magi had been able to effect almost miraculous cures through a deep understanding of the fundamental harmonies of nature, a powerful form of knowledge which was only revealed by God to a few extraordinary spirits. Thus although Paracelsus himself was not a musician, Gohory (who, by contrast, was an enthusiastic musical amateur) could nevertheless associate him with charismatic figures like Orpheus, Pythagoras and David who apparently anticipated Christ's injunction to heal the sick by combining music with their medicine and theology.[41]

By the time that Gohory portrayed Paracelsus as a modern Christian magus, however, many other sources had enriched this syncretic tradition of occult philosophy, which also converged with humanism. For although Gohory wanted to link Paracelsus with Ficino's spiritual magic, he also wanted to show him as being equally well-versed in medieval alchemy and cabbalistic magic, thereby associating him with Roger Bacon, Arnaldus of Villanova, Trithemius, and other wise masters who actually had no connection with Ficino himself. One reason for this was that it made Paracelsus into a learned scholar whose writings conformed

---

40   Kahn, 'Le paracelsisme de Jacques Gohory', pp. 81–2. On the transformations of Paracelsus since his lifetime, see Andrew Cunningham, 'Paracelsus fat and thin: thoughts on reputations and realities', in *Paracelsus*, ed. Grell, pp. 53–77; also Charles Webster, 'The nineteenth-century afterlife of Paracelsus', in R. Cooter, ed., *Studies in the History of Alternative Medicine* (Oxford, 1988), pp. 79–88.

41   On Gohory's skills as a musician and its relation to his alchemy see Walker, *Spiritual and Demonic Magic*, pp. 99–101; also Jeanice Brooks, 'Chivalric romance, courtly love and courtly song: female vocality and feminine desire in the world of Amadis de Gaule', in Thomasin LaMay, ed., *Musical Voices of Early Modern Women: Many-Headed Melodies* (Aldershot, 2005), pp. 63–95.

with the values of contemporary French humanism.[42] Another reason, however, was that it accounted for the obscurity and confusion of Paracelsus's writings, which Gohory believed was a technique for hiding a kind of astrological medicine that made Paracelsus a much more powerful magus than Ficino had ever been. According to Gohory, the drawback with Ficino's planetary songs was that they were limited to drawing down impersonal astral influences into the spirit and imagination of the magus himself, and therefore constituted a timid and private kind of subjective magic, rather than a more powerful kind of transitive magic that could be used to affect others. A further limitation was that Ficino rejected the use of talismans in favour of his astrological medicines; in short, although he well knew the great marvels that the ancient magi could accomplish, he did not dare perform them himself.[43]

There were good reasons why Ficino had confined his attention to drawing down purely 'natural' influences from heavenly bodies into his own body, a process he tried to account for by the affinity of the human spirit and the astral body or world spirit. The problem with his idea of singing hymns to the sun, in imitation of the Orphic mysteries or other pagan rite, was that it could be misunderstood as idolatry, or demonic magic. Many of the effects that the ancient magi were able to accomplish were extremely dangerous: for example, it was by means of vocal and instrumental power that Orpheus brought Eurydice back from the dead (necromancy) and that Hermes was able to attract demons and souls of the dead into statues and amulets (idolatry, theurgy), and even David curing Saul's madness may have been an act of exorcism. Indeed, the whole problem with incantations was that not only could they be used to affect other people's emotions through altering their imagination, but they also had the power to alter minds – to make people, and other intelligent beings (i.e. demons, angels), act against their will. It was no surprise that Ficino was accused of practising magic in 1489, and only narrowly avoided imprisonment, thanks to the intervention of his patron, Lorenzo de' Medici. Yet Ficino did not deny that demons might be summoned, or that invocations or songs might be harnessed for evil ends. He merely asserted his own, purely medical, intentions, and warned that he was not speaking of worshipping stars, but imitating them. Despite such denials, Walker concludes that Ficino did practise a form of magic or theurgy addressed to good planetary demons, on the basis 'that its dangers might be avoided if it remained within a learnèd, philosophical circle, and were kept secret from the ignorant *vulgus*, who would distort it with idolatry and superstition'.[44]

A clearer idea of how such demonic magic might be practised can be found in Agrippa's *De occulta philosophia*, the very source used earlier in this article to

---

42 See Noel Heather, 'Curing man and the cosmos: the power of music in French Renaissance poetry', in Horden, ed., *Music as Medicine*, pp. 195–212, also Yates, *French Academies*.

43 Walker, *Spiritual and Demonic Magic*, pp. 102–6.

44 *Ibid.*, p. 51. For a broader discussion of demonic magic, see Stuart Clark, *Thinking with Demons: the Idea of Witchcraft in Early Modern Europe* (Oxford, 1997).

argue for Khunrath's understanding of the power of sacred music to achieve spiritual harmony and well-being. This work may well have provided the context for Gohory's conflation of Paracelsian and Ficinian magic, as well as being one of Khunrath's sources of inspiration. For here Agrippa indiscriminately affirms the power of 'songs, sounds and musical instruments' to move the affections and to introduce magical impressions, describes the harmony of man's body and soul and their affinity with planetary harmony, lays out Ficino's rules for planetary songs, and also explicitly gives directions for attracting and controlling good demons, his defence being that:

> no man is ignorant that supercelestiall Angels or spirits may be gained by us through good works, a pure minde, secret prayers, devout humiliation, and the like.... So we read that the antient Priests made statues, and images, foretelling things to come, and infused into them the spirits of the stars.[45]

Nowhere in the *Compendium* does Gohory claim that Paracelsus used music for his magical operations along the lines that Agrippa suggests. It is very likely, however, that Gohory himself experimented with this form of musical magic in the private academy that he set up in an apothecary's garden when he retired from public life in 1571. His 'Lycium philosophal [sic] San Marcellin' is recognized as being one of the earliest 'experimental' research institutions which anticipated Francis Bacon's call to investigate and control the secrets of nature by more than a generation.[46] Here Gohory not only devoted himself to alchemy and the preparation of Paracelsian remedies, but also made talismans 'suivant l'opinion de Arnaud de Villeneuve, & de Marsilius Ficinus' and performed vocal and instrumental music in its 'galerie historiée'.[47] There is no proof that this music was intended to draw down astral influences into talismans or enhance other magical operations, but the 'Lycium' certainly provides a context in which Gohory could have experimentally elided Ficino's musical magic with the spiritual medicine of Paracelsus.

Refining Paracelsus

Although intriguing, Gohory's private experiments are of less relevance to this paper than the more public results he effected in the *Compendium*, where Paracelsus appears transformed from an incoherent drunkard into an almost sacred figure. Here (some forty years before Croll achieved a similar effect in his *Basilica Chemica*) Gohory successfully recontextualized Paracelsus so that he no longer

---

45   Agrippa, *Occult Philosophy*, Book I, chap. 39.
46   Debus, *French Paracelsians*, p. 27; Walker, *Spiritual and Demonic Magic*, pp. 100–1. See also William Eamon, *Science and the Secrets of Nature: Books of Secrets in Medieval and Early Modern Culture* (Princeton, 1994).
47   Walker, *Spiritual and Demonic Magic*, p. 100, the quotations being taken from Gohory's *Instruction sur l'herbe Petum* (Paris, 1572).

needed to be seen as a subversive radical bent on bringing down established medicine and religion. Instead, he might be co-opted into membership of an elite group of *illuminati* whose origins went back to the dawn of history but who still constituted a positive force for change in modern times. By power of association, Paracelsus was made into one of a handful of melancholic magi whose inherent nobility legitimated their dangerous pursuit of occult knowledge and power. Since this quest was ultimately divine in inspiration, and was focused as much on improving social health and harmony as individual well-being and personal gain, Renaissance magi were justified in transgressing prevailing cultural norms as they sought to extend the boundaries of human understanding and fulfilled God's divine plan for mankind. We can see these same powerful associations at work a generation later in Khunrath's self-image as a Christian magus: as well as invoking King David, the kneeling alchemist also embodies a refined version of Paracelsus, whose experimental practices and new form of scientific knowledge have now been successfully integrated into the courtly world of occult natural magic.

In conclusion, this paper suggests that music may have provided one of the most important means through which the radical and potentially revolutionary ideas of Paracelsus could be harmonized with established systems of medical and scientific thought, and, especially, made attractive to elite and intellectually sophisticated patrons like Landgraf Moritz of Hessen and even the Emperor Rudolf himself.[48] Music was central to courtly Paracelsianism around 1600 not so much for its own sake (although it was well established as an art and science in its own right) as for its capacity to *refine*.[49] That is to say, music was an important instrument of social as well as spiritual transformation, one which also served as an indicator of high status. Nowhere was this perhaps more true than at the Kassel court, since Moritz himself was an accomplished poet and musician as well as being one of the most enthusiastic promoters of the occult philosophy and Paracelsian alchemy.[50] Khunrath's picture suggests that the 'physician' who practises his kind of alchemy and spiritual medicine is capable of restoring inner harmony within individuals and society – and therefore of potentially eliminating all sickness and disease – through his ability to harness cosmic harmonies. This is not a practice that ordinary doctors can aspire to, even if they have traditional medical qualifications. Only the most noble spirits are capable of practising this divinely inspired medicine, the harmony of sacred psalmody being an outward reflection of, and a means of moving towards, this mystical inner state. Such a message would certainly make sense to a patron like Moritz, whose engagement with the occult sciences was part of his

48 For the broader intellectual context and further bibliography, see Moran, *Alchemical World*, and Gouk, 'Natural philosophy and natural magic'.

49 On the lute song as an expression of courtly identity and an index of nobility see Jeanice Brooks, *Courtly Song in Late Sixteenth-Century France* (Chicago and London, 2000), especially pp. 126–32.

50 Moran, *Alchemical World*, pp. 12, 19–24. See also H. Borggrefe, V. Lüpkes, and H. Ottomeyer, eds, *Moritz Der Gelehrte. Ein Renaissancefürst in Europa* (Eurasburg, 1997).

broader quest to achieve political harmony and religious reconciliation at a time of fragmentation and deepening crisis in the period up to the Thirty Years' War.[51] Whether calling on demons or simply appealing to God's mercy, the practice of 'soul medicine' along the lines I have described would have been recognized as a powerful healing ritual.[52] Thus, far from being peripheral, music was one of the principal means through which the courtly Paracelsians rendered their experimental form of life meaningful to their patrons.

51   Moran, *Alchemical World*, pp. 25–35.
52   On the relationship between war and discourses on the healing powers of music, see Penelope Gouk, 'Sister disciplines? Music and medicine in historical perspective', in Gouk, ed., *Musical Healing*, pp. 171–96 (especially pp. 173–6).

Chapter 3

The Economy of Magic in Early Modern England

Lauren Kassell

When my mistress died, she had under her arm-hole a small scarlet bag full of many things, which, one that was there delivered unto me. There was in this bag several sigils, some of Jupiter in Trine, others of the nature of Venus, some of iron, and one of gold, of pure angel gold, of the bigness of a thirty-three shilling piece of King James' coin. In the circumference of one side was engraven, *Vicit Leo de tribu Judae Tetragramaton* +, within the middle there was engraven a holy lamb. In the other circumference there was Amraphael and three +. In the middle, *Sanctus Petrus, Alpha* and *Omega*.

A sigil is an amulet in the form of a metal seal depicting images or words, often worn around the neck or fixed in a ring. This episode is dated 1624 and appears in the 'autobiography' that William Lilly wrote at the behest of Elias Ashmole in 1668.[1] In 1620 Lilly had moved to London as a servant in the household of Gilbert and Margery Wright, a recently – and unhappily – married couple in their late sixties or early seventies (each had been married before). In 1622 Mrs Wright developed a swelling in her left breast, and Lilly nursed her for the next two years,

I would like to thank Robert Goulding and Anthony Grafton for inviting me to present a version of this paper at a colloquium on 'The Magic of Things' in Princeton in April 2003, and the participants for their comments; members of the early modern seminar at the Institute for Advanced Study, Princeton, for a lively discussion in February 2004; Margaret Pelling, Joad Raymond, Simon Schaffer, and Koen Vermeir for reading drafts; and Wyatt MacGaffey for teaching me about economic anthropology. Some of the research for this paper was supported by the Wellcome Trust.

1   *William Lilly's History of His Life and Times* (London, 1822), p. 32. This text figures briefly in Paul Delany, *British Autobiography in the Seventeenth Century* (London, 1969). For an account of the importance of astrology in the genres of life-writing, see Anthony Grafton, 'Geniture collections, origins and uses of a genre', in Marina Frasca-Spada and Nick Jardine, eds, *Books and Sciences in History* (Cambridge, 2000), pp. 49–68. Lilly appears in most accounts of astrology in early modern England. For a detailed discussion of his art, see Ann Geneva, *Astrology and the Seventeenth Century Mind: William Lilly and the Language of the Stars* (Manchester, 1995).

eventually using a pair of scissors gradually to cut away the mortified breast; she soon died, leaving him the sigil that she had kept in her armpit. Lilly copied down the inscriptions that he describes above, and sold the sigil for thirty-two shillings.[2]

From Margery Wright, Lilly acquired more than experience in the rudiments of surgery and a golden sigil. She introduced him to the occult arts. She had frequently visited cunning men to discover whether her husband would die before her; 'this occasion begot in me [Lilly] a little desire to learn something that way, but wanting money to buy books, I laid aside these notions'.[3] Simon Forman, the astrologer-physician who had died in 1611, had been one of these cunning men, and he had made the sigil that Wright left to Lilly. Wright's previous husband had been haunted by the spirit of a murdered man which entreated him to cut his own throat, and so long as he wore Forman's sigil around his neck the spirit desisted.[4] Lodged in Wright's armpit, the sigil was a token of her encounters with the powers of the occult. When Lilly copied its notations and cashed it in, he redeemed its material value, negated its sentimental value, and stripped it of its magical power, keeping that in the less precious, and less effective, medium of pen and paper. He could do this because the value of the sigil was not inherent to the object.

Ideally Lilly would have re-invested the thirty-two shillings in books of magic, but it was the best part of a decade before he did so. He continued in his service to Mr Wright, who soon remarried a woman called Ellen. During the plague of 1625, Wright fled the city and left Lilly in charge of the household. Lilly bought a bass viol and took lessons on how to play it, and he spent a lot of time bowling in Lincoln's Inn Fields.[5] His master died in 1627 leaving him twenty pounds a year, and Lilly married the widow, Ellen, though she was much older than he. She died in 1633, leaving him more than a thousand pounds. In 1632 Lilly had begun to study astrology under the tutelage of John Evans, and then to buy books to further his studies.[6] In 1634 he spent forty shillings on a manuscript Ars Notoria, a text attributed to Solomon and containing images and orations for invoking angels who endowed one with the understanding of arts and sciences, perfect memory, and the eloquence to convey this knowledge.[7]

---

2   Lilly, *Life*, p. 34.
3   Lilly, *Life*, pp. 28–9.
4   Lilly, *Life*, pp. 33–4.
5   Lilly, *Life*, p. 46.
6   Evans later wrote a treatise on antimonial cups, and perhaps other works including a series of almanacs: Bernard Capp, *Astrology and the Popular Press* (London, 1979); Allen Debus, *The English Paracelsians* (London, 1965), p. 170; Margaret Pelling, *Medical Conflicts in Early Modern London: Patronage, Physicians, and Irregular Practitioners, 1550–1640* (Oxford, 2003), p. 69n.
7   For the importance of the Ars Notoria and its circulation in late medieval England see Frank Klaassen, 'English manuscripts of magic, 1300–1500: a preliminary survey', in Claire Fanger, ed., *Conjuring Spirits: Texts and Traditions of Medieval Ritual Magic* (Thrupp, 1998), pp. 3–31. See also Stephen Clucas, 'John Dee's angelic conversations and the *Ars Notoria*: Renaissance magic and mediaeval theurgy', in Clucas, ed., *John*

This essay is about the definitions and values of magic that are inscribed in sigils like that which Forman made and Lilly sold. Through the activities of Forman, Lilly and Ashmole, it charts the trade in magical objects, texts, and knowledge in England from the 1580s to the 1680s. Sigils, the skills to make them, and the texts that preserved this expertise had a number of values, monetary, practical, natural historical, antiquarian and natural philosophical.[8] I am using the term 'economy' to denote all of these values, and I will explain what I mean by this before returning to Forman, Lilly and Ashmole.

The value of things

By the time that Lilly sold the sigil, in 1634, the world was disenchanted. This is how Max Weber described the process of rationalization and systematization that resulted from the rise of Protestantism and capitalism. Weber used this notion differently at different times. In *The Protestant Ethic*, he described the inner loneliness afflicting Calvinists as the culmination of a process that had been initiated by Hebrew prophets and fostered by Hellenistic science, a process which eliminated magic from the world; salvation and redemption could no longer be found through the magic of the church.[9] In 'Science as a Vocation' he described the outcome of scientific rationalization not as the production of knowledge itself, but as knowing that we can learn through calculation, and thus we need not 'implore the spirits'.[10] In *The Religion of China* he concluded with a comparison of Confucianism and Puritanism, echoing the passage in *The Protestant Ethic*: 'Nowhere has the complete disenchantment of the world been carried through with greater consistency [than in early modern Protestantism], but that did not mean freedom from what we nowadays customarily regard as "superstition".'[11] Rationality does not replace magic; disenchantment is a process within history, not a product of modernity.

It is now unfashionable to pursue universal, monolithic definitions of religion, magic, and science. Robert Merton, following Weber, documented the study of natural philosophy and innovations in technology by Puritans in early modern England, and Charles Webster explored the intellectual fervour of this world, a

Dee: Interdisciplinary Studies in English Renaissance Thought (Dordrecht, forthcoming); Lynn Thorndike, *A History of Magic and Experimental Science*, Vol. 2 (New York, 1934), pp. 281–3.

8   Cf. Brian Copenhaver, 'A tale of two fishes: magical objects in natural history from antiquity through the Scientific Revolution', *Journal of the History of Ideas*, 52–3 (1994), 373–98; Krzysztof Pomian, *Collectors and Curiosities: Paris and Venice, 1500–1800* (Cambridge, 1990).

9   Max Weber, *The Protestant Ethic and the Spirit of Capitalism* (London, 1930), p. 105.

10   H.H. Gerth and C. Wright Mills, *From Max Weber: Essays in Sociology* (New York, 1946), p. 139; see also pp. 148, 155, 357.

11   Max Weber, *The Religion of China* (New York, 1951), p. 226.

world in which science, religion and magic were part of the same project of reformation.[12] Weber kept returning to the notion of the disenchantment of the world, not only because he was studying religion, but because he was concerned for the plight of the individual and the premium on rationality in a world where people, economy, administration, politics and science are systematized. The notion of the rational individual remains problematic in histories of early modern magic, science and religion because we, via nineteenth-century anthropologists, have inherited definitions of these subjects dating from the seventeenth century.[13]

This also holds true for definitions of economy that centre on the rational individual.[14] In the formal sense, economy can be defined as the production, distribution and consumption of goods and services. Were we to explain the history of magic in terms of this formal concept of economy, we would document the production, distribution and consumption of magical goods and services according to the choices of individuals. Capitalism mystifies, or fetishizes wealth, and attributes (or generates) a value inherent to land, labour and capital; this value is defined as 'use value', something intrinsic to the object. The problem with magical objects is that from our perspective they contain a dubitable inherent value. We thus explain the 'belief' in their inherent value, their intrinsic efficacy, in terms of psychological

---

12   R.K. Merton, 'Science, technology and society in seventeenth-century England', *Osiris*, 4 (1938), 360–632; Charles Webster, *The Great Instauration: Science, Medicine and Reform 1626–1660* (London, 1975); Charles Webster, *From Paracelsus to Newton: Magic and the Making of Modern Science* (Cambridge, 1980); see also Christopher Hill, *Intellectual Origins of the English Revolution* (Oxford, 1965). For general discussions of magic, science and religion see Stanley Tambiah, *Magic, Science, Religion and the Scope of Rationality* (Cambridge, 1990); Richard Kieckhefer, *Magic in the Middle Ages* (Cambridge, 1989) and 'The specific rationality of medieval magic', *American Historical Review*, 99 (1994), 813–36; and Robert Scribner, 'The Reformation, popular magic, and the "disenchantment of the world"', *Journal of Interdisciplinary History*, 23 (1993), 475–94. These discussions have been fuelled by Keith Thomas, *Religion and the Decline of Magic* (Harmondsworth, 1971) and Valerie Flint, *The Rise of Magic in Early Medieval Europe* (Princeton, 1991). On Thomas see Hildred Geertz, 'An anthropology of religion and magic, I', *Journal of Interdisciplinary History*, 6 (1975), 71–89 and Thomas's reply, 'An anthropology of religion and magic, II', *Journal of Interdisciplinary History*, 6 (1975), 91–109. On Flint see Kieckhefer, 'Specific rationality' and Brian Vickers, 'On the rise of magic in early mediaeval Europe', *History of European Ideas*, 18 (1994), 275–87. For a call for 'a revival of Weberian-style historical sociology...of the cultural origins and character of scientific rationality', see Lorraine Daston, 'The moral economy of science', *Osiris*, 10 (1995), 2–24.
13   Thomas, *Religion and the Decline of Magic*, p. 69; Tambiah, *Magic, Science, Religion*, p. 24; Kieckhefer, *Magic*, pp. 14–15.
14   See Louis Dumont, *From Mandeville to Marx* (Chicago, 1977); William Pietz, 'Fetishism and materialism: the limits of theory in Marx', in Emily Apter and William Pietz, eds, *Fetishism as Cultural Discourse* (Ithaca, 1993), pp. 119–51; Karl Polanyi, *The Great Transformation* (New York, 1944).

need. In an unpredictable, dangerous, anxiety-ridden world, people flock to the marketplace to purchase magical goods and services. This account, however, sacrifices contemporary ideas about the inherent value and intrinsic power of magical objects in order to preserve a notion of rationality. It also undermines the authority and expertise of the magical practitioner, and neglects the dynamic between him and his clients. Magic is demystified and it becomes quackery or religion.

Historians and anthropologists tracing the emergence of capitalism have noted the tautology implicit in using a formal notion of economy to distinguish between pre- and post-capitalist societies. Following Karl Polanyi, they adopt a version of the substantivist (as opposed to the formal) approach which defines economy as a socially embedded process. Here value is defined as 'exchange value', where it is not intrinsic to a static, reified thing, but accrued, expressed and measured through its process across space and time.[15] Arjun Appadurai describes this as the 'social life of things'.[16] Things, as embodiments of social action, undermine the conceptual categories of religion, economy and social structure (or lineage), categories which themselves became defined in early modern Europe.

This is why this essay is about magical sigils, particularly the one that Forman made.[17] To make a sigil was to stamp the powers of the stars into a piece of metal, creating an object both natural and artificial; to use it was to traffic in the occult powers of nature, the dead, or demons; to record its designs was to collect its meaning; to sell it was to redeem its value either as a piece of precious metal or an object of curiosity; to collect it was to endow it with natural historical or antiquarian value, an object, like a coin or medal, embodying the virtues of the past, or like a shell, the secrets of nature, a token for trading with the invisible, what John Aubrey called 'the Oeconomie of the Invisible World'.[18] The value of a sigil was inherent to the object but it was not constant.[19] Occult powers were subject to the

15   For a clear outline of these ideas see Karl Polanyi, 'The economy as instituted process', reprinted in George Dalton, ed., *Primitive, Archaic and Modern Economies: Essays of Karl Polanyi* (New York, 1968), pp. 139–74. For a survey of the uses of the term 'economic' by anthropologists, with some criticisms of Polanyi for his emphasis on objects, see Robbins Burling, 'Maximization theories and the study of economic anthropology', *American Anthropologist*, 64 (1962), 802–21.

16   Arjun Appadurai, 'Introduction: commodities and the politics of value', in Appadurai, ed., *The Social Life of Things: Commodities in Cultural Perspective* (Cambridge, 1986), pp. 3–63.

17   My approach is especially indebted to Igor Kopytoff's notion of a 'cultural biography of things', for which see his 'The cultural biography of things: commoditization as process', in Appadurai, *Social Life of Things*, pp. 64–91.

18   John Aubrey, *Miscellanies* (London, 1696), sig. A3v.

19   On collecting and the invisible, see Pomian, *Collectors and Curiosities*, especially pp. 7–44. On coins as magical objects, see Henry Maguire, 'Magic and money in the early Middle Ages', *Speculum*, 72 (1997), 1037–54. For gestures towards the importance of economic factors in early modern science see the introduction to Pamela Smith and Paula Findlen, eds, *Merchants and Marvels: Commerce, Science and Art in Early Modern Europe* (New York, 2002). On the preternatural as a subject of natural

vicissitudes of nature, the motions of the stars and planets and the whims of demons, and economic values depended on how an object had been made, where it had come from, and whether it was to be used or collected. A natural and a social history were inscribed in the life of a magical object.

Simon Forman's magic

Lilly showcased the sigil that was made by Forman, worn by Mrs Wright's first husband, kept in Mrs Wright's armpit, left to Lilly, and copied and sold by him. Lilly's history was part of Ashmole's project to record the history of magic, astrology and alchemy in Britain, a project that led him to preserve, even fetishize and idolize, thousands of pages of manuscripts, including Forman's. Forman wrote compulsively, spurred by the need to correlate the motions of the stars and planets with the vicissitudes of life in Elizabethan and early Jacobean London. Between 1580 and his death in 1611 he filled more than fifteen thousand pages with details mundane, celestial and divine. Forman's pursuit of magic is most thoroughly documented in a pair of works dating from his final decade, an alchemical commonplace book 'Of Appoticarie Druges' and a series of incomplete essays on 'the motion of the 3 superiour heavens' (hereafter 'The Motion of the Heavens').[20]

'Of Appoticarie Druges' can be read as a record of Forman's study of 'chymical' and 'hermetical' physic and a compendium of his expertise in using alchemy, astrology and magic in his medical and related practices.[21] Thirty of its three

philosophical inquiry see Lorraine Daston, 'Preternatural philosophy', in Daston, ed., *Biographies of Scientific Objects* (Chicago, 2000), pp. 15–41. On stamping, see Katharine Park, 'Impressed images: reproducing wonders', in Caroline A. Jones and Peter Galison, eds, *Picturing Science, Producing Art* (New York, 1998), pp. 254–71.

20   For more on Forman's magic see my *Medicine and Magic in Elizabethan London: Simon Forman, Astrologer, Alchemist, and Physician* (Oxford, 2005), especially chapter 10. For Forman's life see also A.L. Rowse, *Simon Forman: Sex and Society in Shakespeare's Age* (London, 1974), and Barbara Traister, *The Notorious Astrological Physician of London: Works and Days of Simon Forman* (Chicago, 2001).

21   This is bound in two volumes: Oxford, Bodleian Library, Ashm. 1494 and 1491 respectively. Some pages from this work are now located in Lonodon, British Library, Sloane MS 3822. I am indebted to David Pingree for assembling a copy in which the pages from Sloane 3822 are reinstated in the volumes, and to Carol Kaske for providing me with a copy of this text. Forman seems to be modelling this work on Josephus Quercetanus [Duchesne], *The Practise of Chymicall, and Hermeticall Physicke*, trans. Thomas Tymme (London, 1605), and his title perhaps echoes sigs BB3v–BB4 of this work. On Paracelsianism see especially Charles Webster, 'Alchemical and Paracelsian Medicine', in Charles Webster, ed., *Health, Medicine and Mortality in the Sixteenth Century* (Cambridge, 1979), pp. 301–34; cf. Debus, *English Paracelsians* and Paul Kocher, 'Paracelsian medicine in England: the first 30 years', *Journal of the History of Medicine*, 2 (1947), 451–80. On commonplace books see William Sherman, *John Dee: The Politics of Reading and Writing in the English Renaissance* (Amherst,

hundred entries mention magical operations or principles specifically and a handful ('magia naturalis', 'ars magnetica', 'homunculus') address magic directly. A majority of these operations were to effect love magic or more malicious influences on a person's will, and some were for healing. In the entry on 'Electrum', a mixture of two or more metals, Forman described the correlation between types of magic and metals:

> Quicksilver hath power of and over enchanting & enchanted. Led hath power over witchcrafte. Copper hath powere of bindinge. Gould against poison & to comforte the harte. Tyne against thunder lightining & diseases. Silver doth preserve & hath power in magik & enchantment. Yron doth bind & command & threton.[22]

Under the entry for 'Spiritus' he described a hierarchy of spirits corresponding to the elements that could be used to bind, loose, curse, bless, and do harm.[23] Sometimes Forman appealed to occult forces in nature, sometimes to spirits; he never mentioned demons. Many entries described astral magic that worked through objects inscribed with images and words. Others described entities typically alchemical, such as the homunculus, mandrake and speaking statue; classically occult natural objects (loadstone, poison from plants, spiders, snakes, toads, and menstrual blood); images made from wax and metals; amulets made from metals, gems, stones and herbs; potions in which such images were soaked or stones and minerals dissolved; human ingredients (urine, hair, blood, menstrual blood, turds, semen); animal ingredients (bones, snakes and eggs); plants and herbs; and manufactured items such as nails, bells and ink. Occasionally Forman recorded incantations and in quite a few entries he discussed the power of words and writing.[24] He designated some practices as traditional or old-fashioned, such as determining how well a garment would last according to the phase of the moon when it was first worn. Under 'Observances and old rulles' he discussed the meaning of thunder.[25] Very few operations were divinatory, except a brief account of hazel rods and a device made with a loadstone that could be used to communicate with someone hundreds of miles away. An entry on 'Prophetes and

---

1995), pp. 59–65; Ann Moss, *Printed Common-place Books and the Structuring of Renaissance Thought* (Oxford, 1996); Kevin Sharpe, *Reading Revolutions: The Politics of Reading in Early Modern England* (New Haven, 2000).

22   Ashm. 1494, pp. 483–4; on electrum see also Sloane 3822, fol.7.

23   Ashm. 1491, pp. 1127–8. This scheme followed Michael Psellus, the eleventh-century Byzantine scholar, though Forman attributed it to himself. See also Ashm. 244, fols 73ᵛ–5.

24   See Ashm. 1494, pp. 398–404, 490, 586–96; Ashm. 1491, pp. 1214, 1216, 1220–3, 1304–5, 1306–9.

25   Ashm. 1494, p. 272; Ashm. 1491, p. 830.

prophesyinge' described the need for a diviner to be physically pure.[26]

Forman also collected testimonials about the uses of magical objects and substances. Occasionally he had experienced these powers himself: he boiled snakes in a strong water and when he drank it his grey hair turned red again; he drew characters on his left arm and right breast in a semi-permanent ink in order to alter his destiny; the angel Raziel advised him about the virtues of mistletoe that grew on oak trees; and he had to give away the taffeta britches that he first wore during a waning moon.[27] Sometimes he noted gossip, such as when in 1603 a man in Westminster reported that 'he sawe a mandrake of 7 inches longe with hair down to the feet and under the arm holes, like unto a man in form which was taken by on head [one Head] a constable in turtell street from a witch which was carried to prison for bewitching of Sr Jhon Harizes sonn'.[28] But most of the information in these volumes does not contain verification or instruction. Forman did not privilege experience as a measure of whether or not a power or substance existed, and this compendium documents his collection of details about magic, informed through a lens of alchemical and Paracelsian medicine refined in the final decade of his life. This volume could be read as Forman's contribution to Baconian natural history, but instead magical pursuits dominated his legacy.

Forman was especially devoted to the study and practice of astral magic, the use of sigils, laminas, rings, and 'characts' to harness the powers of the stars. These objects 'enclosed som parte of the vertue of heaven and of the plannets according to the tyme that it is stamped caste or engraven or writen in'.[29] Throughout the 1590s Forman designed numerous magical objects, some for his own use, some for his friends and clients, some to cure disease, some to empower their bearer.[30] In 1597 he prescribed for Jackemyne Vampena, a Dutch woman married to an English merchant, a series of potions, including one in which a ring engraved with the symbol of Jupiter had been immersed.[31] That year he thought he had lost a gold lamina, a flat, metal amulet, which he had worn on his chest, but he found it

---

26   Sloane 3822, fol. 90v; Ashm. 1491, pp. 1358, 884. For evidence that Forman made such rods, see a record of his wife Jean (still a virgin) cutting eight hazel rods at the appointed hour which were then immediately whitened and inscribed on 8 February 1598: Ashm. 226, fol. 303. The same long-distance communication device, constructed slightly differently, was described in a text appended to *Ars Notoria: the Notary Art of Solomon*, trans. Robert Tanner (London, 1657), pp. 136–8.

27   Ashm. 1491, p. 1278 (mistletoe); Ashm. 1494, pp. 938 (hair), 586v (tattooing), 272 (britches). For a recipe for the ink see Ashm. 1494, p. 402.

28   Ashm. 1494, p. 679.

29   Ashm. 392, fol. 46; see also Ashm. 390, fol. 30.

30   For various laminas see Ashm. 234, fols 96, 99; Ashm. 226, fols 148, 152, 310. For sigils see Ashm. 219, fol. 48; Ashm. 226, fols 148, 249v; Ashm. 363, fols 69v–71. Sloane 3822 is a collection of sigils and texts about them by Forman, Napier, Lilly and Ashmole.

31   Ashm. 411, fols 95, 99v, 115, 118v.

'behind my back in my doublet'.[32] In 1598 and 1599 he designed a series of rings and sigils made at the requisite times to capture the desired astral properties.[33] One of these rings had a golden setting holding a large coral stone engraved with the sign of Jupiter, under which was wedged a piece of parchment bearing Forman's name and an inscription of the words and symbols for Virgo and Mercury, the astrological house and its ruling planet at the time of his birth. It was to be worn on the little finger of his left hand, and would protect him against witchcraft and other ills as well as giving 'favour & credit & to mak on famouse in his profession & to overcom enimies'.[34] In 1601 he designed a sigil made under the sign of Scorpio for one Martha Shackleton.[35] The following year he designed a golden lamina for Jean Sherly that took four days to make and cost £4 13s.[36] In 1611 he sent Richard Napier some brass moulds to make symbols of the planets.[37] Sometime during these years Forman made the sigil that Lilly inherited from Mrs Wright, and in the entry for 'Sigilla' in 'Of Appoticarie Druges' Forman recorded the design for the type of sigil that Lilly later described.[38]

Forman recorded incidental details about his use of sigils, and he also wrote about the powers of astral magic. 'The Motion of the Heavens', the incomplete essays that he drafted at the same time as compiling 'Of Appoticarie Druges', is a sustained treatment of this subject, combining medieval cosmology, Arabic astral magic and Neoplatonic natural philosophy.[39] Forman explained the analogy between the three superior, celestial heavens, known as the eight, ninth and tenth spheres, the Trinity, and man. The tenth sphere, or *primum mobile*, moves naturally from east to west, and carries all of the spheres 'against their own proper and naturalle motions'. The ninth sphere has no natural motion of its own, and as the soul obeys the spirit so the ninth sphere follows the tenth. The eighth sphere contains the fixed stars and has two motions, 'unnaturally' from east to west

32   Ashm. 205, fol. 23; Ashm. 226, fol. 166.
33   Ashm. 195, fols 29v, 56v–7v, 58. See Ashm. 219, fol. 48, for details of the timing and costs of a ring and a sigil, one of which was made for Forman's close friend Alice Blague, and for evidence that Forman might have paid for these partly in kind with his laminas.
34   Sloane 3822, fol. 11. For Forman's description of how to make an 'imperialle' ring or lamina of gold by inserting a piece of peony, bay or vervain and images of a lion, ram and goat and their related astrological symbols on parchment or leather under a ruby, diamond and heliotrope, then suffumigating it and praying, see Sloane 3822, fol. 77v.
35   Ashm. 411, fol. 58v. This might be the same Mrs Shackleton whose coat of arms Forman described as having been made for her burial on 7 January 1608: Ashm. 802, fol. 207v. For Forman's account of a sigil of similar design, see Sloane 3822, fol. 96.
36   Sloane 3822, fols 13–15. For details of the other rings and sigils that he made that year and the next see Sloane 3822, fols 16–19.
37   Ashm. 240, fol. 106. Forman indicated that someone else would have made the sigils.
38   Sloane 3822, fol. 94.
39   Edward Grant, *Planets, Stars, and Orbs: The Medieval Cosmos, 1200–1687* (Cambridge, 1994), chaps 13, 18, esp. pp. 315–23; S.K. Heninger, *The Cosmographical Glass: Renaissance Diagrams of the Universe* (San Marino, CA, 1977), chaps 3, 4.

following the tenth sphere, and 'naturally' such that its equinoxes vary by eight degrees.[40] Forman stressed that a proper understanding of these motions was essential for making astrological calculations and enacting magical operations. While the ninth sphere is filled with symbols and spirits, he argued, 'the influences operations and effects magicalle are in and done by the 8 heaven and not by the 9 heaven and primo mobile'. This is why the distinction between the natural and unnatural motions of the eighth sphere was important: 'all influences natural do come from and proceed from the 8 heaven and from the fixed stars therein, and from the plannets moving under the 8 heaven according to nature and natural workinge'.[41] Forman made detailed calculations about the differing motions of the eighth sphere because they were essential for determining the timing at which to make rings, images, sigils, and swords that could be used to cure diseases, expel vermin, dogs and wolves, vanquish a man's enemies, and improve or hinder his fortune.[42] He also specified that the hours of the day could be calculated by dividing the period from midnight to midnight into 24 equal periods, the hours of daylight into twelve, or by basing one's calculations on the ascension of the ecliptic line of the eighth heaven. The first sort were natural hours, the second artificial, and the third magical; sigils were to be made according to the magical hours.[43] Seven decades later Ashmole collected Forman's papers, had them bound in leather into thick volumes with brass clasps, and carefully studied his writings on sigils.[44]

Forman's legacy: alchemy, astrology and magic

In 'Of Appoticarie Druges' and 'The Motion of the Heavens' Forman records information old and new, from books and experience, an eclecticism informed by Paracelsianism and years of experience as an astrologer-physician and student of magic and alchemy in London. When he died in 1611, Richard Napier, his astrological protégé, soon acquired most of his papers.[45] Within a month of receiving them, Napier tested a recipe for potable gold from 'Of Appoticarie Druges', noting his approval in the margin.[46] He often shared his books, and 'Of Appoticarie Druges' bears evidence of other readers. For instance, in an entry on

---

40   Ashm. 244, fols 35–47.
41   Ashm. 244, fols 40v, 46.
42   Ashm. 244, fol. 48.
43   Ashm. 244, fols 91–2.
44   C.H. Josten, ed., *Elias Ashmole, Autobiographical and Historical Notes, Correspondence, and Other Sources* (5 vols, Oxford, 1966), i, p. 210; iii, p. 1208; iv, pp. 1454–5, 1809.
45   Kassell, *Medicine and Magic*, Introduction; Michael MacDonald, *Mystical Bedlam: Madness, Anxiety, and Healing in Seventeenth–Century England* (Cambridge, 1981), p. 290n; Traister, *Notorious Astrological Physician*, p. xiv.
46   Ashm. 1494, p. 145.

antimony Thomas Robson made a correction which he marked with his name.[47] Robson probably also wrote the hash marks in the margins to denote which passages he had copied from these volumes into other notebooks.[48] Others occasionally added their hands to the text without recording their identities or purposes in reading. Decades later Ashmole inserted a brief entry describing how to make a disappearing re-appearing ink.[49]

When Lilly wrote the history of his life in 1668, at the request of Ashmole, he drew on the legacy of Forman, a legacy traced through rumour and manuscripts and linking himself and Ashmole in their pursuit of the natural and social histories of astrology, alchemy and magic in early modern England. Lilly read many of Forman's manuscripts, probably either when he visited Napier in Great Linford, Buckinghamshire throughout 1632–3, or after Sir Richard Napier, Napier's nephew, had inherited them in the 1630s.[50] He also heard about Forman from Margery Wright and from Forman's widow, known as Ann, Jean, and Forman's pet name for her, 'Tronco'. Lilly's story of his life as an astrologer is punctuated with digressions about the skill and integrity of other practitioners in astrology and alchemy and the successes of various scryers, including John Dee's assistant, Edward Kelley.[51] The story of the sigil in the armpit sparks the first digression, and Forman is its subject. Lilly praised Forman's astrological integrity; but he insinuated that Forman was an old-fashioned, ill-educated magician, noting that Margery Wright had habitually consulted cunning or wise men 'as were then called'. Forman was 'judicious and fortunate' in horary questions such as thefts, and sickness was his 'masterpiece'. He was meticulous and thorough in his calculations, and 'had he lived to methodize his own papers, I doubt but that he would have advanced the Iatromathematical part thereof very completely'. Despite his calculations, Lilly continues, Forman had difficulty in his pursuit of the philosophers' stone and his own preferment. Elsewhere Lilly noted that according to Margery Wright, Forman was very successful in his conferences with spirits; he also, according to Lilly, had a book that he 'made the devil write with his own hand in Lambeth Fields 1596' and he predicted his own death.[52]

About his own life, Lilly reports that he himself first began to study magic in

47 Ashm. 1494, p. 62.
48 Many volumes of Robson's notes on alchemical texts are preserved in the Ashmole and Sloane collections.
49 Ashm. 1494, p. 552. For notes probably by Ashmole see Ashm. 1494, p. 85; Sloane 3822, fol. 84v. Ashmole might also have book-marked items, as the entry on 'Karacters' is presently marked with a slip of paper bearing numbers and astrological houses seemingly in Ashmole's hand: Ashm. 1494, p. 586.
50 Lilly, *Life*, p. 79. On the nexus of astrologers including Dee, Forman, Napier and Lilly see Michael MacDonald, 'The career of astrological medicine in England', in Ole Grell and Andrew Cunningham, eds, *Religio Medici: Medicine and Religion in Seventeenth Century England* (Aldershot, 1996), pp. 62–90.
51 Lilly, *Life*, pp. 221–7.
52 Lilly, *Life*, pp. 42–4.

1634, the year after his first wife died. He bought a copy of the Ars Notoria, and he admits ('I do ingenuously acknowledge') that he used the art briefly before giving it up.[53] His disillusionment with magic began when he went on a hunt for treasure in a ruined abbey using dowsing rods, but too many people were present, demons were let loose and had Lilly not dismissed them the abbey would have collapsed.[54] Then he advised a woman in matters of love, divining where she might meet her estranged lover, and she nearly poisoned herself. Following these mishaps, Lilly 'burned his books which instructed in these curiosities' and moved to the country.[55] But Lilly tells us that in 1634–5 he taught John Hegenius, a Dutch physician and astrologer, his 'art in framing Sigils, Lames &c. and the use of the Mosaical rod'.[56] Lilly had probably learned about sigils from some books and moulds that had been stashed by one Mathias Evans in the wall of his house, only to be discovered by a later occupant; Ashmole noted that Lilly had bought these for five shillings.[57]

Lilly, Ashmole, and antiquarianism

Lilly recounted the story of Forman's amulet, noted his lack of method (at which Lilly excelled) but extreme diligence in the science of astrology, and described the interest in spirits to which he too, briefly, had succumbed. Without saying any more about Forman's sigil, he quietly reported his own expertise in the casting of sigils, stressing, like Forman, that astrology was essential to all other arts. He noted his and Ashmole's pursuit of books and manuscripts, and reported on his study of Forman's astrological figures and accounts of his life. Through stories about the occult practitioners that he had known or heard about and the curious events that he had experienced, Lilly, like Forman, portrayed astrology, alchemy and magic as related arts. Lilly, however, did not people his account with mandrakes and homunculi, or even magnets and menstrual blood. At the request of Ashmole he recorded the materials for a social history of magic in England, and in so doing he stressed his own practices, said nothing about the natural history of magic, and perhaps taunted Ashmole with details such as his having sold Forman's golden sigil, burned some books, and visited a wood filled with fairies.[58] Perhaps Lilly was suggesting that the antiquarian pursuit of magic was no more than the stuff of romance.

53   Lilly, *Life*, p. 76.
54   Lilly, *Life*, pp. 78–81.
55   Lilly, *Life*, p. 83.
56   Lilly, *Life*, p. 221.
57   Lilly, *Life*, pp. 152–3. Evans was known for his magical and astrological practices and he was a friend of Richard Napier's and an enemy of John Lambe's: Kassell, *Medicine and Magic*, chaps 3 and 4; Macdonald, 'Career of astrological medicine', p. 85; Pelling, *Medical Conflicts*, p. 112; Thomas, *Religion and the Decline of Magic*, pp. 297, 413.
58   Lilly, *Life*, pp. 34, 83, 228.

Lilly and Ashmole had met in 1646, soon after Ashmole had begun to study astrology, alchemy, natural history and other subjects and to acquire related books and manuscripts. Ashmole's fortune improved in 1649 with his marriage to Lady Manwaring, and he began to collect coins and medals, then from the 1650s to study heraldry and collect portraits, antiquities and curiosities artificial and natural. Through texts, images and objects, Ashmole preserved the relics of the history of Britain and the lives of his countrymen, materials forgotten or desecrated by his contemporaries.[59] His collection of magical texts dates from 1648 at the latest, when he and Lilly swapped their copies of the Picatrix, an Arabic book of magic circulating in manuscript.[60] In 1649 Ashmole transcribed a treatise entitled 'Three books on natural magic'.[61] He also used these texts: in July 1650, for instance, following directions attributed to Paracelsus, he made a magic speculum to see things in the past and present.[62] A few days later he made four sigils to drive away caterpillars, flies, fleas and toads, and in September he made sigils against the pox.[63] Those against vermin were made from lead, took the shape of the creature, were void of characters, and were cast during a conjunction of Saturn and Mars. Those against the pox took the form of genitalia and were cast during a conjunction of Venus and Mars.[64]

That same year Ashmole acquired a number of magical books and manuscripts, including one on Arabic talismans and another on calling spirits.[65] In 1651 he prepared *Theatrum Chemicum Britannicum* for publication. This included

59   Cf. Pomian, *Collectors and Curiosities*, p. 34. On Ashmole see Josten, *Ashmole* and Michael Hunter, *Elias Ashmole, 1617–1692: The Founder of the Ashmolean Museum and His World* (Oxford, 1983), reprinted in Hunter, *Science and the Shape of Orthodoxy: Intellectual Change in Late Seventeenth-Century Britain* (Woodbridge, 1995), pp. 21–44. On Ashmole's collection of books and manuscripts see Josten, *Ashmole*, i, p. 210; iii, p. 1208; iv, pp. 1454–5, 1809. Most of these manuscripts are now in the Ashmole collection in the Bodleian Library, though it is unclear why some of Ashmole's papers, particularly those containing magical material, are now in the Sloane Collection in the British Library. For the Ashmole collection see William Black, *A Descriptive, Analytical and Critical Catalogue of the Manuscripts Bequeathed Unto the University of Oxford by Elias Ashmole* (Oxford, 1845) and W.D. Macray, *Index to the Catalogue of Manuscripts of Elias Ashmole* (Oxford, 1866). On coins and medals see Josten, *Ashmole*, ii, p. 684; iv, pp. 1717, 1727, 1864 and Hunter, *Ashmole*, pp. 37–8, 40.

60   Josten, *Ashmole*, i, p. 53; ii, p. 466. Lilly's copy might have come from Sir Richard Napier.

61   Ashm. 358. Black attributes this text to Ashmole and Josten disagrees: Josten, *Ashmole*, ii, p. 490.

62   Josten, *Ashmole*, i, p. 72; ii, p. 536.

63   Josten, *Ashmole*, ii, pp. 537, 545–9.

64   Josten, *Ashmole*, ii, pp. 594, 608, 619. He also describes sigils with embracing couples on one side and words (Hagiel, Graphiell) on the other: Josten, *Ashmole*, ii, p. 608. For Forman's description of a sigil against rats, see Sloane 3822, fol. 102v.

65   Josten, *Ashmole*, ii, p. 537n.

Thomas Norton's 'Ordinal of Alchemy', and Ashmole glossed the line 'But the chief Mistris among sciences all/for the helpe of this art, is magic naturall' with a five-page essay on the subject. Following Paracelsus, Agrippa, Francis Bacon and others he distinguished 'True Magicians' from 'Conjurers, Necromancers and Witches'. He lamented the false accusations of demonic magic made against scholars in previous centuries, and he stressed that natural magic did not require incantations, words, circles, charms or other 'invented fopperies'; but he did not proscribe the use of magical objects.[66]

Around 1668 Ashmole and Lilly swapped stories about their lives and their experiences with magic. Lilly studied Ashmole's nativity and noted that though an educated gentleman, Ashmole was expert in casting medals and sigils. Ashmole asked Lilly to write an account of his life and times, which he did.[67] Then Ashmole asked Lilly to elaborate on the details of who was present and what happened during the magical activities that he described.[68] Around this time Lilly also sent Ashmole a trunk full of sigils that had belonged to one 'Lord Bothwell', then Sir Robert Holborn, the lawyer and astrological enthusiast who had died in 1648. Ashmole recorded the designs of several sigils, rings and stones by impressing them in wax.[69] When Sir Richard Napier died in 1676 Ashmole bought his collection, including Forman's papers, from his son, Thomas. He studied Forman's writings, and from 1677 he made dozens of sigils, some to improve his fortune, some to stop his wife from vomiting, and most to drive vermin from his house and garden.[70] He compiled lists of titles of Forman's treatises, noted works that he cited, re-copied damaged pages, and indexed figures that he had cast about the weather and the making of sigils.[71] Ashmole studied Forman's notes on sigils with particular care. For instance, throughout the entry on 'Amulets' in 'Of Appoticarie Druges' he systematically noted whether Forman's calculations were based on natural or artificial hours, and Ashmole likewise included these two sorts of time throughout his records for making sigils from late in 1677.[72] He also annotated Forman's essays in 'The Motion of the Heavens', paraphrased them, and checked

---

66 Elias Ashmole, ed., *Theatrum Chemicum Britannicum* (London, 1652), pp. 443–7.
67 Josten, *Ashmole*, iii, pp. 1072–3; ii, p. 538n. On images of famous men, identities of collectors, autobiographies, and medals see Paula Findlen, *Possessing Nature: Museums, Collecting, and Scientific Culture in Early Modern Italy* (Berkeley, 1994), pp. 291–392.
68 Josten, *Ashmole*, i, p. 62; iii, pp. 1113–15.
69 On the trunk of sigils see Josten, *Ashmole*, iii, p. 1076; Thomas, *Religion and the Decline of Magic*, pp. 634–5. On Holborn, see Josten, *Ashmole*, ii, p. 471. On impressions: Josten, *Ashmole*, iv, pp. 1233, 1288. The former example is explicitly magical, while the latter might have had magical or heraldic values.
70 Josten, *Ashmole*, ii, pp. 537, 538, 545–9, 567, 578–9, 584, 594, 595, 608, 619; iv, pp. 1508, 1513, 1523, 1533, 1538–40, 1608–32, 1616, 1624, 1629, 1656–7, 1662–3, 1679, 1681, 1688–97, 1738.
71 Ashm. 421, fol. 152; Ashm. 1790, fol. 102; Sloane 3822, fol. 20.
72 Sloane 3822, fols 6–19; Josten, *Ashmole*, iv, p. 1508.

Forman's figures against other sources, at one point finding Forman's calculations lacking in comparison with those included in Edward Sherburne's *The Sphere of M. Manilius* (1675).[73] In a letter to Anthony Wood a decade later, Ashmole described Forman as 'a very able Astrologer and Phisitian, as appears by the manuscript bookes he left behinde him, which are now in my possession'.[74] Hundreds of sigils were probably numbered amongst the almost nine thousand silver, brass and copper coins and medals that Ashmole lost, along with impressions of heraldic seals, printed portraits, notes on history and heraldry and other antiquities and curiosities, in the fire in the Middle Temple in 1679. That his collection of manuscripts and gold coins (less precious but more valuable) survived because Ashmole kept them at his house in South Lambeth was an irony that neither he nor Lilly could have foreseen.[75]

Lilly had inherited a tradition of magic from Forman that was tied to astrology and dominated by the uses of sigils and a curiosity about scrying. Ashmole collected the relics of Forman's and Lilly's expertise. From Lilly he received stories to chronicle the progress of astrology and encounters with spirits, demons and fairies. Forman's reputation and papers might have inspired him to perfect the art of making sigils and certainly informed his understanding of the motions of the heavens and their importance for magical operations. For Ashmole, Lilly, and Forman, the value of magic inhered in knowledge and expertise, knowledge most often used to make sigils that harnessed astral powers. Magical objects, the texts that described them and documented their uses, and knowledge about how they worked, followed distinct paths of transmission between practitioners, clients and friends, and across generations. Objects might shed occult powers and they and their legacies acquire historical value; the meaning of texts and the expertise they conveyed was more enduring. Whether magic was distinguished from religion in terms of coercion or supplication; whether a new type of contemplative, spiritual magic was defined that achieved divine enlightenment instead of Faust's mundane powers and pleasures; whether the magus, no longer a priest, aspired to a clerical role; whether religion and magic together were moved from the church to the home; in seventeenth-century England magical objects were disenchanted not only because of Baconian natural histories, but because of Ashmole's antiquarianism. He knew that his collections were channels for conversations with the dead and that his sigils worked by magic.

---

73   Ashm. 1790, fols 78–100; Ashm. 421, fols 149r–v. For his annotations, see especially Ashm. 244, fols 50, 51v, 92, 96–7v, 99v, 107v.

74   Josten, *Ashmole*, iv, p. 1809.

75   Josten, *Ashmole*, i, pp. 229–30; iv, pp. 1726–7; Hunter, *Ashmole*, pp. 37–40. Sloane 3822 preserves Ashmole's records of sigils, including at least one impression in wax (fol. 159; cited in Josten, iii, p. 1233).

Chapter 4

Chemical Medicine and Paracelsianism in Italy, 1550–1650

Antonio Clericuzio

Historians of Italian Renaissance medicine have investigated the relationship of medicine and humanism, as well as the introduction of anatomy and botany in the medical curriculum, but they have paid little attention to chemistry and to its impact on medical theories and practice. Italian Paracelsianism is still little known, despite the fact that, as we shall see, Paracelsus's theories and practices can be traced all over the Peninsula. Studies of the Paracelsian movement have assessed the importance and impact of the chemical medicine propounded by Paracelsus and his followers in various countries, but have entirely ignored Italy.[1] The only exceptions are the pioneering contributions of Paolo Galluzzi and Giancarlo Zanier, who investigated specific regional contexts – respectively Bologna and Venice (Zanier) and Tuscany (Galluzzi).[2] Zanier has underestimated the impact of Paracelsianism in Italy, stating that no major contribution to medical theory and to natural philosophy came from Italian Paracelsians. It is my contention that the supposed lack of systematic and original contributions to Paracelsianism is not a good reason to dismiss Italian Paracelsian physicians as marginal characters in the

I wish to thank Maria Conforti, Silvia de Renzi, and Margaret Pelling for their useful comments on previous drafts of this paper.

1   See for instance Allen G. Debus, *The Chemical Philosophy: Paracelsian Science and Medicine in the Sixteenth and Seventeenth Centuries* (New York, 1977); Walter Pagel, *The Smiling Spleen. Paracelsianism in Storm and Stress* (Basel and London, 1984); Hugh Trevor-Roper, 'The Paracelsian movement', in Trevor-Roper, *Renaissance Essays* (London, 1986), pp. 149–99; Ole P. Grell, ed., *Paracelsus: The Man and His Reputation, His Ideas and Their Transformation* (Leiden, 1998).

2   Paolo Galluzzi, 'Motivi paracelsiani nella Toscana di Cosimo II e di Don Antonio dei Medici: alchimia, medicina "chimica" e riforma del sapere', in *Scienze, credenze occulte, livelli di cultura* (Florence, 1982), pp. 31–62; Giancarlo Zanier, 'La medicina paracelsiana in Italia: aspetti di un'accoglienza particolare', *Rivista di Storia della Filosofia*, 4 (1985), 627–53. For useful information see Richard Palmer, 'Pharmacy in the Republic of Venice in the sixteenth century', in A. Wear, R. French and I.M. Lonie, eds, *The Medical Renaissance of the Sixteenth Century* (Cambridge, 1985), pp. 100–17 and 303–12.

history of medicine. As we shall see, Paracelsian ideas and practices played a prominent part in Italy and contributed to the establishment of innovative theories in physiology, for example those espoused by Pietro Castelli and Giovanni Alfonso Borelli.

Paracelsianism and iatrochemistry made their way into Italy later than in northern European lands, notably France, Germany, and England. The delay that affected the diffusion of Paracelsianism in Italy can be explained as the outcome of two main factors. The first was the strong influence of humanism and of the Galenical tradition; the second was religious censorship. It is apparent that in post-Tridentine Italy many Paracelsian ideas were seen as dangerous to religion and in the event various Paracelsian books were put on the *Index*.[3] The association of some Italian Protestants with Paracelsianism contributed to make Paracelsianism suspect to the religious authorities. Religious refugees became involved in the diffusion of Paracelsian books and ideas in Switzerland and Germany: the printer and publisher Pietro Perna (d. 1582), from Lucca, published a great number of Paracelsian works in Basel, Giuseppe Micheli (c.1530–1600) advocated Paracelsian chemcal medicine in opposition to Libavius, and Angelo Sala (1576–1637), from Vicenza, adopted Paracelsian views and became one of the champions of iatrochemistry in Germany.[4]

It is apparent that in Italy Paracelsianism did not bring about any dramatic confrontation with traditional medicine, as happened in France.[5] This might be due to the fact that although Italian Paracelsians, like their colleagues elsewhere, promoted the study of the 'living anatomy', that is, the chemical investigation of the human body, they did not rule out anatomy. In the present study I set out to investigate Italian Paracelsianism and chemical medicine from the mid-sixteenth century to the mid-seventeenth century, namely before the diffusion of Joan Baptista van Helmont's medicine in Italy. I will first briefly put chemical medicine and Paracelsianism into an institutional and intellectual framework, then I will investigate the introduction of chemical remedies in Italy, and finally, I will deal with the emergence of what can be called physiological chemistry, namely, the view that chemistry provides the key to the understanding of physiology.

3   See Jesus Martinez de Bujanda, *Index des livres interdits* (11 vols, Geneva and Montreal, 1984–2002), ix (Geneva, 1994): *Index de Rome, 1590, 1593, 1596*, pp. 27, 131, 163, 177, 395.

4   On Perna, see Antonio Rotondò, *Studi e ricerche di storia ereticale italiana del Cinquecento* (Turin, 1974), pp. 273–391. Giuseppe Micheli was the author of *Apologia chymica, adversus invectivas Andreae Libavi calumnias* (Middlebourg, 1597). On Angelo Sala, see Zahkar E. Gelman, 'Angelo Sala, an iatrochemist of the late Renaissance', *Ambix*, 41 (1994), 142–60.

5   Cf. Allen G. Debus, *The French Paracelsians* (Cambridge, 1991) and Didier Kahn, *Paracelsisme et alchimie en France à la fin de la Renaissance* (Geneva, 2005).

Chemical medicine and Paracelsianism in courts and academies

Paracelsian views were adopted in contexts where interest in alchemy and practical chemistry was particularly strong, as attested by the Medici court in Florence.[6] In Italy, like in other parts of Europe (Germany, England and France), court patronage gave substantial support to alchemy and promoted the diffusion of Paracelsianism.[7] Medici patronage, which has been studied by Galluzzi and Perifano, contributed to the dissemination of Paracelsianism and chemistry. Cosimo I gave support to alchemists, supervised the production of the *Ricettario Fiorentino* of 1567, and was personally involved in chemical experiments, which were performed in the *Fonderia*, the chemical laboratory located in the *Palazzo degli Uffizi*. Though Paracelsian works do not seem to have circulated in his court, there is evidence of his links with Adam von Bodenstein – a central character of the Paracelsian movement.[8] Von Bodenstein, who in 1560 dedicated his edition of Paracelsus's *De vita longa* (1560) to the Doge and Senate of Venice, dedicated his edition of Paracelsus's *De tartaro* (1563) to Cosimo I. Bodenstein's later dedication bears evidence of his travel to Italy, and contains an epitome of Paracelsus's philosophy and medicine, as well as an appeal to the Medici family for support for chemical medicine.[9]

Several members of the Medici family were interested in alchemy and in practical chemistry. Francesco I and Ferdinando I patronized alchemy, and employed Leonhart Thurneisser (1531–1596), the wandering Paracelsian alchemist, who

6   François Secret, 'Notes sur quelques alchimistes italiens de la Renaissance', *Rinascimento*, 13 (1973), 197–217; Alfredo Perifano, *L'Alchimie à la Cour de Côme Ier de Médicis: savoirs, culture et politique* (Paris, 1997); Perifano, 'Considérations autour de la question du paracelsisme en Italie au XVIe siècle: les dédicaces d'Adam de Bodenstein au Doge de Venise et à Côme Ier de Médicis', *Bibliothèque d'humanisme et Renaissance*, 62 (2000), 49–61.

7   On patronage and Paracelsianism, see B.T. Moran, *The Alchemical World of the German Court: Occult Philosophy and Chemical Medicine in the Circle of Moritz of Hessen, 1572–1632* (Stuttgart, 2001). See also Vivian Nutton, ed., *Medicine at the Courts of Europe, 1500–1837* (London, 1989). On patronage and science in Renaissance Italy, see William Eamon, 'Court, academy, and printing house: patronage and scientific careers in late Renaissance Italy', in Bruce T. Moran, ed., *Patronage and Institutions: Science, Technology and Medicine at the European Courts, 1500–1750* (Woodbridge, 1991).

8   Perifano, *L'Alchimie*, pp. 131–41.

9   *Ibid.*, pp. 151–70; Perifano, 'Les Deux dédicaces d'Adam de Bodenstein au *De vita longa* de Paracelse', *Chrysopoeia*, 5 (1996), 471–91, and Wilhelm Kühlmann and Joachim Telle, eds, *Corpus Paracelsisticum*, Vol. I: *Der Frueparacelsismus*, Part I (Tübingen, 2001), pp. 104–46.

performed the trick of transmuting half an iron nail into gold for Francesco I.[10] Cosimo II purchased a number of Paracelsian works which became part of the library of the Pisan Botanical Garden (*Giardino dei Semplici*). The most active patron of Paracelsianism was Don Antonio dei Medici, the son of Francesco I and Bianca Cappello. He patronized alchemists, made chemical experiments, and owned Paracelsian books and manuscripts.[11] In *La fonderia del Signor Don Antonio dei Medici* there is evidence of his chemical views: he extolled chemistry as the pillar of medicine, praised Paracelsus's remedies and described the medical uses of antimony, nitre and potable gold.[12] Following a pattern that became common in late Renaissance Italy, Don Antonio combined Paracelsianism, alchemy, Neo-platonism and Hermeticism.[13] In Don Antonio's laboratory worked Antonio Neri, alchemist and author of the renowned *Arte Vetraria*, who followed Paracelsian medicine and rejected both Galenism and scholastic philosophy.[14] Paracelsian views were also shared by two other members of Don Antonio's circle, namely, the Florentine alchemist Agnolo della Casa, who left a huge amount of alchemical manuscripts, and Raffaello Gualterotti, who adopted the chemical theory of principles.[15] Furthermore, Carlo Ponicelli and Benedetto Punta, both of them physicians to Cristina di Lorena (1565–1636), Ferdinando's wife, adhered to Paracelsianism.[16]

Paracelsians found support in several Italian courts, especially Mantua and Ferrara. As we shall see, a number of chemical works inspired by Paracelsus were dedicated to Vincenzo (1587–1612) and to Ferdinando (1612–26) Gonzaga. The former chose the Paracelsian Francesco Bruschi as his physician; the latter appointed Fabrizio Bartoletti, the author of *Encyclopaedia hermetico-dogmatica* (1615), at the newly founded university in Mantua.[17] In Ferrara, Alfonso II d'Este (1559–97) appointed as distiller at court Luigi Squalermo, known as Anguillara (1512–70), who moved to Ferrara in 1561, after serving for fifteen years as *Prefetto* of the botanical garden in Padua.

Rome offered greater career opportunities than other cities and attracted eminent physicians and natural philosophers – some of them contributing to chemistry and to Paracelsian medicine. In 1534 Vannoccio Biringuccio

---

10   For Leonhart Thurneisser see J.R. Partington, *A History of Chemistry* (4 vols, London, 1961–70), ii (1961), pp. 152–5; *Dictionary of Scientific Biography* (hereafter *DSB*); Wolf-Dieter Müller-Jahncke's entry in Claus Priesner and Karin Figala, eds, *Alchemie. Lexicon einer hermetischen Wissenschaft* (Munich, 1998), pp. 360–1.

11   Galluzzi, 'Motivi paracelsiani', pp. 38–40.

12   *La fonderia dell'Ill.mo et Ecc.mo Sig. Don Antonio Medici Principe di Capistrano, etc. Nella quale si contiene tutta l'arte spagirica di Teofrasto Paracelso, & sue medicine* (Florence, 1604), pp. 1–51, 69, 82, 99.

13   Galluzzi, 'Motivi paracelsiani', pp. 36–46.

14   *Ibid.*, pp. 49–56. On Neri, see *DSB*.

15   Galluzzi, 'Motivi paracelsiani', pp. 52–5.

16   *Ibid.*, pp. 58–61.

17   On Bruschi and Bartoletti, see below.

(1480–1539), who had travelled to Germany and had been employed in several Italian courts (Siena, Milan, Ferrara and Parma), was appointed head of the papal foundry, director of papal munitions, and captain of the papal artillery. In his *Pirotechnia*, published posthumously in 1540, Biringuccio dismissed schoolmen on the grounds that their knowledge was only speculative, and praised the chemists who pursued the knowledge of nature.[18] Following Biringuccio, chemistry made headway in Rome. Girolamo Rossi (1539–1608), from Ravenna, physician to Pope Clement VIII, wrote a book on distillation, which was meant to promote chemistry by means of reason and experiment.[19] Andrea Bacci (1524–1600), professor of botany at *La Sapienza* (the University of Rome), and physician to Sixtus V, wrote on poisons and on mineral waters, of which he gave detailed chemical analyses.[20] In 1592, Andrea Cesalpino (1519–1603), who was professor of medicine in Pisa, was appointed to the post of physician to Pope Clement VIII and of professor at *La Sapienza*. Besides medicine and botany, Cesalpino contributed to chemistry with a tract devoted to metals. His *De metallicis*, dedicated to his patron Clement VIII, dealt with the theory and practice of mineralogy and metallurgy, namely, the generation and composition of metals and the extraction of alum in the papal state, as well as a number of remedies that were relevant to chemical medicine: antimony, sal ammoniac, red precipitate (made with mercury) and a mercurial ointment for the cure of venereal diseases.[21]

In Rome, chemistry attracted the support of cardinals and prominent families. Michele Mercati (1541–1593), a former student of Cesalpino in Pisa, was in the service of Cardinal Ippolito Aldobrandini (later Clement VIII). Mercati, who was superintendent of the Vatican gardens and physician to Clement, combined interests in medicine and chemistry. Besides publishing a book on the plague, the *Instruttione sopra la peste* (Rome, 1576), he wrote a tract devoted to metals, the *Metallotheca*, which was published posthumously in 1717. Cardinal Odoardo Farnese (1573–1626) appointed Tobia Aldini of Cesena as keeper of the Farnese Gardens on the Palatine Hill. Chemical investigations evidently took place in the *Horti Farnesiani*, since Aldini styled himself 'chemical physician' and was mentioned by Pietro Castelli for his chemical remedies. Finally, Pietro Castelli, who

18 Vannoccio Biringuccio, *De la Pirotechnia libri X* (Venice, 1540). For Biringuccio, see *Dizionario Biografico degli Italiani* (Rome, 1960–, in progress) (hereafter *DBI*); *DSB*, and Partington, *History*, ii, pp. 31–7.

19 Girolamo Rossi, *De Destillatione... liber in quo... chemicae artis veritas, ratione & experimento comprobatur* (Ravenna, 1582; 2nd edn, Venice, 1604).

20 Andrea Bacci, *De venenis et antidotis* (Rome, 1586); *idem*, *De thermis* (Venice, 1571).

21 Andrea Cesalpino, *De metallicis* (Rome, 1596), pp. 182–95.

promoted iatrochemistry in Rome and in Southern Italy, made his early career through the patronage of the Barberini family. [22]

A central part in the diffusion of chemical medicine was played by the Roman *Accademia dei Lincei*, founded in 1603 by the young Federico Cesi, a member of one of Rome's most powerful families. The *Accademia dei Lincei* has traditionally been associated with Galileo, but it is apparent that the activities of the *Lincei* were not confined to the study of mathematical sciences. Natural history, chemistry and medicine played a substantial part in the work of the *Lincei*, who also contributed to the dissemination of Paracelsian medicine. [23] At the very beginning of the Academy's life, the *Lincei* styled themselves 'searchers of the arcane sciences and dedicated to the doctrine of Paracelsus' (*arcanarum sagacissimi indagatores scientiarum et Paracelsicae dediti disciplinae*). [24]

Indeed the works and correspondence of Johannes Eck (1579–c.1620), one of the founders of the Academy, and of two German *Lincei*, Johann Faber (1574–1629), and Johann Schreck (1576–1630), unambiguously show that Paracelsianism was well entrenched in the early *Accademia dei Lincei*. It appears that in 1604 Eck wrote a book dealing with spagyric medicine ('De triplici medicina, magica humorali spagyrica'), which was never published; the manuscript has not been found. In 1605 he published at Deventer *Disputatio unica de peste*, drawing from Petrus Severinus's *Idea medicinae* (1571). Schreck was evidently in Prague before 1609, when he met Oswald Croll (c.1580–1609), who informed him of the transmutation that Edward Kelley (1555–post-1597) achieved in Prague for the

---

22   Tobia Aldini, *Exactissima descriptio rariorum quarundam plantarum, quae continentur Romae in Horto Farnesiano* (Rome, 1625). The authorship of this work has been debated. The title states that Aldini, of Cesena and curator of the gardens, was the author. However, the dedicatory poem contains an acrostic hiding the name 'Petrus Castellus Romanus' and the printer's address to the reader contains the same acrostic (without 'Romanus') followed by the phrase 'In gratiam Tobiae Aldini scripsi cuncta' in capitals which seems to be Castelli's acknowledgement of Aldini's help in writing the work. Aldini's medicines are mentioned in Pietro Castelli, *Calcanthinum dodecaphorion, sive duodecim dubitationes in usu olei vitrioli et defensio antiquorum in arsenici atque sandarachae potu, ad Raymundum Mindererum* (Rome, 1619), p. 33. For Castelli, see *DBI*.

23   See Giuseppe Gabrieli, *Contributi alla storia della Accademia dei Lincei* (2 vols, Rome, 1989); Giuseppe Olmi, 'In esercitio universale di contemplatione e prattica. Federico Cesi e i Lincei', in Letizia Boehm and Ezio Raimondi, eds, *Università, Accademie e Società Scientifiche in Italia e in Germania dal Cinquecento al Seicento* (Bologna, 1981), pp. 169–235; Silvia de Renzi, 'Il progetto e il fatto. Nuovi studi sull'Accademia dei Lincei', *Intersezioni*, 9 (1989), 501–17.

24   Letter of Johannes Eck to Tommaso Mermann, 17 February 1604, in Giuseppe Gabrieli, ed., *Il Carteggio Linceo* (Roma, 1996), pp. 30–1. On Eck, see *DBI*, and Antonio Clericuzio and Silvia de Renzi, 'Medicine, alchemy and natural philosophy in the early Accademia dei Lincei', in D.S. Chambers and F. Quiviger, eds, *Italian Academies of the Sixteenth Century* (London, 1995), pp. 175–94: pp. 178–84.

Emperor Rudolf II.[25] In 1616 Schreck put together a collection of passages taken from Paracelsus's works, 'Compendium eorum quae a Philippo Paracelso suis inscriptis dispersa sunt', that was never published. Schreck's Paracelsian 'Compendium' dealt with the microcosm theory and the magnetic cure of wounds, as well as with the controversial doctrine of the homunculus – a topic that also attracted the interest of Tomasso Campanella.[26] Federico Cesi, who had established close contacts with Neapolitan natural philosophers like Giovan Battista della Porta and Ferrante Imperato, planned to found a branch of the *Accademia dei Lincei* in Naples, which however never materialized.[27] In Naples the *Accademia dei Segreti* of Girolamo Ruscelli (c.1500–1565/6), which flourished sporadically in the 1540s, had spurred interest in chemistry. In the *Accademia dei Segreti* worked apothecaries, goldsmiths and perfumers, and there was also a laboratory, where some artisans were employed.[28] The programme of the Neapolitan branch, which was discussed in 1612, included both a library and a chemical laboratory.[29] After Cesi's death (1630), Cassiano dal Pozzo (1588–1657), nobleman and virtuoso, secretary to Cardinal Francesco Barberini, and well known for his collection of drawings and prints (*Museo Cartaceo*), played an important part in the patronage of science and medicine. Himself a *Linceo*, Cassiano corresponded with and patronized several physicians who gave a strong impulse to iatrochemistry, for example Johannes Faber, Pietro Castelli, Pierre Potier, and Marco Aurelio Severino.[30]

Chemical medicines and pharmacy

The early influence of Paracelsus in Italy was mainly associated with the introduction of new medicines, which were adopted by a number of distillers and apothecaries. Though chemical medicines were not exclusively Paracelsian (for instance, book five of Dioscorides's *Materia Medica* dealt with mineral drugs for internal and external use), it is apparent that chemically prepared medicines were clearly perceived as alternatives to traditional medical practice and soon became a distinctive sign of Paracelsianism. In the first part of the sixteenth century, chemical medicines were adopted by Antonio Musa Brasavola, professor at Ferrara, and

25 Schreck to Faber, 22 April 1622, published in Gabrieli, *Contributi*, ii, pp. 1040–7. For Kelley, see John Ferguson, *Bibliotheca Chemica* (2 vols, London, 1954), i, pp. 453–5; Julian Paulus's entry in Priesner and Figala, *Alchemie*, pp. 192–3.
26 See Clericuzio and de Renzi, 'Medicine, alchemy and natural philosophy', pp. 175–94. For Severino, see below.
27 For della Porta and Imperato, see below.
28 William Eamon and Françoise Paheau, 'The Accademia Segreta of Girolamo Ruscelli. A sixteenth-century Italian scientific society', *Isis*, 75 (1984), 327–42.
29 Federico Cesi to Galileo Galilei, 9 June 1612, in Gabrieli, *Il Carteggio Linceo*, pp. 236–8.
30 On Cassiano dal Pozzo see Francesco Solinas, ed., *Cassiano dal Pozzo. Atti del seminario internazionale di studi* (Rome, 1989).

then physician to Pope Paolo III, and by Angelo Forte from Corfù, active in Venice in the first half of the sixteenth century. Though Brasavola criticized alchemists and rejected many medicines made with metals, he adopted several chemical remedies, including oil of vitriol, tartar, arsenic, bezoar, quicksilver and corrosive sublimate.[31] Forte's interest in chemical remedies was stronger than Brasavola's and it is possible that he had some direct knowledge of Paracelsus, as the latter was in Venice as a military surgeon in 1522.[32] Giovanni Bratti of Capodistria, who graduated in medicine at Padua in 1579 and then settled in Venice, promoted alchemy and chemical medicine in a book that he dedicated to the famous alchemist Marco Bragadino.[33]

An outspoken advocate of the Paracelsian medicines was Zaccaria dal Pozzo, from Feltre, who studied in Padua and graduated at Venice in 1593. He served at Fiume as *Provveditore alla Sanità* and as *Medico Condotto* until about 1620, and joined the Venetian College of Physicians in 1617.[34] His *Clavis medica rationalis, spagyrica et chyrurgica* (Venice, 1612) draws on Paracelsian authors such as Quercetanus, Croll, and Ruland and promotes a number of spagyrical remedies, like quintessence of human blood, oil of lead, and oil of mercury. Dal Pozzo collaborated with Venetian apothecaries, for example Girolamo Brochino, apothecary at the *Grifo*, and Alberto Stecchini, at the *Struzzo*. Stecchini was involved in the preparation of Paracelsian remedies and planned a collection of chemical remedies that he never published.[35] In Verona, Zeffirele Tommaso Bovio (1521–1609), a medical practitioner who became acquainted with Paracelsus's works in 1566, produced and sold his own chemical medicines. His medicines soon became popular and were sold both in Verona, and in Venice, notably by the Fenari brothers and by Francesco Teofanio, at the *Dio Padre* pharmacy.[36] Bovio's new remedies gained the support of Francesco Calzolari, pharmacist in Verona, who is known for his museum, where he prepared mineral remedies, including oil of vitriol – a Paracelsian medicine used as a narcotic.[37]

The diffusion of chemical medicines prompted the Veronese Giovanni Balcianelli to publish a work against the use of antimony and other medicines made by chemists. For Balcianelli, who advocated learned medicine and attacked both empirics and apothecaries, it was foolish to replace the old medicines, based on long-term experience, with the dangerous new chemical remedies. Antimony, mercury, and other substances employed in the new medicines – wrote Balcianelli

31   Antonio Musa Brasavola, *Examen omnium simplicium* (Rome, 1536).
32   Palmer, 'Pharmacy', p. 111.
33   Giovanni Bratti, *Discorso della vecchia e nova medicina...nel qual si ragiona dell'oro* (Venice, 1590). For Bragadino (1545/50–1591), see Karin Figala's entry in Priesner and Figala, *Alchemie*, pp. 91–2.
34   Richard Palmer, *The Studio of Venice and its Graduates in the Sixteenth Century* (Trieste, 1983), p. 187.
35   Palmer, 'Pharmacy', pp. 116–17.
36   *Ibid.*, p. 114.
37   On Calzolari see Giuseppe Olmi, *L'inventario del mondo* (Bologna, 1992), pp. 271–3.

– were too hot and dry and therefore noxious to the natural heat.[38] The case of Balcianelli seems to be rather isolated, as no major confrontation took place between Galenists and chemical physicians, at least at an early stage. Indeed, chemical investigations, as well as the preparation of chemical remedies, went ahead in the universities, notably in Padua, Bologna and Pisa. There is strong evidence that in Padua, the botanical garden (founded in 1544–5) gave an impulse to research on chemical medicines. Its director, the Paduan nobleman Giacomo Antonio Cortuso (1513–1603), built rooms to contain distilleries and praised Paracelsus for his investigations of simples.[39] Cortuso corresponded with Aldrovandi and Mattioli, who were both interested in chemical medicine. Ulisse Aldrovandi owned books by Paracelsus, and Pietro Andrea Mattioli prepared chemical medicines, including antimony and potable gold.[40]

Chemical remedies were also advocated by several university professors in Bologna: Camillo Baldi (1550–1637), Fabrizio Bartoletti (1576–1630), and Pierre Potier (1582–1643). Baldi's unpublished 'Trattato dell'alchimia e sua medicina' extolled Paracelsian medicine, while Bartoletti drew on Paracelsus and promoted chemical medicines in his *Encyclopaedia*.[41] Pierre Potier's *Pharmacopoea Spagirica* (Bologna, 1622), dedicated to Cassiano dal Pozzo, is a collection of chemical remedies mainly taken from Paracelsus and Quercetanus, which starts by pointing out the ancient origins of chemical medicine.[42] The famous surgeon Cesare Magati (1579–1647), who taught at Ferrara, made use of Paracelsian remedies, including the so-called *mumia* (made from human blood).[43] As in Padua,

---

38 Giovanni Balcianelli, *Discorso contro l'abuso dell'antimonio preparato* (Verona, 1603), pp. 6–22.

39 Giacomo Antonio Cortuso was appointed *Prefetto* of the botanical garden in 1590. See *DBI*, and Alessandro Minelli, ed., *L'orto botanico di Padova 1545–1995* (Venice, 1995), pp. 62–4.

40 On Ulisse Aldrovandi (1522–1605) see *DBI*; Olmi, *L'inventario*, pp. 21–161; Marco Ferrari, 'Alcune vie di diffusione in Italia di idee e di testi di Paracelso', in *Scienze, credenze occulte*, pp. 21–9.

41 On Baldi, see *DBI*, and Zanier, 'Medicina Paracelsiana in Italia', pp. 638–9. Fabrizio Bartoletti, *Encyclopaedia hermetico-dogmatica, siue Orbis doctrinarum medicarum physiologiae, hygiinae pathologiae, simioticae, et therapeuticae* (Bologna, 1619). On Bartoletti, see *DBI*, and Zanier, 'Medicina Paracelsiana in Italia', pp. 640–1.

42 Little is known of Potier's life. He was a native of Anjou and settled in Italy at the beginning of the seventeenth century. See Ferguson, *Bibliotheca Chemica*, s.v. The date of Potier's birth is revealed by his portrait included in the 1635 edition of his *Pharmacopoea Spagyrica*.

43 Cesare Magati, *De rara medicatione vulnerum* (Venice, 1616), pp. 62, 79. On Cesare Magati see Ladislao Münster and Giovanni Romagnoli, *Cesare Magati (1579–1647), lettore di chirurgia nello studi ferrarese* (Ferrara, 1968) and Zanier, 'La medicina paracelsiana in Italia', pp. 648–9. On the Paracelsian *mumia*, see Partington, *History*, ii, p. 126.

in Pisa too chemistry made its way in the botanical garden.[44] The Scot James Macollo directed the botanical garden from 1614 to 1616 and his brother John was in charge of the chemical laboratory. Macollo's chemical investigations are complemented by the fact that the library of the botanical garden contained several chemical books, including works of Paracelsus and of his followers. John wrote a tract on syphilis (*Theoria chymica luis venereae*, 1616), where he recommended Paracelsian remedies.[45] Marco Cornacchini (c.1550–1626), professor of medicine in Pisa, in his *Methodus* (1619), advocated the use of chemical medicines, including antimony.[46] A strong impulse to the diffusion of chemical medicines came from the pharmaceutical work of Joseph Duchesne (Quercetanus) (1544–1609). Many editions of Quercetanus's *Pharmacopoea dogmaticorum restituta* appeared in Venice, namely in 1619, 1638, 1646, 1655, 1665, and 1684, while an Italian translation, made by Giacomo Ferrari, *protomedico* and professor of medicine in Mantua, was published in 1619. Ferrari, who dedicated his translation of Quercetanus to Ferdinando Gonzaga, was acquainted with the French and German Paracelsians and collaborated with Count Francesco Bruschi, physician to the Duke of Mantua, and himself a student of Quercetanus in Paris. In 1623 Bruschi published *Promachomachia iatrochymica* (Mantua, 1623), a work based on Paracelsian medicine.[47]

In 1628, an anonymous tract extolling the use of antimony appeared in Turin. The author seems to have been Vincenzo Solombrino (c.1577–?), a Jesuit from Forlì. Solombrino appears as the author of annotations to the text, and it is likely that he was also the author. He sold his medicines made with antimony in Turin, and for this reason he was expelled from the order in 1629. Solombrino, who was familiar with the works of Paracelsus, Croll, Quercetanus, and Libavius, as well as of Basilius Valentinus, described antimony as a substance that purges humours as well as metals by means of the celestial virtue it contains.[48]

It is apparent that chemical medicines were attracting increasing interest in Rome and in southern Italy. In Rome, chemical remedies were adopted by Pietro

---

44   Ciro Sbrana, 'Per una ricostruzione dell' antica biblioteca del Giardino dei Semplici di Pisa: nuovi elementi', *Physis*, 24 (1982), 423–34.

45   For John (1576–1622) and James Macollo (1574–before 1623), see R.W. Innes Smith, *English-speaking Students of Medicine at the University of Leyden* (Edinburgh, 1932), pp. 149–50.

46   Marco Cornacchini, *Methodus qua omnes humani corporis affectiones* (Florence, 1619).

47   *Le ricchezze della riformata farmacopea del sig Giuseppe Quercetano* (Venice, 1619). For Bruschi, see Zanier, 'La medicina paracelsiana in Italia', pp. 642–3.

48   *L'antimonio, cioè trattato delle meravigliose virtù dell'antimonio commune* (Turin, 1628). On Solombrino, see Sergio Tira, '1628: l'antimonio di Torino ed il suo Autore', in Franco Calascibetta and Eugenio Torraca, eds, *Atti del II Convegno Nazionale di Storia e Fondamenti della Chimica* (Rome, 1988), pp. 69–78.

Castelli, Johannes Faber, Tobia Aldini, Camillo Gorio, and Enrico Corvino.[49] In Naples, Giovan Battista della Porta highlighted Paracelsian medicines, as did the pharmacist and naturalist Ferrante Imperato (*Historia Naturale*, 1599), who praised the therapeutic power of antimony and explicitly aligned himself with the Paracelsian Gerard Dorn.[50] Chemical medicines found their way into the pharmacies of monasteries, as attested by Fra Donato d'Eremita (died c.1629), the Dominican keeper of the pharmacy at the Convento of Santa Caterina in Formello (Naples). Fra Donato, who had been working in the Grand Duke's *Fonderia* in Florence for several years, moved to Naples in 1611 and in 1613 opened a pharmacy in the monastery of Santa Caterina. There he made spagyric remedies, dedicating his *Elixir di lunga vita* (1624) to Ferdinando II dei Medici, whom he praised as a patron of chemical medicine. The *Elixir*, which contains numerous images of chemical apparatus from Fra Donato's laboratory, places special emphasis on the distillation of the quintessence, described as a celestial substance, being able to heal all diseases. Following a syncretic pattern that was common among Neapolitan physicians and natural philosophers, the author presented his work as a development of that of Paracelsus, as well as of those of Johannes de Rupescissa, Philipp Ulstadt, Girolamo Cardano, Michele Savonarola, and Guglielmo Gratorolo. Fra Donato also adopted Paracelsian theories, namely the theory of signatures and the macro-microcosm analogy.[51] Chemical medicines played a relevant part in Fra Donato's *Antidotario* of 1639, of which only one out of four parts was published. In the *Antidotario* we find several Paracelsian remedies, such as antimony, vitriol, *crocus martis* (obtained by calcining iron with

49   For Tobia Aldini and Enrico Corvino, see below. Camillo Gorio wrote *Disceptatio unica de Chalcantho* (Rome, 1616).
50   The index of Giovan Battista della Porta's unpublished 'Taumatologia' is in Luisa Muraro, *Giambattista della Porta mago e scienziato* (Milan, 1978), pp. 187–99. In the second edition of his *Magia Naturalis* (1589) della Porta advocated the magnetic cure of wounds, which he attributed to Paracelsus. In fact this idea was not Paracelsus's, but it was associated with him at the outset, since it appeared in the pseudo-Paracelsian *Archidoxis Magica*, first published in 1570 as part of *De Summis Naturae Mysteriis*, a collection of tracts edited by Gerard Dorn. On della Porta see *DBI*; Nicola Badaloni, 'I Fratelli Della Porta e la cultura magica e astrologica a Napoli nel '500', *Studi Storici*, 1 (1959–60), 677–715; William Eamon, *Science and the Secrets of Nature. Books of Secrets in Medieval and Early Modern Culture* (Princeton, 1994), pp. 206–33. Ferrante Imperato, *Historia naturale* (Naples, 1599), pp. 438–41. For Ferrante Imperato (1550–1625), see *DBI*; Enrica Stendardo, *Ferrante Imperato: collezionismo e studio della natura a Napoli tra Cinque e Seicento* (Naples, 2001).
51   See Fra Donato d'Eremita, *Elixir vitae* (Naples, 1624), pp. 1–22, 40. On Fra Donato d'Eremita see Gabrieli, *Contributi*, ii, pp. 1487–95, 1533–8; Andrea Russo, *L' arte degli speziali in Napoli* (Naples, 1966), p. 77.

sulphur), mercury, *mumia,* and *bezoar minerale* (an oxide of antimony made with *aqua fortis*).[52]

The slow but steady progress of chemical medicines in Italy is also evidenced by the *Antidotarium* of Messina, written by Giovanni Battista Cortesi (1554– c.1636), professor at Messina, who did not question traditional medicine, but introduced into the pharmacopoeia a number of chemical remedies, mainly taken from Quercetanus.[53]

It is apparent that, after 1630, an increasing number of Italian physicians adopted chemical medicines. A turning point was the plague that in 1630 swept across Lombardy and the Republic of Venice. Thereafter, chemical remedies became more popular and tended to replace traditional ones. The Venetian physician Valerio Martini, deputed to care for the sick during the plague of 1630, promoted the remedies of Paracelsians like Quercetanus, Croll, Libavius, and Wecker.[54] The Bolognese physician Giovanni Antonio Vignati in his *Antidotario contro la peste* (1630) urged his readers to adopt chemical medicines, like bezoar, mercury, antimony and spirit of human blood.[55] Ludovico Locatelli (c.1600–1657), a medical practitioner from Bergamo, sold chemical remedies in Milan, Verona and Vicenza in 1630, and wrote a chemical tract based on Paracelsus and Petrus Severinus.[56]

The emergence of iatrochemistry

The evidence given above illustrates the degree to which chemical medicines entered Italy in the second half of the sixteenth and in the early decades of the seventeenth century. Not only did chemical remedies enter Italian medicine; Paracelsian theories did as well. There is evidence that Paracelsian medical philosophy and medicine appealed to many Italian physicians and natural

52   Fra Donato D'Eremita, *Antidotario* (Naples, 1639), pp. 20–9, 72–3, 94–135. According to Thomas Bartholin, who had visited Naples in 1644, the two works published under Fra Donato's name were actually written by Pietro Castelli. See Thomas Bartholin, *Epistolae Medicinales* (Copenhagen, 1663), p. 202. There is no evidence to assess what was Castelli's role in the production of the two books in question. Castelli was on good terms with Fra Donato, and certainly collaborated with him in Naples in 1626. See Gabrieli, *Contributi,* ii, p. 1495.

53   Giovanni Battista Cortesi, *Pharmacopoeia, sive Antidotarium messanense* (Messina, 1629). On Cortesi, see *DBI,* and Corrado Dollo, *Modelli scientifici e filosofici nella Sicilia spagnola* (Naples, 1984), pp. 145–8.

54   Valerio Martini, *Trattato della Curatione* (Venice, 1630). See Palmer, 'Pharmacy', p. 117.

55   Antonio Vignati, *Antidotario contro la peste* (Bologna, 1630), pp. 7–27.

56   Lodovico Locatelli, *Teatro d'Arcani* (Milan, 1644), p. 179. Little is known of Locatelli's life. He was born at the end of the sixteenth century and died in 1637. See A. Hirsch, *Biographisches Lexikon der hervorragenden Aerzte* (6 vols, 3rd edn, Munich, 1962), *s.v.*

philosophers, but no major confrontation between Galenists and Paracelsians took place in Italy. Outside official medicine, interest in alchemical medicine was widespread and was certainly reinforced by Paracelsian attacks on traditional medicine. The appeal of Paracelsus to the lower ranks of the medical profession has been documented for England and is also evident in Italy.[57] Currents of heterodox medicine, which were particularly strong in Venice, prepared the way and were drawn into Paracelsianism. Thanks to Eamon's work, we are now well informed on heterodox medicine in Italy, as well as on the role and contents of books of secrets, which dealt extensively with alchemy and medicine.[58] The most popular champion of Italian heterodox medicine was Leonardo Fioravanti, an eclectic writer, whose attacks on the medical establishment, and quest for a radical reform of medicine, were very close to Paracelsus's views. Like Paracelsus, Fioravanti maintained that unlettered experience was to be preferred to bookish medical learning, and adopted a number of chemically prepared medicines. Whether or not Fioravanti was influenced by Paracelsus, it is difficult to say. It is however a matter of fact that his works were often associated with those of Paracelsus and were praised by the Paracelsians, like John Hester in England.[59] Fioravanti himself admired Paracelsus, though he did not share relevant aspects of the latter's philosophy, such as the macro-microcosm analogy and the doctrine of signatures.[60] There can however be little doubt that Fioravanti's works paved the way for the diffusion of Paracelsian medicine in Italy.

The earliest impact of Paracelsian medicine occurred in the Republic of Venice. In Venice, Angelo Forte attacked Galenic medicine with arguments analogous to those of Paracelsus. Forte, who was a medical practitioner in Venice and fierce enemy of the Venetian College of Physicians, rejected the doctrines of humours and of natural heat, and condemned venesection. Like Paracelsus, Forte maintained that the physician had to develop a personal knowledge of nature and diseases by travelling and studying local people in different countries.[61] Later in the century, at the opposite end of the medical profession, we find Paracelsian views adopted by Alberto Cimerlino of Verona, rector of the arts university at Padua 1567–9.[62] The strongest attacks on Galenic medicine came from Verona, notably from the pen of Zeffirele Tommaso Bovio, a lawyer who turned medical practitioner. Bovio, who travelled to Bohemia, Germany, and France, corresponded with Fioravanti and styled himself 'physician to those who are sunk in despair' (*medico dei disperati*). He cured the poor and claimed that he successfully treated more than a thousand people during the plague that spread in Verona in 1576. Bovio was skilled in practical chemistry and often attacked the traditional

---

57   For England, see C. Webster, 'Alchemical and Paracelsian Medicine', in *idem*, ed., *Health, Medicine and Mortality in the Sixteenth Century* (Cambridge, 1979), p. 327.
58   Eamon, *Science and the Secrets of Nature*, pp. 134–93.
59   *Ibid.*, p. 254.
60   *Ibid.*, p. 191.
61   Palmer, 'Pharmacy', pp. 111–12.
62   Palmer, *The Studio of Venice*, pp. 24–30.

physicians (*medici razionali*) for their incompetence and greed.[63] True medicine – he claimed – was a gift from God and was only available to humble people and to those who cultivated empirical knowledge. Bovio, who stated that he had read up to 37 works of Paracelsus, stressed the importance of astrology and alchemy as the foundations of medicine.[64]

Galenic medicine was also criticized in 1615 by Fabrizio Bartoletti, who followed the Paracelsian theory of *semina* as the agents of diseases.[65] Like Bartoletti, Camillo Baldi taught in Bologna. Baldi adopted numerous aspects of Paracelsian medicine and opposed Galenic medicine as based on useless reasoning and devoid of empirical knowledge. To Baldi, the new medicine was to be rooted in chemistry and had to endorse the theory of the spagyrical principles.[66] The aforementioned Mantuan physician Francesco Bruschi, *archiatra* to the Duke of Mantua, in his *Promachomachia iatrochymica* (1623), attacked traditional medicine and espoused the chemical theory of principles and Petrus Severinus's view of spirits. During the early decades of the seventeenth century Paracelsian medicine (and in particular Petrus Severinus's *Idea Medicinae*) diffused more widely in Pisa, as attested by the aforementioned John Macollo, who followed Severinus's theory that *semina* were the origin of all natural bodies, and the cause of diseases.[67] Like Macollo, the Pisan professor Marco Cornacchini criticized the traditional Galenic therapies and also ruled out the use of venesection.[68] The Portuguese Estêvão Rodrigues de Castro (c.1559–1638), who in 1610 settled in Florence, where he worked as physician to the Grand Duke Cosimo II, and was appointed professor at Pisa, adhered to the doctrine of signatures (*Quæ ex quibus, opusculum in quatuor libros divisum medicinæ studiosis valde utile*, Florence, 1627) as well as to the Paracelsian analogy between macrocosm and microcosm (*De meteoris microcosmi*, Florence, 1621). Castro's work on meteors contains a long digression on atoms and a chemical account of the physiology of the human body.[69] For Castro, both the natural world and the human body worked as chemical laboratories, in which

63 Zeffirele Tommaso Bovio, *Flagello de' medici rationali* (1583; 2nd edn, Milan, 1617), pp. 50–1. On Bovio see *DBI*; Zanier, 'La medicina paracelsiana', pp. 633–5.

64 Bovio, *Fulmine contro de' medici putatitii rationali* (1592; 2nd edn, Milan, 1617), p. 203, and *idem, Melampigo overo confusione de' medici sofisti* (1585; 2nd edn, Milan, 1617). Bovio dedicated his *Fulmine* to Vincenzo Gonzaga, Duke of Mantua.

65 Fabrizio Bartoletti, *Encyclopaedia hermetico-dogmatica* (Bologna, 1615).

66 On Baldi, see Zanier, 'La medicina paracelsiana', pp. 638–9. His work on physiognomy is a commentary on pseudo-Aristotelian physiognomy: *In physiognomica Aristotelis commentarii* (Bologna, 1621). His Paracelsian views are contained in a manuscript tract entitled 'Trattato dell'alchimia e sua medicina': Bologna, Archiginnasio, MS B 1397, fols 124v–125r.

67 Macollo, *Theoria chymica*.

68 Cornacchini, *Methodus*.

69 Rodrigues Estêvão de Castro, *De Meteoris Microcosmi* (1st edn, Florence, 1621; 2nd revd edn, Venice, 1624), pp. 41–50, 100. For biographical details, see Hirsch, *s.v.* For Castro's atomism, see Pietro Redondi, 'Atomi, indivisibili e dogma', *Quaderni storici*, 20 (1985), 529–71.

distillations and circulations are continuously produced.[70] He explained fevers by means of the three chemical principles and by their interactions.[71]

In Southern Italy, Paracelsian views were widely adopted, though before 1650 they seldom brought about open opposition to Galenic medicine. Neapolitan physicians adopted Paracelsian ideas and practices. In his *Historia Naturale*, Ferrante Imperato stressed the importance of chemistry as the foundation of medicine, sought for the universal medicine, and adopted the macro-microcosm analogy.[72] In *De distillatione* (1608), Giovan Battista della Porta, following medieval alchemists, aimed at discovering secret and active principles contained in natural bodies, as, in his view, the four Aristotelian elements acted according to a force to be identified with the alchemists' quintessence.[73] In the *Phytognomonica* (1588), della Porta developed the doctrine of signatures – a cornerstone of Paracelsus's philosophy of nature – establishing correspondences between the forms and the therapeutic properties of plants.[74] Chemical investigations played a relevant part in the work of Colantonio Stelliola (1547–1623) and Fabio Colonna (1567–1640), who opposed scholasticism and stressed the importance of experimental knowledge.[75]

As we have seen, the *Accademia dei Lincei* contributed to the diffusion of iatrochemistry, notably through Schreck and Faber, the two German members of the *Accademia*, who were responsible for the dissemination of Paracelsianism among the *Lincei* and Roman physicians. Schreck, who in 1611 left the *Accademia* because he became a Jesuit, kept up his contacts with the *Lincei*, especially with Faber, to whom he sent information on Paracelsian books.[76] Faber was a central character in Roman medicine and natural philosophy at the beginning of the seventeenth century.[77] He replaced Michele Mercati and Bacci respectively as keeper of the papal garden and as professor of botany at *La Sapienza*. In 1608 he spent two months in Naples, where he became familiar with Imperato, della Porta, Fra Donato d'Eremita, Colonna, Stelliola and Marco Aurelio Severino. On 20 November 1622 Faber delivered, possibly at *La Sapienza*, an oration dealing with

70   Castro, *De Meteoris*, p. 112.
71   *Ibid.*, p. 233.
72   Ferrante Imperato, *Historia naturale*, pp. 432–41, 568–77.
73   Giovan Battista della Porta, *De distillatione* (Rome, 1608), pp. 2, 32–4.
74   See Massimo Bianchi, *Signatura Rerum. Segni, magia e conoscenza da Paracelso a Leibniz* (Rome, 1987), pp. 90–2.
75   On Stelliola, see Saverio Ricci, 'Nicola Antonio Stigliola enciclopedista Linceo', in *Atti della Accademia nazionale dei Lincei*, ser. 9, vol. 8, fasc. 1 (1996), 3–147. See also Nicola Badaloni, *Introduzione a Vico* (Milan, 1961), pp. 13–24.
76   Gabrieli, *Carteggio Linceo*, pp. 598–9, 605–6. The inventory of Faber's library shows that he owned several iatrochemical works: see Silvia de Renzi, 'La biblioteca di Johann Faber Linceo', in Eugenio Canone, ed., *Bibliothecae selectae: da Cusano a Leopardi* (Florence, 1993), pp. 517–24.
77   For Faber, see Gabrieli, *Contributi*, ii, pp. 1177–253; *DBI*; Clericuzio and de Renzi, 'Medicine, alchemy and natural philosophy', pp. 184–93.

the nature of fire and the origin of metals, in which he rejected the Aristotelian theory of elements and qualities. Faber's 'Oratio' tells us much about his chemical experiments, particularly those on the action of solvents, such as aqua regia and aqua fortis, and on the nature and possible transmutations of mercury. He recognized the possibility of extracting mercury from different compounds, and this suggests he regarded mercury as one of the basic elements of all matter.[78]

Besides his personal contributions to chemistry and Paracelsian medicine, Faber developed a network of correspondence with physicians and natural philosophers from various countries. One of his friends was the German iatrochemist Raymund Minderer (c.1570–1621), of Augsburg.[79] Faber was also in touch with the Dutch inventor Cornelis Drebbel (1572–1633), and with Drebbel's brothers-in-law, namely the Küffeler brothers, Jacob (1600–1622) and Abraham (1598–1657), both skilled in chemistry. The former died in Rome in 1622, while Abraham, after a brief stay in Rome, settled in Naples, where he met Fra Donato d'Eremita.[80] In Rome, Faber collaborated with Giulio Mancini, *Archiatra Pontificio*, and an advocate of chemical medicines.[81] Among Faber's acquaintances we find the group of physicians and apothecaries who met in the pharmacy at the sign of the Imperial Eagle (*All'Aquila Imperiale*) in Rome, who were renowned for their chemical medicines. Hendrik Cornelizen de Raeff (1554–1639), italianized as Enrico Corvino, an apothecary from Delft, and member of the *Accademia dei Lincei* from 1611, owned that pharmacy and built a celebrated botanical garden.[82] He was the brother-in-law of Pietro Castelli, one of the most innovative physicians and botanists in Rome in the 1620s and 1630s. Born in 1575, Castelli taught first in Rome and then in Messina, where he died in 1662.[83] In Rome, Castelli was a student of Andrea Bacci, Marsilio Cagnati, and Andrea Cesalpino and started his career by giving private lessons in chemistry and botany.[84] He was part of the influential circle of Cassiano dal Pozzo and Francesco Barberini, and was connected with powerful physicians, notably Paolo Zacchia (1584–1659), well known for his contributions to forensic medicine. Castelli was *lettore dei semplici*

78   'Oratio qua ignis et metallorum exemplo, quam parvum sciamus demonstratur': Naples, Biblioteca Nazionale, MS VIII.D.13.
79   See Gabrieli, *Contributi*, i, p. 541; ii, p. 1182.
80   Letters of Faber to Federico Cesi, 22 March 1625 and 13 April 1625, in Gabrieli, *Carteggio Linceo*, pp. 1033, 1038. For Drebbel, see *DSB*; for the Küffelers, see *Nieuw Nederlandisch Biografisch Woordenboek*, Vol. 2 (Leiden, 1912), cols 735–6.
81   See Clericuzio and de Renzi, 'Medicine, alchemy and natural philosophy', p. 191.
82   For Corvino, see Godefridus J. Hoogwerf, 'Henricus Corvinus', *Mededeelingen van het Nederlandisch Historisch Instituut te Rome*, 6 (1936), 91–109; 10 (1940), 123–7.
83   On Pietro Castelli, see *DBI*; Alessandro Ottaviani, 'Da Fabio Colonna a Paolo Boccone: momenti di storia della botanica tra Napoli e la Sicilia', in Corrado Dollo, ed., *Filosofia e scienze nella Sicilia dei secoli XVI e XVII* (Catania, 1996), pp. 137–66: pp. 137–54; Oreste Trabucco, '*Delle cagioni delle febbri maligne* di G.A. Borelli. Una lettura contestuale', *Giornale Critico della Filosofia Italiana*, 20 (2000), 236–80.
84   On Marsilio Cagnati (1543–1612), physician at Santo Spirito and professor of medicine at *La Sapienza*, see *DBI*.

at *La Sapienza*, and, after Johannes Faber's death (1629), became professor of medicine and keeper of the Vatican Garden.

In 1634 Castelli moved to Messina, where he taught medicine, founded the botanical garden, and unsuccessfully tried to introduce chemistry into the medical curriculum. Castelli's proposal of establishing chemical lectures in the University of Messina was part of his broader project to reform medical teaching. As shown by a letter he sent to Cassiano dal Pozzo on 1 March 1641, Castelli practised and taught chemistry in a laboratory built in the botanical garden.[85] He investigated the chemical properties of oil of vitriol, its preparation and uses in medicine, which he discussed in letters to Minderer.[86] He also prepared an electuary (made with tartar) that he used against diseases of the nervous system. His project of reforming medicine is articulated in his *Optimus Medicus* (1637), containing a chapter aimed at legitimizing chemistry as part of the medical curriculum. By rejecting the objections of traditional physicians, such as Francesco Avellino, a colleague of his in Messina, Castelli tried to demonstrate that chemistry could confer many benefits on medicine.[87] Following Libavius, he rejected Paracelsus's philosophy while extolling his medicines. Castelli quoted Libavius's definition of chemistry as contained in *Alchemia*: 'alchemy is the art of perfecting magisteries, and of extracting pure essences from compounds by separating them from their corporeal matrix'.[88] In order to make chemical medicine palatable to those who were not prepared to reject traditional medicine, Castelli argued that much of what Paracelsus wrote was by no means new, as he had often given new names to old notions.

Although Castelli would appear here to have adopted a cautious position that did not question traditional medicine, he was providing a rationale for a major reform of medicine that – in his view – could be accepted by academic physicians. In referring to Libavius's defence of chemistry against the Parisian medical faculty (*Alchymia triumphans*, 1607), Castelli stated that chemistry was to be recognized as indispensable to medicine. Thanks to chemistry – he stated – the physician would be able to prepare medicines that were more powerful than traditional ones.[89] His solution in this work was to establish a compromise between Galenic and Paracelsian medicine. However, if we consider Castelli's other works, we find

---

85   Rome, Biblioteca Corsiniana, Archivio dal Pozzo, MS. XII, fol. 17r–v. Castelli's letter is published in Ottaviani, 'Da Fabio Colonna', p. 159. Castelli's chemical investigations in Messina are also attested by his nephew Giovanni Pietro Corvino and by Borelli: see Dollo, *Modelli scientifici*, p. 153.

86   Pietro Castelli, *Calcanthinum dodecaphorion* (Rome, 1619). See also Castelli, *Epistolae Medicinales* (Rome, 1626).

87   Castelli, *Optimus medicus* (Messina, 1637), pp. 25–32. On Avellino and his attacks on chemistry see Dollo, *Modelli*, pp. 143–5, 153.

88   Castelli, *Optimus medicus*, p. 25. Castelli explicitly refrains from discussing transmutational alchemy. He quotes from Andreas Libavius, *Alchemia* (Frankfurt, 1597), p. 1. For Libavius see Owen Hannaway, *The Chemists and the Word* (Baltimore, 1975), pp. 75–151.

89   Castelli, *Optimus medicus*, p. 26.

that his views were much more innovative than it would appear from the *Optimus medicus*, which pursued the difficult task of making chemistry part of the academic medical curriculum. It is apparent that Castelli did not confine himself to introducing chemical remedies; he also questioned one of the pillars of Galenic therapeutics, namely, phlebotomy, by using arguments taken from classical authors and from Martin Ruland the younger (1569–1611).[90]

The most advanced aspect of Castelli's thought was his chemical interpretation of human physiology – mostly contained in a series of letters published in 1626. Castelli, who adopted the Paracelsian analogy between macrocosm and microcosm, maintained that an acid spirit was responsible for most physiological phenomena. Such a spirit was not made of the four elements and did not work according to the elementary qualities. Following Severinus, Castelli ruled out the Aristotelian doctrine of qualities and described the spirit as an active principle, of celestial origin. Castelli identified spirit with Paracelsus's alchemist, namely, the spiritual directing force located in the body.[91] Castelli's boldest move was his rejection of the Galenic theory of digestion as *concoctio* of food – that is, produced by heat. He explained digestion in chemical terms, namely, as a process produced by an acid ferment contained in the stomach. It is notable that Castelli adopted the chemical explanation of digestion before Joan Baptista van Helmont published his own theory of digestion in the *Ortus Medicinae* (1648). For Castelli, the bodily ferment was the same as those to be found in nature and producing all sorts of fermentation.[92] He described digestion as a fermentation originating from an acid spirit communicating its movement to the sulphurous, saline and mercurial parts contained in food.[93]

Castelli's letter on fermentation was addressed to Marco Aurelio Severino (1580–1656), who was then physician at the *Ospedale degli Incurabili* in Naples.[94] A student of Stelliola and follower of Campanella, Severino was connected with the botanist Fabio Colonna and Cassiano dal Pozzo.[95] Severino is mainly known for his contributions to anatomy and surgery; however, his works show that he pursued chemical investigations and applied chemistry to medicine. This is particularly evident in his book on vipers, which deals with the therapeutic use of the viper's

---

90   Castelli, *De Abusu Phlebotomiae* (Rome, 1628), pp. 77, 89–90. Castelli's reference
      was to Martin Ruland, *Thesaurus Rulandinus* (Basel, 1628).
91   Castelli, *Epistolae*, pp. 121–2, 154.
92   *Ibid.*, pp. 133–41.
93   *Ibid.*, p. 142.
94   The correspondence between Castelli and Severino is in Rome, Biblioteca Lancisiana.
      See Oreste Trabucco, 'La corrispondenza tra Pietro Castelli e Marco Aurelio
      Severino', in Dollo, *Filosofia e scienze nella Sicilia*, pp. 109–31. For Severino, see
      DSB, and Charles Schmitt and Charles Webster, 'Harvey and M.A. Severino: a
      neglected medical relationship', *Bulletin of the History of Medicine*, 45 (1971), 49–75.
95   See Oreste Trabucco, 'Scienza e comunicazione epistolare: il carteggio fra Marco
      Aurelio Severino e Cassiano dal Pozzo', *Giornale Critico della Filosofia Italiana*, 16
      (1996), 204–45.

poison. Following Paracelsus, Severino believed that poisons could be powerful remedies if deprived of their lethal properties by chemical treatment.[96] Like Castelli, Severino placed special emphasis on fermentation, which in his view was the cause of digestion and of generation.[97]

Severino's iatrochemical views were shared by other physicians in Naples, notably by Giovan Battista Capucci, whom Severino referred to as a chemical physician who adopted Paracelsian views. Filippo Finella (1584–c.1650) was also active in Naples; in 1649 he issued a tract on salts, dealing extensively with the extraction of salts and their medical uses. Finella's work clearly shows that in Naples the use of chemical remedies was widely accepted and that physicians and apothecaries were engaged in chemical investigations on substances (salt of tartar, salt of mercury and salt of lead) that Paracelsian physicians had long been promoting.[98]

It is apparent that by the 1640s Paracelsian medicine had gained momentum in Italy and that iatrochemical theories were being adopted by a number of Italian physicians. In 1643 the Genoese physician Girolamo Bardi, who was a correspondent of Pierre Gassendi, adopted Daniel Sennert's view of Paracelsus, namely, he defended Paracelsian iatrochemistry, but rejected the philosophy of the Swiss physician.[99] In 1644 there appeared the first Italian translation from Paracelsus, made by the aforementioned Ludovico Locatelli, who included a version of Paracelsus's *Erklärung über etliche Aphorismen des Hippokrates* in his *Teatro d'arcani*.[100] Unlike Bardi, Locatelli was a fervent Paracelsian; he espoused Paracelsus's medicine and philosophy, and explicitly rejected traditional medicine. Locatelli, who travelled to Germany in 1642, maintained that chemical reactions took place in the human body that were the same as those produced in the laboratory.[101] Natural bodies contained a subtle and pure spiritual substance that chemists could extract and use for their remedies.[102] Following Bovio, Locatelli attacked Galenists as ignorant and greedy, and promoted a great number of chemical remedies, like *arcanum corallinum*, tartar, vitriol, *mercurius vitae*, and *aurum potabile*, most of them taken from Paracelsus, Martin Ruland and Quercetanus.[103]

96   Marco Aurelio Severino, *Vipera Pythia* (Padua, 1651), pp. 511–13.
97   Severino, *Vipera*, pp. 354–5.
98   Filippo Finella, *Soliloquium Salium* (Naples, 1649), pp. 71, 101, 106–27.
99   Girolamo Bardi, *Medicus politico-catholicus* (Genoa, 1644), pp. 25, 380.
100   Locatelli, *Teatro d'arcani*, pp. 308–402 (Karl Sudhoff, *Bibliographia Paracelsica* (Graz, 1958), no. 361). In order to publish his *Teatro*, Locatelli obtained a special permission from the *Sant'Uffizio* in 1643, as he quoted from books on the *Index*, namely those of Paracelsus, Lull, and Arnald of Villanova.
101   Locatelli, *Teatro d'arcani*, p. 6.
102   *Ibid.*, pp. 34–9.
103   *Ibid.*, pp. 54–254.

In 1648, Castelli's plea for a reform of medicine based on chemistry found the support of Giovanni Galeano, physician in Palermo.[104] In the following year Giovanni Alfonso Borelli, who had settled in Messina in 1636, published the lectures he gave at the *Accademia della Fucina* in Messina in 1648.[105] The subject of Borelli's lectures was the 'malignant fevers' (possibly typhus) that spread in Sicily in 1647 and 1648 – a subject that Castelli too had dealt with in 1648. Castelli's explanation of the fevers was very close to Paracelsus: he maintained that fevers were produced by the *ens deale* (that is, the wrath of God), *ens spirituale* (acting through the spirits, and originating from unclean spirits), and finally, by the *ens naturale* (that is, natural causes, including air) – but dismissed Paracelsus's astrological explanation (that is, his *ens astrale*) as impious.[106] For his part, Borelli omitted both the *ens deale* and the *ens spirituale* and also rejected humoralism and astrology, explaining fevers by means of chemical and corpuscular theories. He argued that the sun drew poisonous and corrosive exhalations from the bowels of the earth, which he styled seeds of the plague (*semi pestilenziali*).[107] For Borelli, chemistry accounted for both the origin of malignant fevers and their cure, so he recommended the use of a remedy made with sulphur that he prepared with the help of Pietro Castelli.[108] In Borelli's view, fevers were not to be confused with the disease, as they were the outcome of the motion of blood and spirits, which was aimed at combating the external poisonous agents.[109] Borelli's work included a section on digestion, where he developed Castelli's views. Digestion, Borelli maintained, is both a chemical and a mechanical process by which food is minced into small parts, which are acted upon by the acid juice contained in the stomach. This was confirmed by what was observable in nature, where vitriols and other acids could dissolve the hardest bodies.[110]

Conclusions

It is apparent that in Italy Paracelsianism promoted new approaches in medical theory and practice, in a variety of social and intellectual contexts: in courts and academies, as well as in pharmacies and in universities. Paracelsus and his followers were initially seen as proponents of new chemically prepared medicines

104 Giovanni Galeano, *Epistola medica* (Palermo, 1648). See Trabuco, 'Delle cagioni', pp. 258–9.
105 On Borelli, see *DSB*; *DBI*; Ugo Baldini, 'Borelli e la rivoluzione scientifica', *Physis*, 16 (1974), 97–128.
106 Castelli, *Preservatio corporum sanorum* (Messina, 1648), pp. 10–20. Cf. Trabucco, 'Delle cagioni', pp. 261–2.
107 Giovanni Alfonso Borelli, *Delle cagioni delle febbri maligna della Sicilia negli anni 1647 e 1648* (Cosenza, 1649), pp. 106–7, 113–15, 126–8.
108 *Ibid.*, pp. 137–44.
109 *Ibid.*, pp. 157–73.
110 *Ibid.*, pp. 206–16.

– which indeed by 1630 were accepted all over the Peninsula. As we have seen, frontal attacks on Galenic medicine, like those of Bovio and Locatelli, were rather isolated. Paracelsian medical theories were adopted by many physicians, who tried to establish a compromise with traditional medicine. As evidenced by Castelli, this attitude to compromise did not prevent Italian physicians from introducing radical changes in medicine, notably in physiology. Both Castelli and de Castro pursued new approaches to medicine giving chemistry a central role. From the *Accademia dei Lincei*, at the beginning of the seventeenth century, to Borelli's work on malignant fevers, there runs a continuous thread of interests in those problems defined by the Paracelsians, especially the chemical foundation of medicine. When Joan Baptista van Helmont's *Ortus Medicinae* was published in 1648, a substantial number of Italian physicians had already adopted both chemical medicines and Paracelsian views. Van Helmont's iatrochemistry, together with Harvey's circulation physiology and corpuscularianism, provided Italian physicians with an articulated set of theories that enabled them to redefine the main physiological functions of the human body, and to reject many Galenical assumptions that the previous generation of physicians did not question.

Chapter 5

Politics, Medicine, and Masculinity: Physicians and Office-bearing in Early Modern England

Margaret Pelling

In Charles Webster's *The Great Instauration*, science and medicine are shown to be integrally connected to religious convictions among Puritan reformers. These seventeenth-century idealists had political aims which were practical as well as visionary. Their schemes involved harnessing medical and scientific discoveries to improve the nation's health as well as its wealth, within a framework of religious conviction. They sought political influence in order to achieve their aims, and some of them held representative office. Nonetheless, Webster's argument does not require that this involvement occurred as a result of either their medical and scientific qualifications, or the greater respect being accorded to science or medicine in the modern professional sense. Webster's later work on the National Health Service analyses the evolution, in practice as well as principle, of a unique political effort aimed at bringing the benefits of modern medicine to the population as a whole.[1] However, although the medical profession was essential to this process, few of the political actors involved were doctors. Thus, even in circumstances most fruitful for the interaction of medicine and politics, the role of medical practitioners themselves was not definitive and could of course also be antagonistic rather than supportive.

For comments on the text, I should like to thank Anne Laurence (especially for guidance on Irish and Scottish Parliaments), and Scott Mandelbrote. I also owe thanks to Carole Rawcliffe, for information on John Somerset and other early physician-MPs; Christine Churches and Martin Holt, for advice on cases in King's Bench; John Pickstone, for the Cooter reference; and Ian Mortimer, for allowing me to cite his thesis.

1   Charles Webster, *The Great Instauration: Science, Medicine and Reform 1626-1660* (London, 1975); idem, *The Health Services since the War. Volume I, Problems of Health Care: the British National Health Service before 1957* (London, 1988); idem, *The Health Services since the War. Volume I, Government and Health Care: the National Health Service 1958-1979* (London, 1996); idem, *The National Health Service: A Political History* (Oxford, 1998).

What then, if any, is the accustomed relationship between medicine and politics in the British Isles? This question is not widely considered, suggesting that the instinctive response is likely to be in negative terms – that is, it is assumed that the two are independent of each other, or more simply that there is little relationship at all. There may be a number of possible reasons for this, though all of them are open to challenge. First, the professional ethos attributed to medicine requires detachment, objectivity, and a commitment to the individual human person regardless of his or her beliefs, political and otherwise. This ethos is underwritten by medicine's claims to be securely anchored in scientific principles. Secondly, and more pragmatically, it could be assumed that medical practitioners were, and are, simply too busy to involve themselves in rival activities likely to make appreciable demands on their time; moreover, they are obliged to respond to calls from ill and injured people as a first priority.[2] Thirdly, they can be located in the same position as publicans and shopkeepers: reluctant to avow political allegiance for fear of alienating their preferred clientele. Lastly, medical practitioners tend to be seen as individualistic. In spite of contrary indications such as the effectiveness of some of their organizations (like the British Medical Association), the development of joint practices, and the tribal loyalties fostered in medical schools and hospitals, medical men appear, in literature and elsewhere, as detached, necessarily competitive, socially somewhat rootless or even isolated, often free-thinking, and difficult to enlist for any common purpose.

Obviously, a positive response to the question is also possible. This would most commonly be in terms of medicine's integral role in liberal reforms, especially from the Enlightenment onwards.[3] Such an account transforms into positive virtues some of the features suggested above for the negative case. Thus politics, like medicine, can devote itself to the health and well-being of the individual in secular society; scientific medicine can offer models for social transformation. A central concept in this area of discussion is 'medical police', which can however be located in absolutist as well as liberal regimes, and which has been detected, for England, as early as the Jacobean period.[4] In the second place, many would equate

2   For a succinct discussion, in terms of the 'peculiarly professional belief system' of a cohesive, 'very successful [American] social elite', see W.A. Glaser, 'Doctors and politics', *American Journal of Sociology*, 66 (1960), 230–45, at p. 230.

3   Cf. for example Peter Gay, 'The Enlightenment as medicine and as cure', in W.H. Barber et al., eds, *The Age of the Enlightenment: Studies Presented to Theodore Besterman* (Edinburgh, 1967), pp. 375–86; A.C. Vila, *Enlightenment and Pathology: Sensibility in the Literature and Medicine of Eighteenth-Century France* (Baltimore, 1998); L.W.B. Brockliss, *Calvet's Web: Enlightenment and the Republic of Letters in Eighteenth-Century France* (Oxford, 2002).

4   George Rosen, *From Medical Police to Social Medicine: Essays on the History of Health Care* (New York, 1974); H.J. Cook, 'Policing the health of London: the College of Physicians and the early Stuart monarchy', *Social History of Medicine*, 2 (1989), 1–33; Dorothy Porter, *Health, Civilization and the State: A History of Public Health from Ancient to Modern Times* (London, 1999), pp. 52–4.

medicine and politics with medical reform, which has received a good deal of attention from historians.[5] This is the attempt by medicine to reform itself by political means, leading to educational specifications, a qualifying process, and a register of authenticated practitioners recognized by the state. The assumption would be that the aims of medical reform and the interests of society were one and the same. A third major argument could be constructed on the basis of the public health movement, and subsequently, the relationship between doctors and the state in the context of the rise of welfare. Whether medical men as a group were active or passive participants in these movements is debatable, but they are currently given the benefit of the doubt by many historians.[6]

As already suggested, the positive and the negative cases have certain features in common. Chronologically, both place their emphasis on more recent periods, when medicine had gained in authority and acquired something like professional status. Both grant medicine a good deal of autonomy, and accord it the right to suggest how politics should be conducted and for what purposes. Hence, in these contexts, where medical practitioners are seen as political actors in any sense they are medical first, and political second, if at all. In the Webbs' analysis of the relationship between doctors and the state, for example, actual participation by doctors in politics was not an issue. In terms of providing a recent overview of the topic, the current benchmark is perhaps the collected volume edited by Porter and Porter, *Doctors, Politics and Society*. Chronologically, the contributors begin with the Utilitarian philosopher Jeremy Bentham, moving on to sanitary reform and public health, notable twentieth-century medical politicians (Viscount Addison, Lord Dawson of Penn), interwar movements (social medicine and Nazism), and medically qualified historians of medicine with strong political views (Henry Sigerist, George Rosen). Many of the individuals considered in these essays had only a relatively tenuous connection with medicine and medical practice, but the

5   Royston Lambert, *Sir John Simon 1816–1904 and English Social Administration* (London, 1963); Irvine Loudon, *Medical Care and the General Practitioner 1750–1850* (Oxford, 1986); Hilary Marland, *Medicine and Society in Wakefield and Huddersfield 1780–1870* (Cambridge, 1987), esp. chap. 8.

6   Cf. M.E. Rose, 'The doctor in the Industrial Revolution', *British Journal of Industrial Medicine*, 28 (1971), 22–6; Margaret Pelling, *Cholera, Fever and English Medicine 1825–1865* (Oxford, 1978); J.V. Pickstone, *Medicine and Industrial Society: A History of Hospital Development in Manchester and its Region, 1752–1946* (Manchester, 1985); Simon Szreter, 'The importance of social intervention in Britain's mortality decline c.1850–1914: a re-interpretation of the role of public health', *Social History of Medicine*, 1 (1988), 1–37, and the ensuing debate between Szreter and Sumit Guha in that journal, 7 (1994), 89–113, 269–82; Jane Lewis, 'The medical journals and the politics of public health 1918–90', in W.F. Bynum, Stephen Lock and Roy Porter, eds, *Medical Journals and Medical Knowledge: Historical Essays* (London, 1992), pp. 207–27; Dorothy Porter, ed., *The History of Public Health and the Modern State* (Amsterdam, 1994); Paul Weindling, ed., *International Health Organisations and Movements 1918–1939* (Cambridge, 1995).

overall framework is in terms of what medicine has to say to the state. *Doctors, Politics and Society* focuses mainly on the British Isles, as the present chapter intends to do. The excellent monograph by Ellis, on late nineteenth-century France, amply demonstrates how different the results can be if we look elsewhere. Ellis's work is particularly relevant here because he considers medical practitioners who were actively engaged in representative politics, as opposed to being agents and advisers of the state in less visible or more subsidiary ways. Nonetheless, Ellis's physician-legislators belong to a period when medicine was rapidly gaining in authority and status.[7]

Office-bearing: functions, burdens, and inducements

The issues involved in the positive and negative cases as outlined above are all of course extremely important. Nevertheless, it is hard to escape the impression that direct involvement by medical practitioners in the political system in the British Isles was (and is) relatively limited. The purpose here is to provide some hard evidence for this view, by approaching the original question in a rather different way and for a period arguably pre-dating medicine's emergence as a profession. My main concern is neither the overlap between medicine and the public interest, nor with the issue of the political convictions held by medical men. Rather, I would like to look at the politically-related functioning of medical practitioners as members of a given society – in particular, their willingness to take on the public and representative roles which can be roughly grouped together under the heading of office-bearing. With respect to office-bearing itself, this will perforce imply a certain conceptual shift from the voluntary to the obligatory. The voluntary principle must dominate the consideration of office-bearing in the modern period, but for earlier centuries, while many offices were coveted and competed for, many others, particularly at the parish level, were imposed or seen as the inescapable duty of every householder. Equally, 'politics' is being used here in a broad sense as overlapping with 'government', rather than implying party politics, which is not a relevant concept until the later seventeenth century. The focus for present purposes will be on offices above the parish level, partly because of problems of evidence, partly because of the effect of exemptions for the middling sorts and above, and partly to place the stress on offices which were more desirable and more closely related to government.

7   Sidney Webb and Beatrice Webb, *The State and the Doctor* (London, 1910), preface; Dorothy Porter and Roy Porter, eds, *Doctors, Politics and Society: Historical Essays*, Clio Medica 23 (Amsterdam, 1993); J.D. Ellis, *The Physician-Legislators of France: Medicine and Politics in the Early Third Republic, 1870–1914* (Cambridge, 1990). For information on medical practitioners as members of the US Senate and House of Representatives, see 'Doctors in government', *Journal of the American Medical Association*, 163 (1957), 361–4.

The approach taken here arises from earlier work which suggested that early modern medical practitioners faced considerable difficulties in terms of their status in society, which could be related, in part, to the gendered nature of the work they did.[8] Physicians were perhaps the most vulnerable to gender-related disadvantage, and also the most ambitious, and the most anxious, in status terms. They can be detected as following strategies designed to compensate for their equivocal position, which were partly successful but which also led them into the pitfalls of over-compensation. This ambivalence is epitomized in the remarkable degree to which they were isolated from the normal structures of male authority. They might have been expected to behave like other groups seeking to establish themselves, by seeking and accepting office whenever it was offered. Instead, they seem to have avoided office-bearing at almost every level. For example, although in some towns physicians were included in barber-surgeons' companies, their role in civic life was extremely limited. They claimed exemption from all military, policing, and jury duties as a right of privilege, while offering little in return in terms of public service.[9] As already indicated, a retrospective view might find this detachment unsurprising. However, if we set aside retrospection, and examine the phenomenon on its merits, it becomes both interesting and extremely unusual.

Office-bearing as a whole is clearly a major subject, involving almost infinite local variation as well as changing religious and political circumstances. It is hardly possible to consider it fully here. However, the scholarly consensus is firm enough to supply a context for the present discussion in which office-holding was pervasive at all levels of early modern English society.[10] Bearing office, like

8 See Pelling, *Medical Conflicts in Early Modern London: Patronage, Physicians and Irregular Practitioners 1550–1640* (Oxford, 2003), and references there cited.

9 For physicians in companies, see Pelling, *The Common Lot: Sickness, Medical Occupations and the Urban Poor in Early Modern England* (London, 1998), pp. 209ff, 237. On exemption, claimed first by surgeons but for different reasons and with different consequences, see G.N. Clark, *A History of the Royal College of Physicians of London* (2 vols, Oxford, 1964–6), i, pp. 81–4, 138, 190, 281, and ii, p. 533; Sidney Young, *Annals of the Barber-Surgeons of London* (1890; repr. New York, 1978), pp. 60, 97–100; Jessie Dobson and R. Milnes Walker, *Barbers and Barber-Surgeons of London* (Oxford, 1979), pp. 20, 27–8, 66.

10 The consensus about office-bearing is closely related to the perceived need to explain the relative stability of early modern English society, and has been reached with particular reference to London: see for example Jeremy Boulton, *Neighbourhood and Society: A London Suburb in the Seventeenth Century* (Cambridge, 1987); Steve Rappaport, *Worlds Within Worlds: Structures of Life in Sixteenth-Century London* (Cambridge, 1989). In the process of this revision, office-bearing itself has been revalued: Peter Clark, 'The civic leaders of Gloucester 1580–1800', in Peter Clark, ed., *The Transformation of English Provincial Towns 1600–1800* (London, 1984), pp. 311–45. For valuable overviews, see I.A. Archer, 'Politics and government 1540–1700', in Peter Clark, ed., *The Cambridge Urban History of Britain: Vol. II, 1540–1840* (Cambridge, 2000), pp. 235–62; Alison Wall, *Power and Protest in England 1525–1640* (London, 2000).

marriage, signified adult maturity and fitness to head a household. Although oligarchical or dynastic tendencies can be identified in some places or situations, these were seen not as the norm but as a departure from it.[11] Most offices were held on an annual basis or 'at the pleasure' of higher authority, and there was a high rate of turnover of incumbents.[12] Virtually universal office-bearing was also in many respects a necessity, given the absence of regular police, a standing army, or a fully developed civil service. The Tudor period saw an increase of governance and the offices to effect it, from poor law officials up to the lords lieutenant of shires.[13] Some offices paid expenses or attracted fees and perquisites, including bribes, but most were unpaid and dependent upon their holders having sufficient property to make dishonesty look dishonourable.[14] For individuals, bearing office was a means of consolidating their position in the community, or of improving it. For authority, every link in the chain of office, however small, strengthened stability, religious conformity, and awareness of mutual social obligations. This is not to deny that office was frequently seen as onerous, expensive, and something to avoid if at all possible.[15] Office-holding could also be self-interested in its aims, and socially divisive in its effects. But the essential point is how broadly the burden of responsibility was felt and carried. That is, holding office was normal for adult males; never holding office, in the absence of some disqualification such as idiocy or extreme poverty, was not.

Eligibility is an obvious factor to take into account with respect to particular offices. Barriers did exist, such as oaths, bearing mainly on matters of religion. Higher offices required the incumbent to hold substantial property, preferably in land, and residence was a frequent prerequisite. Even parish offices involved versions of these requirements.[16] Perceived conflicts of interest could disqualify

---

11   J.T. Evans, 'The decline of oligarchy in seventeenth-century Norwich', *Journal of British Studies*, 14 (1974), 46–76. Cf., on Parliament, Ellis Wasson, *Born to Rule: British Political Elites* (Stroud, 2000).

12   See Alison Wall, '"The greatest disgrace": the making and unmaking of JPs in Elizabethan and Jacobean England', *English Historical Review*, 119 (2004), 312–32.

13   See for example Norman Bell, 'Representation in the English House of Commons: the new boroughs, 1485–1640', *Parliament, Estates and Representation*, 15 (1995), 117–24; Gary Gibbs, 'New duties for the parish community in Tudor London', in K.L. French, Gary Gibbs and B.A. Kümin, eds, *The Parish in English Life 1400–1600* (Manchester, 1997), pp. 163–77.

14   R.C. Braddock, 'The rewards of office-holding in Tudor England', *Journal of British Studies*, 14 (1975), 29–47; R.C. Latham, 'The payment of parliamentary wages – the last phase', *English Historical Review*, 66 (1951), 27–50.

15   See for example J.I. Kermode, 'Urban decline? The flight from office in late medieval York', *Economic History Review*, 35 (1982), 179–98; R.M. Wunderli, 'Evasion of the office of alderman in London, 1523–1672', *London Journal*, 15 (1990), 3–18.

16   See Charles Drew, *Early Parochial Organisation in England: the Origins of the Office of Churchwarden* (York, 1954), pp. 10ff.

certain occupations, for example victuallers.[17] Nonetheless, it can be said that there was virtually no form of disqualification of this kind that could not be set aside if the conditions were right, or the influences in favour of it sufficiently strong. Similarly, criteria for eligibility could appear most prominently when competition for office was most fierce, as in localities where there was factional in-fighting or an unstable balance of power. Self-disqualification is also important here because exemption from offices at the bottom end of the ladder – for example, in the parishes – was often sought by claimants to higher status. However, refusing an office usually meant paying a fine or appointing a proxy, which again required certain levels of available income.

Proving the case with respect to medical practitioners requires the evidence to be systematic as well as comprehensive. Here, it is possible to provide only a provisional overview, and to suggest some hypotheses for future testing.[18] These will necessarily be based on a somewhat scattered sample, and only certain offices can be considered. There are also, of course, definite limitations as to sources. Even official lists of Members of Parliament (MPs) and justices of the peace (JPs) are imperfect, and these problems are compounded by the fact that in such contexts, status, including land-holding, was far more important as a signifier than was occupation. Official lists often gave names alone, so that the historian's attention is pushed towards those who are readily recognizable.[19] Even minor gentry can be surprisingly difficult to identify with certainty. Where more information is given, a prosperous physician is less likely to be identified as such than to be hidden behind status descriptors such as gentleman and esquire, descriptors which the physician might equally prefer to use of himself in drawing up his own will. Even at the parish level, it was more relevant to indicate the individual's sufficiency for office than his occupation. Problems also arise with anecdotal evidence. Some claims in older sources are impossible to substantiate. Many contemporaries reporting on office-bearing wanted to push a case about burdens, interference, or decline, and such reports, like the polemics against intruders into medicine, could be misleading about the social status of those being used as examples. Similarly, for many standard secondary works, especially older ones, occupation is irrelevant compared with status, and occupation in any case relates mainly to exceptions which can be so few in number that they are disregarded. For the same

---

17 Francis Blomefield, *An Essay Towards a Topographical History of the County of Norfolk* (11 vols, London, 1805–10), iii, p. 129; S.L. Adams, 'Office-holders of the borough of Denbigh and the stewards of the Lordships of Denbighshire in the reign of Elizabeth I', *Denbighshire Historical Society Transactions*, 25 (1976), 92–113, at p. 103.

18 It is hoped that the present essay will form the basis of a full-length study. If readers have instances or counter-instances to suggest, these would be most gratefully received.

19 See for example *The Roll of the Mayors of Bath* (Bath, [1926]), in which additional information is first given for 1801.

reason, grounds for exemption from office are most frequently mentioned only in passing.

Close to the Crown: lieutenants and sheriffs

Thus both the question being asked here, and the evidence needed to answer it, are in general well below the surface of both record-keeping and historical discussion. For this reason, if for no other, *a priori* assumptions should be kept to a minimum. However, there are offices at the highest levels which can be ruled out for medical practitioners almost by definition; that is, the absence of medical holders is insignificant because they would never have been seen as eligible. These include, in the early modern period at least, the lords lieutenant of the shires, and their deputies.[20] It is worth noting nonetheless that these major offices suggest a theme which will recur with respect to lesser ones, namely the connection between office-holding and military responsibilities, and the detachment of physicians from both. With respect to the great offices of state, we might expect the same as with lords lieutenant; but this expectation is complicated by the few exceptions, which include John Somerset (d. 1454), who was Chancellor of the Exchequer in 1439 as well as Warden of the Mint. Somerset was a court physician, and his rare eminence illustrates how proximity to the Crown could produce single exceptions that prove the rule.[21] From 1500 until the twentieth century, officers of state with medical qualifications were rare to non-existent. The very different kind of influence (rather than power) commonly exerted by practitioners close to government is illustrated by Henry VIII's physicians Sir William Butts (c.1485–1545) and Augustine de Augustinis (d. 1551), Sir Alexander Fraizer (1607?–1681), physician and political adviser to Charles II, or, at the end of the eighteenth century, Lord Chatham's friend and physician, Anthony Addington (1713–90). Addington was the father of Viscount Sidmouth who, as prime minister, was nicknamed 'the Doctor' by satirists, in reference to his middling origins.[22] A telling case of similar date is that of Sir William Knighton (1776–1836, MD Aberdeen 1806), who began in practice as a naval surgeon and accoucheur. Knighton's personal qualities enabled him to become physician and then chief man of business to the Prince of Wales, later George IV. His role seems to have been entirely honourable but he was prevented from becoming a privy councillor and private secretary to the king by Lord

---

20　Wall, *Power and Protest*, pp. 40–1, 106–7.
21　H.C.G. Matthew and Brian Harrison, eds, *Oxford Dictionary of National Biography* (60 vols and online Oxford, 2004) [hereafter *OxfordDNB*].
22　E.A. Hammond, 'Doctor Augustine, physician to Cardinal Wolsey and King Henry VIII', *Medical History*, 19 (1975), 215–49; W.H. Helfand, 'Medicine and pharmacy in British political prints – the example of Lord Sidmouth', *Medical History*, 29 (1985), 375–85. For Butts, Fraizer and Addington, see *OxfordDNB*.

Liverpool, on the grounds of his having been intimate, as a man-midwife, with 'all the ladies in London'.[23]

The office of sheriff is another that might be ruled out on first principles, but this would be, at least partially, a mistake. Sheriffs represented the Crown in their localities, especially with respect to law and order, and transmitted the summons to Parliament. However, their powers had waned by the early modern period, and the position became first less prestigious, and then, by the nineteenth century, increasingly nominal and honorific.[24] Medical practitioners were chosen for the office even before 1700, but very much in a civic context: the locations are the largest towns, the office is usually the prelude to the mayoralty, and the practitioners involved are not physicians, but apothecaries and barber-surgeons. Not surprisingly, apothecaries predominate overall, since they were positioned near the top of the civic hierarchy; barber-surgeons had only a middling position among the crafts. However, a series of eminent London barber-surgeons served as sheriff, starting with John Ayliffe (d. 1556), surgeon to Henry VIII, Master of the Barber-Surgeons' Company in 1538 and elected sheriff ten years later. The exceptional Peter Proby (d. 1625), a London barber-surgeon who (necessarily) translated to the Grocers' Company in 1622 in order to take on the mayoralty, had been elected alderman and sheriff in 1614. Ayliffe and Proby were both knighted, Ayliffe in 1549 and Proby in 1623.[25] A cluster of similar figures can be found in the second half of the seventeenth century, interlocked through apprenticeship, business, marriage, and (to some extent) Nonconformity and stranger origins: (Sir) John Frederick (1601–1685), Master of the Barber-Surgeons in 1654 and 1658, and sheriff in 1655; (Sir) Nathaniel Herne (c.1629–1679) Master in 1674 and sheriff in the same year; (Sir) John Lethieullier (1632/3–1719), Master in 1676 and sheriff two years earlier; and (Sir) Thomas Challoner (d. 1766), Master in 1761 and sheriff in 1762.[26] These individuals might be seen as barber-surgeons only in name, as they were also successful merchants, but, even when they had to translate elsewhere to stand for the mayoralty, their loyalty to their original, middle-ranking company seems to have been strong. Only Frederick may not himself have served an apprenticeship. Mercantile interests were not unusual among barber-surgeons in major towns, especially those with links overseas: Lethieullier's interests in textiles, dyeing and metals were traditional diversifications for barber-surgeons.

---

23   *OxfordDNB.*

24   Roger Virgoe, 'The crown, magnates, and local government in fifteenth-century East Anglia', in J.R.L. Highfield and Robin Jeffs, eds, *The Crown and Local Communities in England and France in the Fifteenth Century* (Gloucester, 1981), pp. 73–6; Irene Gladwin, *The Sheriff: The Man and his Office* (London, 1974); J.B. Payen-Payne, *The Roll of the High Sheriffs of England and Wales, for the Year of Grace 1878* (London, 1879).

25   Young, *Annals*, pp. 516–21, 532–5. See also A.B. Beaven, *The Aldermen of the City of London* (2 vols, London, 1908–1913).

26   See Young, *Annals*, pp. 550–7, 567; for Lethieullier, see also *OxfordDNB*; for Herne, see also *OxfordDNB*, art. 'Herne, Sir Joseph'.

Ayliffe was also a merchant, but his career was first advanced by his curing Henry VIII of a fistula. Apparently cognate with this group is (Sir) Humphrey Edwin (1642–1707), who was elected Master of the Barber-Surgeons' Company in 1688, sheriff in the same year, and mayor in 1697. However Edwin, the son of a Welsh feltmaker who became mayor of Hereford, was also, more unusually, sheriff of Glamorganshire, having bought estates there, and he was made alderman in London on the direct appointment of James II. His profile is further complicated by his Nonconformity: he caused considerable controversy by attending conventicles in full civic state as London's mayor.[27]

Among the apothecaries, Edmund Phillips senior, of London, alderman from 1621, and first Master of the Society of Apothecaries, was called to be sheriff, but declined the office.[28] In Norwich, the second city after London in this period, for which there is also considerable information, we find a thin trickle of 'medical' sheriffs beginning with the apothecary John Mingay (1556–1625), who was sheriff in 1602 and mayor in 1617, and the apothecary George Birch (d. c.1632), sheriff in 1604 and mayor in 1621. Both appear to have been active as apothecaries; Birch certainly practised medicine.[29] Later apothecary-sheriffs in Norwich include Roger Hawes, sheriff in 1658 and mayor ten years later, and John Pell, mayor in 1730. Hawes was forbidden from keeping an apothecary's shop during the plague in 1631, not long after taking out his freedom, and was ejected from the aldermanry in 1677.[30] Medical sheriffs in Norwich in the eighteenth century, by contrast, tended to be surgeons, serving during a period of major political upheaval, and notable for their strong political views. James Crowe (1750–1807), son of a mayor of Norwich, was an 'ardent' Whig who was himself mayor (twice, in 1774 and 1797) after serving as sheriff in 1771.[31] Another Whiggish surgeon, Elias Norgate (d. 1803), was sheriff in 1781 and mayor in 1785.[32] A third, Edward Rigby (1747–1821), sheriff in 1803 and mayor a year later, was said to have danced round a

27   Young, *Annals*, pp. 516–17, 560–2; for Edwin, see also *OxfordDNB*.
28   T.D. Whittet, 'The charter members of the Society of Apothecaries', unpublished paper (summarized in *Proceedings of the Royal Society of Medicine (Section of the History of Medicine)*, 64 (1971), 30), p. 2.
29   B. Cozens-Hardy and E.A. Kent, *The Mayors of Norwich 1403 to 1835* (Norwich, 1938), pp. 73, 75; *Correspondence of Lady Katherine Paston 1603-1627*, ed. Ruth Hughey, Norfolk Record Society XIV (1941), pp. 100, 101; Margaret Pelling and Charles Webster, 'Medical practitioners', in Charles Webster, ed., *Health, Medicine and Mortality in the Sixteenth Century* (Cambridge, 1979), pp. 214, 221–2.
30   Cozens-Hardy and Kent, *Mayors of Norwich*, pp. 93, 118; W.L. Sachse, ed., *Minutes of the Norwich Court of Mayoralty 1630–1631*, Norwich Record Society XV (1942), p. 157.
31   Cozens-Hardy and Kent, *Mayors of Norwich*, p. 134. On Norwich politics, see Nicholas Rogers, *Whigs and Cities: Popular Politics in the Age of Walpole and Pitt* (Oxford, 2001).
32   Cozens-Hardy and Kent, *Mayors of Norwich*, pp. 138–9; A. Batty Shaw, *Norfolk and Norwich Hospital. Lives of the Medical Staff 1771–1971* (Norwich, 1971), p. 40.

'Tree of Liberty' singing the Marseillaise. Rigby had been educated at Joseph Priestley's school in Warrington, and visited France in 1789. He is described as a physician, but he trained as a surgeon, practised as a lithotomist, and was surgeon to the Norfolk and Norwich Hospital for over 40 years before being appointed as a physician there in 1814.[33] Similar figures – surgeons or surgeon-apothecaries – can be found in Newcastle during the same period.[34]

An interesting break in the line of politically active Norwich surgeons is the physician John Beevor (1726–1815, MD Cambridge 1764). Beevor was born in Norwich, and was not isolated from his more radical surgical colleagues in that one of his daughters married James Crowe, while a brother, who inherited the family's brewing business, married a daughter of Edward Rigby. Beevor was 'pricked' for sheriff in 1789, but refused to serve, 'being a doctor of physic, in extensive practice'. He applied to the court of King's Bench for exemption, and his plea was admitted. Beevor had county connections, made a good second marriage, and claimed the status of 'esquire'.[35] His resistance to civic office-bearing contrasts with the enthusiasm detectable in physicians by the end of the following century. (Sir) Frederic Bateman (d. 1904, MD Aberdeen 1850), house-surgeon and then physician at the Norfolk and Norwich Hospital, 'took a full part in civic affairs', becoming sheriff in 1872 as well as a magistrate. He was born in Norwich and his father had also been sheriff.[36] A positive relish for office, especially its ceremonial aspects, was shown by (Sir) Peter Eade (1825–1915, MD London 1850), who was elected to Norwich City Council in 1869, aged about 44, just over ten years after his first appointment as physician to the Norfolk and Norwich Hospital. Eade, 'one of the best known provincial physicians in the country', was sheriff in 1880, mayor three times, and knighted in 1885. Eade noted of himself that, before 1915, he was the only member of the medical staff of the Hospital to serve as mayor more than once, or, for over a hundred years, to serve in the two offices of mayor and sheriff.[37]

Medicine and law: the magistracy

The shrievalty might perhaps be dismissed, as having become too peripheral to government or political engagement. The same could not be said of the magistracy.

33   *Oxford DNB*; Batty Shaw, *Norfolk and Norwich Hospital*, pp. 23–5; Cozens-Hardy and Kent, *Mayors of Norwich*, pp. 146–7.

34   T.R. Knox, 'Wilkism and the Newcastle election of 1774', *Durham University Journal*, 72, new ser. 41 (1979), 23–37, esp. pp. 29, 30.

35   Batty Shaw, *Norfolk and Norwich Hospital*, pp. 15–16; P. Browne, *History of Norwich* (Norwich, [1814]), p. 62. For the legal position on exemptions by the early nineteenth century, see J.W. Willcock, *The Laws Relating to the Medical Profession* (London, 1830), chap. 8.

36   Batty Shaw, *Norfolk and Norwich Hospital*, pp. 57–8.

37   *Ibid.*, pp. 55–6; Peter Eade, *Autobiography*, ed. S.H. Long (London, 1916), p. 11.

As is well known, the workhorses of administration and adjudication throughout the early modern period were the justices of the peace for the counties and boroughs. These varied in number under different reigns – Elizabethan policy favoured small, efficient benches, which were allowed to expand under James I – and there are longstanding debates about the degree to which the commissions for the peace were subject to political influence, as opposed to representing the shifting balance of power among men of property in their localities.[38] Such men could exercise influence on the bench by proxy, through their relatives and connections, as well as in their own persons. Complaints about central interference were usually associated with claims that property qualifications were being ignored or that the new justices were men of no account. By the eighteenth century justices had increased in numbers and it was not uncommon for members of the professions as well as the lesser clergy to be selected. Given also that a justice might be appointed but never become active, this is not then a case in which medical practitioners can be ruled out as possible incumbents *a priori*. Instances found so far are nonetheless very few for earlier periods, enough to prove that it was possible, but so few as to indicate that it was rare. Somerset was a justice, as was the royal physician John Hamond (d. 1617, MD Cambridge), for Surrey;[39] the royal physician (and royalist historian) Robert Brady (c.1627–1700, MD Cambridge by royal mandate 1660), for Middlesex and Westminster;[40] Thomas Arris (MD Oxford 1651), son of Edward Arris, serjeant-surgeon to the king, for Hertfordshire;[41] and the royalist John Lamphire (1614–1688, created MD Oxford 1660) for Oxford. The pleasure-loving Lamphire was described by Wood, whose physician he was, as 'a public-spirited man but not fit to govern'.[42] These were all physicians, but a (royal) surgeon could be a justice: Alexander Baker (d. 1635, Master of the London Barber-Surgeons' Company in 1622), serjeant-surgeon to James and Charles I, and son of the well-known surgeon George Baker, was JP for Middlesex.[43] The royalist

---

38   There is a considerable literature on justices of the peace, but see M.L. Zell, 'Early Tudor JPs at work', *Archaeologia Cantiana*, 93 (1977), 125–43; J.R. Lander, *English Justices of the Peace, 1461–1509* (Gloucester, 1989); Wall, *Power and Protest*; A. Hassell Smith, *County and Court: Government and Politics in Norfolk 1558–1603* (Oxford, 1974); J.H. Gleason, *The Justices of the Peace in England 1558–1640: A Later Eirenarcha* (Oxford, 1969); L.K.J. Glassey, *Politics and the Appointment of Justices of the Peace 1675–1720* (Oxford, 1979); Norma Landau, *The Justices of the Peace, 1679–1760* (Berkeley, 1984). The role of JPs in Scotland, initiated by James I and VI, developed much later than in England.

39   *Oxford DNB*; Gleason, *Justices of the Peace*, p. 259.

40   *Oxford DNB*.

41   Young, *Annals*, p. 549; William Munk, *Roll of the Royal College of Physicians of London*, Vol. I (2nd edn, London, 1878), p. 342.

42   *Oxford DNB*.

43   *Ibid.*, art. 'Baker, George'; Young, *Annals*, pp. 8, 495; J.L. Chester, ed., *The Marriage, Baptismal and Burial Registers of the Collegiate Church or Abbey of St Peter, Westminster*, Harleian Society X (1876), p. 131.

Sir Thomas Bludder (d. 1655), MP for Reigate as well as JP for Surrey, can hardly be counted among the surgeons, although he sought the freedom of the London company in 1621.[44]

Other medical justices include Thomas Jeesop (MD Oxford 1569, d. 1615), in his home county of Devon;[45] and, in Yorkshire during the Commonwealth, Joseph Micklethwaite (1594–1658, MD Basel 1620), whose father Elias was an alderman of York.[46] An interesting instance from Scotland illustrating the effect of patronage is the well-known chemist and clinical teacher William Cullen (1710–1790), who served as a magistrate and surgeon in Hamilton, under the aegis of the Duke of Hamilton, before graduating MD at Glasgow in 1740.[47] Later examples include the 'leading Norwich physician of his time', Warner Wright (1775–1845), who was born in Norwich, and Richard Woosnam (1815–1888, MRCS), JP for Brecon and high sheriff of Montgomeryshire. Although Woosnam travelled as a surgeon (and diplomatic secretary) in India and China, both his parents were born in Montgomeryshire.[48] What these scanty examples suggest is, again, the influence of proximity to the Crown, and to the capital; and secondly, the force of local connections, relevant for justices at all periods, but having its main effect somewhat belatedly with respect to medical practitioners.

Over the course of the nineteenth century, both the medical profession, and the role of justices of the peace, changed considerably.[49] With the growth in public administration (police, poor law, public health, local government) the duties of justices became at once less comprehensive and more purely honorific. By this time, at least in the towns, the occupational catchment-area for justices was relatively wide. In a list of the names and professions of justices drawn up in the 1890s for England and Wales, based on returns made by the localities, 78 boroughs out of 113 (69 per cent) named at least one medical practitioner as a member of their commission for the peace. (Benches did of course vary considerably in size.) Medical justices were present in the English counties and peculiars in about the same proportion as for the boroughs of England and Wales (34 out of 55, or 62 per cent).[50] However, there are striking contrasts with the boroughs. For the counties,

44   Young, *Annals*, p. 545.
45   Munk, *Roll*, pp. 74–5; Gleason, *Justices of the Peace*, p. 249.
46   R.W. Innes Smith, *English-Speaking Students of Medicine at the University of Leyden* (Edinburgh, 1932), p. 158.
47   *OxfordDNB*.
48   Batty Shaw, *Norfolk and Norwich Hospital*, p. 31 (for Wright); Payen-Payne, *Roll of the High Sheriffs*, p. 94 (Woosnam is the sole medical sheriff in this list); J.A. Venn, *Alumni Cantabrigienses...from 1752 to 1900*, Vol. VI (Cambridge, 1954).
49   See C.H.E. Zangerl, 'The social composition of the county magistracy in England and Wales, 1831–1887', *Journal of British Studies*, 11 (1971–2), 113–25.
50   Calculated from: 'Return giving the names and professions, or descriptions, of all justices of the peace for the counties of England and Wales...for cities and boroughs of England and Wales...', *Parliamentary Papers*, 1893–4, LXXIV, Pt I, pp. 229–475. I hope to provide a more detailed analysis at a later date.

the lists of justices still have an *ancien régime* look about them. Counties lacking medical JPs were, roughly speaking, those where the bench was still dominated by the gentry, the church, the military, and the law, for example Oxfordshire.

These later lists which provide occupational information tend to confirm first, that medical practitioners seldom held office until the office concerned had faded in importance in political (but not necessarily status) terms; secondly, that office-bearing only became common when the status of practitioners was more assured; thirdly, that where higher-status groups were dominant, medical men were likely to be squeezed out; and lastly, that medical practitioners were at a disadvantage *vis-à-vis* office-bearing because their careers involved little contact with the civil law. This last point can be taken further, and has parallels with what was said earlier about military obligations being intimately connected with higher office. Blackstone, writing in the mid-eighteenth century, took it for granted that medical men had scant use for legal knowledge except to support the character of a gentleman, and Gisborne's later handbook of the 'duties' of different walks of life gives the same impression.[51] This is not to say that all JPs were, by contrast, well trained in the law. Men of property however tended to have some stake in it, and some direct contact, starting with the Inns of Court as young men, and going on to their own law suits.[52] Legal knowledge was perhaps the most useful acquirement in someone seeking a patron or employer among the elite. Towns also valued legal expertise, and service as a legal adviser of any kind was a regular route to representative office. Medical practitioners were largely excluded from this pervasive network of posts and influence, and this, combined with their self-imposed exclusion from military obligations, cut them off from much of the male world in which authority was exercised.

Mayors and aldermen: the *cursus honorum* of towns

We have already seen, in various examples, that offices such as that of sheriff could be staging posts on the *cursus honorum* of office-bearing in towns. The basis of such office-bearing, as of urban representative politics in general, was the freedom, and from this world too physicians were almost entirely barred, by a process of self-exclusion. It is true that in many places only a proportion of

---

51   William Blackstone, *Commentaries on the Laws of England* (2 vols, Dublin, 1766–7), i, p. 14; Thomas Gisborne, *On the Duties of Physicians, Resulting from their Profession* (Oxford, 1847), pp. 9, 36; repr. from 6th edn (1811) of his *An Enquiry into the Duties of Men in the Higher and Middle Classes of Society in Great Britain* (Dublin, 1795).

52   Lawrence Stone, *The Crisis of the Aristocracy 1558–1641* (abridged edn, Oxford, 1967), pp. 312–13; C.W. Brooks, *Pettyfoggers and Vipers of the Commonwealth* (Cambridge, 1986), chaps 4 and 5.

members in a given craft or trade took out the freedom,[53] that a man could become free without having served an apprenticeship, and that physicians did, as already noted, belong to craft companies in a few of the larger provincial towns. However, physicians hardly saw themselves as on a par with the humbler crafts and trades which seldom produced a mayor or even an alderman. They were deeply reluctant to associate on equal terms even with those at the upper levels of the urban hierarchy, such as merchants, goldsmiths, and (especially) apothecaries, essentially because these groups were too close for comfort.[54] Thus, the invisibility of physicians in urban contexts seems to be a measure of their disengagement from civic life in its public dimensions. This also limited their presence as justices of the peace, as they did not have that standing in corporate towns which entitled them to act as magistrates by virtue of their position as alderman or mayor. The readiness of physicians to leave for the country during plague epidemics may have been only one facet of their ambivalent relationship with towns. In the earlier period at any rate, physicians give the impression of mobility, or at least of not wanting to identify with a particular urban locality.[55]

It is therefore unsurprising that physicians are almost never found as mayors in earlier periods, even in the eighteenth century. Surgeons on the other hand do occasionally appear in high civic office. William Gale (d. 1610), Thomas Thorney (d. 1614) and John Richmond were members of London's common council;[56] Edward Arris, mentioned above, was a London alderman in the 1660s. Of those already noted as serving as sheriff of London, Proby (1622/3), Frederick (1661), and Edwin (1697) completed the *cursus* to become mayors, as did another merchant member of the Barber-Surgeons, (Sir) William Stewart (d. 1723), sheriff in 1711 and mayor in 1721.[57] As we have already seen for Norwich and London, aldermanic apothecaries were relatively common from an early date. Robert Maskew of York, in the 1570s and 1580s, had a fairly typical identity as grocer, apothecary, alderman, and surgeon.[58] The prominent apothecary Gideon Delaune

---

53   For overall figures, see Joyce Ellis, 'A dynamic society: social relations in Newcastle-upon-Tyne, 1660–1760', in Peter Clark, ed., *The Transformation of English Provincial Towns 1600-1800* (London, 1984), pp. 201, 223.

54   See Pelling, *Medical Conflicts*, esp. chap. 5.

55   On London physicians, mobility and urban plague, see *ibid.*, chap. 2. On the importance of local roots see for example Clark, 'Civic leaders of Gloucester'. Interestingly, Ellis's physician-legislators mostly originated not in major towns but in small market towns and villages: *Physician-Legislators of France*, p. 21; cf. however p. 24.

56   Young, *Annals*, pp. 7, 538–9, 574 and *passim*; F.F. Foster, *The Politics of Stability: A Portrait of the Rulers in Elizabethan London* (London, 1977), pp. 170, 171.

57   Young, *Annals*, pp. 19, 562–3.

58   Margaret Barnet, 'The Barber-Surgeons of York', *Medical History*, 12 (1968), 24; David Palliser, 'Civic mentality and the environment in Tudor York', *Northern History*, 18 (1982), 92. On practitioners of this type, see Pelling, *Common Lot*, chaps 4 and 9.

(1564/5–1659) was elected for Dowgate ward in London; he had to decline on account of his alien birth, paying a fine of £30, but he gained precedence in the Society of Apothecaries.[59] A centre like Canterbury produced aldermanic apothecaries from the later sixteenth century on a routine basis.[60] More controversially, the 'arch dissenting apothecary' John Greenwood was installed as mayor in Lancaster in 1688, offending Tory opinion in a similar manner to the London Barber-Surgeon Humphrey Edwin.[61] In the next century, Philip Potter, apothecary and son of an apothecary of the same name, was mayor of Great Torrington in Devon three times between 1705 and 1719.[62] The exception among physicians so far is Francis Banister (MD Oxford 1620), member of a largely surgical dynasty, who is said to have been mayor of Bedford in 1635 and 1645.[63] The timing might suggest unusual political circumstances attributable to revolutionary conditions, as in the case of the Yorkshireman John Webster (1611–1682), an ordained schoolmaster, who was a surgeon and possibly chaplain in the Parliamentary army, and in-bailiff of Clitheroe in Lancashire 1657–9; Webster did however hold this last office again after the Restoration, in 1665 and 1675.[64]

Slightly later, and on the other side of the political divide, we find the Tory John Tarleton (b. 1650), son and heir of a Liverpool gentleman. Tarleton began as a surgeon, took out a licence as a physician, and became mayor of Lancaster before returning to his inheritance (augmented by marrying an East India Company heiress) in Liverpool. A second, and native, Lancaster example is the Catholic Tory Henry Bracken (1697–1764), who practised as a surgeon and also wrote on farriery. Bracken was, perhaps wrongly, imprisoned for abetting Jacobites; shortly afterwards, in 1748, he was elected mayor, and was elected again a decade later.[65] A third, somewhat later instance from the north is the surgeon John Drake Bainbridge (1725–1814), who was elected mayor of Durham at least five times between 1761 and 1794.[66] Enduring local connections were also exhibited by the naval surgeon and diarist James Yonge (1647–1721), born in Plymouth, a royalist and Tory who travelled widely but returned to became alderman and mayor of Plymouth in 1694. Yonge took out an ecclesiastical licence to practise physic, and became an extra-licentiate of the Royal College of Physicians just before his

59 See F.N.L. Poynter, *Gideon Delaune and his Family Circle* (London, 1965), pp. 20–1 and *OxfordDNB*, which disagree as to the date of election.

60 See I.J.F. Mortimer, 'Medical assistance to the dying in provincial southern England, *c.*1570–1720', unpublished Exeter University Ph.D. thesis (2 vols, 2004), i, pp. 197, 200; ii, pp. 183, 194, 215, 230, 240, 289.

61 M.A. Mullett, 'Conflict, politics and elections in Lancaster, 1660–1688', *Northern History*, 19 (1983), 81.

62 J.J. Alexander and W.R. Hooper, *The History of Great Torrington in the County of Devon* (Sutton, 1948), pp. 133, 223.

63 I owe this information to Michael Cooke.

64 *OxfordDNB*.

65 Mullett, 'Conflict, politics and elections in Lancaster', pp. 75, 79; *OxfordDNB*.

66 *OxfordDNB*, art. 'Fothergill, Anthony'.

retirement from practice in 1703. A similar, but later, west-country case is Stephen Luke (1763–1829, MD Aberdeen 1792, MD Cambridge 1821), born in Penzance, who did well in London but returned to practise as a physician in Falmouth, and published on the diseases of Cornwall. Luke was mayor of Falmouth in 1797 and, interestingly, captain of a volunteer cavalry regiment at the same date. Some thirty years later, he became physician-extraordinary to George IV.[67]

A correlation with west-country or south-coast naval and military ports is also shown by the surgeon-apothecary Edward Linzee, father-in-law and effectively patron of the prominent naval officer Samuel (later 1st Viscount) Hood; Linzee was mayor of Portsmouth for the fifth time in 1766.[68] Still in the west country, but not a port, was Great Torrington, where 'Mr William Craddock', also called Dr Craddock or Cradock, was mayor three times between 1720 and 1738. Craddock was employed by the town to provide medical poor relief, which does not necessarily reflect on his status as a medical practitioner, but his being called 'doctor' in this context does not guarantee that he was a physician.[69] Similarly, Totnes in Devon produced a surgeon-mayor, Benjamin Amyatt, member of a 'leading burgess family' and father of an MP.[70] Several of these medical mayors – Tarleton, Yonge, Luke, and perhaps Linzee – illustrate a pursuit of upward social mobility as well as Tory leanings. To them may be added John Matthews (1755–1826, MD Oxford 1782) who, after a medical career in London and having married an heiress, returned to his native county of Herefordshire and became a leading county figure, building a mansion, and writing bad verse with partly political intent. Matthews served as colonel of militia, magistrate, alderman, mayor of Hereford (1793), and county MP in the 1800s.[71]

The town of Bath might be supposed to provide an exception to the paucity of physician-mayors, along with other health resorts or spa towns. However, even Bath's first examples occur at a relatively late date (Henry Harington, 1793; John Ford Davis, 1830; Randle Wilbraham Falconer, 1857), and it is perhaps more notable that it is apothecaries, above all other occupations, who dominate the mayoral list. Fifteen different apothecaries were mayors of Bath. It should also be noted that a barber, Walter Hicks, was mayor three times between 1683 and 1705.[72] The resort effect might be suggested for Brighton by (Sir) John Cordy Burrows

---

67 *OxfordDNB*.

68 *Ibid.*, art. 'Hood, Samuel'.

69 See Alexander and Hooper, *History of Great Torrington*, pp. 133, 191, 193, which distinguishes the elder Craddock from the younger, also 'doctor', a surgeon and mayor.

70 I.R. Christie, *British Non-Elite MPs, 1715–1820* (Oxford, 1995), p. 73; Lewis Namier and John Brooke, eds, *The House of Commons 1754–1790* (2nd edn, 3 vols, London, 1985), ii, pp. 21–2.

71 *OxfordDNB*.

72 *Roll of the Mayors of Bath*; Trevor Fawcett, *Bath Administer'd: Corporation Affairs in the 18th-Century Spa* (Bath, 2001), p. 78; John Wroughton, *Stuart Bath: Life in the Forgotten City, 1603–1714* (Bath, 2004), pp. 34–7.

(1813–1876, MRCS 1836), who was involved in the purchase of the Royal Pavilion by the municipality, and was twice mayor of Brighton (newly chartered in 1854) in the 1850s. However Burrows, the son of an Ipswich silversmith, was a surgeon, his posts including that of brigade surgeon to an artillery corps. Among his other public activities were contributions towards the founding of a mechanics' institution, and the adoption of the Health of Towns Act. The profile of a physician-mayor of Stratford-upon-Avon of the same period, John Conolly (1794–1866, MD Edinburgh 1821), is closer to that of Burrows than those of the Bath physicians. Conolly was first an ensign in a militia company, and married the daughter of a naval captain. He was popular in Stratford, where he was twice mayor and a supporter of sanitary reform and similar causes; however he was less successful in practice and for this reason took up the asylum work for which he became best known.[73] The examples of Burrows and Conolly suggest some continuity in the civic orientation of surgeons as opposed to physicians.

Medicine in Parliament

What about Members of Parliament? It should be stressed that the duties of a MP were sporadic, depending upon the frequency of parliaments, and were by no means as onerous as those of a justice of the peace. However, as with justices of the peace, there is continued debate among historians about the balance of forces involved in the selection of MPs, which could be reflected in changes in numbers. In the earlier period, contested elections were rare, and have been seen as evidence of breakdown in the normal consensual process of selection, but the degree to which MPs in the Commons were mere appendages of the ruling elite has also been questioned.[74] Recently, more attention has been given to non-elite MPs, and the publications of the History of Parliament Trust are also invaluable in giving some access to these lower-status groups.[75] However it can still be difficult to identify small minorities with any certainty, and discrepancies exist between the Trust's listings and other sources. That said, enough examples are available to suggest that the number of medical MPs is greater than might be expected, from the discussion so far, even for the earlier period.

Nonetheless, on a comparative basis, the numbers of medical MPs remain small. The higher clergy, as of right (in the House of Lords), and the law, in terms

73   *Oxford DNB*.
74   See for example Derek Hirst, *The Representative of the People? Voters and Voting in England Under the Early Stuarts* (Cambridge, 1975); M.A. Kishlansky, *Parliamentary Selection, Social and Political Choice in Early Modern England* (Cambridge, 1986); Bell, 'Representation in the English House of Commons'.
75   Christie, *British Non-Elite MPs*. The publications of the Trust over 60 years are now available as a CD-ROM (1998); five further volumes, for 1690–1715, have since been published. For present purposes the main gaps in coverage are 1604–1659, and 1422–1508.

of backgrounds, training, and occupation, were of course far better represented among MPs than medicine. Being a cleric as well as physician seems to have made office-bearing more likely. Lack of interest in the law, and detachment from civic life, were two reasons why physicians were unlikely to be selected to represent boroughs. Two of the seventeenth-century Barber-Surgeon mayors of London already mentioned, Frederick and his son-in-law Herne, were both MPs, each of them for Dartmouth, and Frederick also for the City of London. Lack of status, it might be presumed, would equally prohibit physicians from being selected as county representatives. The question then arises of how far these limitations could be counterbalanced by the close attachment often found between physicians and elite households (and the Crown), which as has been indicated shows itself in a range of services performed by physicians which could loosely (and sometimes euphemistically) be described as political. Such attachments should not be over-simplified. Medical men might join the following of a particular magnate from religious conviction, which could be of the reforming variety.

Henry VI's physician and Chancellor John Somerset is the first medical practitioner known to have been a MP.[76] The eight medical MPs provisionally identified for the sixteenth century, all of them physicians, provide a variety of illustrations. Robert Harridans or Harrydaunce (c. 1464–1514, MD Cambridge 1499/1500) was a MP in 1512, but he was also a citizen and mercer of Norwich who, while paying to avoid the offices of mayor, sheriff and constable, was active as a common councilman.[77] Certain civic tendencies are also present for Richard Patrick (d. 1566, MD Cambridge 1553), who was MP for his home town of Hunt-ingdon in 1559, being bailiff there in 1554 and 1559. Seemingly very different, but also influenced by local connections, is Humphrey Llwyd or Lloyd (1527–68, MA Oxford 1551), who was for most of his life in the service of the 12th Earl of Arundel, to whom he became connected by marriage. Llwyd was chiefly distin-guished as a Welsh antiquarian, but was MP for East Grinstead in 1559, and for Denbigh Boroughs, in his home county, in 1563. Arundel was a steward of the duchy of Lancaster, and East Grinstead was a duchy borough.[78] Patrick and Llwyd may both have had Catholic sympathies, but two more of the sixteenth-century medical MPs were strongly Protestant. The well-travelled Paracelsian Thomas Moffet (1553–1604, MD Basel 1579) was the son of a London haberdasher; Moffet became physician to the 2nd Earl of Pembroke and, through his influence and that of his wife Mary Herbert, was elected MP for Wilton in 1597. Another London practitioner, Moffet's friend and fellow Paracelsian Peter Turner (1542–1614, MD

76   *OxfordDNB*. In what follows, MPs are allocated to a century according to their date of first election.
77   S.T. Bindoff, ed., *History of Parliament: The House of Commons 1509–1558* (3 vols, London, 1982), ii, p. 313 (as Harydance); C.H. Talbot and E.A. Hammond, *The Medical Practitioners in Medieval England. A Biographical Register* (London, 1965), pp. 70, 423–4.
78   P.W. Hasler, ed., *History of Parliament: The House of Commons 1558–1603* (3 vols, London, 1981), iii, p. 186; ii, pp. 481–2; *OxfordDNB*, art. 'Llwyd, Humphrey'.

Heidelberg 1571), was the son of the botanist and Marian exile William Turner. Peter Turner served as MP for Bridport, and was active in advocating Presbyterian forms of worship.[79] His son Samuel (d. c.1647) was also a medical MP, and attached to the Pembroke circle. He is best known as the outspoken opponent of the Duke of Buckingham in the House of Commons, but later sat in Charles I's Parliament in Oxford.[80] The other sixteenth-century medical MPs were the Paracelsian Richard Bostocke (d. 1606), a gentleman-landowner whose career exhibits the standard features of patronage links, legal experience and service as a justice; the royal physician and government record-keeper John James (d. 1601, MD Cambridge 1578); and Thomas Lake (d. 1595, MD Cambridge 1571), who, according to a later judgement which could be seen as characteristic, 'blended politics with Medicine in a somewhat odd fashion'.[81]

Slightly more (twelve) medical MPs can be found for the seventeenth century.[82] This group is characterized by two additional features: university representation, and Commonwealth politics, which were intimately connected in mid-century because of Oxford's position as a royalist stronghold.[83] Besides the twelve, others, most notably Thomas Sydenham (1624–1689, MD Cambridge 1676), either stood for Parliament or were promoted as possible members. It has been claimed that parliamentary representation in mid-century shows the effects of increased respect for scientific qualifications.[84] This seems true only on the basis first, that medicine and science were seen as having utility in the public interest, and secondly, that the individuals concerned were politically engaged rather than adopting the neutral stance later thought proper to scientific pursuits. This is illustrated both by Sydenham, who saw active military service and also sought public appointments, and stood for his native county of Dorset in 1658; and by (Sir) William Petty (1683–1687, MD Oxford 1650), who became physician-general to the army in Ireland. Petty was most active in public life in Ireland, and was returned for both the Irish and the English Parliaments.[85]

The university representatives include Robert Brady, already mentioned, who was MP for Cambridge in the 1680s. Brady, the son of an attorney, was Master of

79   *OxfordDNB*.
80   *DNB*; *OxfordDNB*; V.A. Rowe, 'The influence of the Earls of Pembroke on parliamentary elections, 1625–41', *English Historical Review*, 50 (1935), 248, 251 ff.
81   David Harley, 'Rychard Bostok of Tandridge, Surrey (c.1530–1605), MP, Paracelsian propagandist and friend of John Dee', *Ambix*, 47 (2000), 29–36; *OxfordDNB* (for James); T.A. Walker, *A Biographical Register of Peterhouse Men* (2 pts, Cambridge, 1927–1930), i, p. 225; Hasler, *History of Parliament*, i, pp. 457–8; ii, p. 374. The identity of Lake remains in some doubt: cf. Hasler, ii, pp. 428–9.
82   This total includes Samuel Turner, and excludes Thomas Bludder, both mentioned above. It currently also excludes a thirteenth potential MP, William Bell, Master of the London Society of Apothecaries 1641–1644.
83   See M.B. Rex, *University Representation in England 1604–1690* (London, 1954).
84   *Ibid.*, pp. 185, 187 (but cf. p. 186).
85   *OxfordDNB*; Rex, *University Representation*, pp. 194, 207.

Caius College and Regius Professor of Physic, but he was active in London as a custodian of the Tower records and supporter of James II.[86] Of a more mixed political complexion, but essentially Tory and anti-Catholic, was (Sir) Thomas Clarges (?1617–1695), brother-in-law of General Monck. Contemporaries pointed to Clarges's low origins as an apothecary and son of a London blacksmith. His role as Monck's agent and emissary was typical of medical men of a certain type – Petty was also a bearer of secret despatches between Ireland and England – but it was unusual in its prominence. As with Samuel Turner, Clarges's active connection with medicine appears to have been negligible over his lifetime compared with his political career. He had a well-defined Parliamentary identity as 'Dr Clarges', but this need not imply that he ever gained formal qualifications as a physician. He first entered Parliament in the 1650s, for a Scottish constituency, and became a university member only from 1689.[87] (Sir) Thomas Sclater (1615–1684, MD Oxford 1649), son of a physician, and a Parliamentary sympathizer who was elected MP for Cambridge University in 1658/9, was assessed by Ralph Cudworth as 'a very ingenious person, of very good abilities'. In spite of the contrary opinion expressed of him by Francis Turner, Master of St John's College, as a 'man of ease' and a 'dumb burgess', Sclater is much more obviously a university member than was Clarges.[88] So too, in spite of his unpopularity among his colleagues, is (Sir) Thomas Clayton the younger (1612–1693, MD Oxford 1639), Warden of Merton from 1661 to his death, and Regius Professor of Medicine from 1647 to 1665, who was elected MP for his university in 1660. Clayton's father held the Regius professorship before him, and he enjoyed useful court connections.[89] He appears as a kind of inverted image of his predecessor, Jonathan Goddard (1617–1675, MD Cambridge 1643), son of a wealthy London shipbuilder, who was Warden of Merton from 1651 until the Restoration. Goddard accompanied Cromwell to Scotland, and was nominated as member for Oxford University in Barebone's Parliament in 1653.[90] Another physician close to Cromwell, John

---

86   See also B.D. Henning, ed., *History of Parliament: The House of Commons 1660–1690* (3 vols, London, 1983), i, pp. 706–7.

87   *OxfordDNB*; Rex, *University Representation*, pp. 372 and *passim*; Henning, *History of Parliament*, ii, pp. 74–81.

88   Rex, *University Representation*, p. 369; W.M. Palmer, 'A biographical note of Sir Thomas Sclater, Bart.', *Proceedings of the Cambridge Antiquarian Society*, 17, new ser. 11 (1913), 124–7.

89   Rex, *University Representation*, p. 369; Joseph Foster, *Alumni Oxonienses*, Vol. I (Oxford, 1891); G.C. Brodrick, *Memorials of Merton College* (Oxford, 1885), pp. 110–22; G.H. Martin and J.R.L. Highfield, *A History of Merton College, Oxford* (Oxford, 1997), pp. 212–16, 220–1; Henning, *History of Parliament*, ii, pp. 87–8.

90   *OxfordDNB*; Webster, *Great Instauration*, pp. 79, 499. Edward Reynolds was briefly Warden of Merton between the tenures of Goddard and Clayton. Brodrick's claim that Goddard was a member of Cromwell's Council of State in 1653 is not confirmed in later sources: Brodrick, *Memorials*, p. 168.

Palmer, was, like Petty, mooted as a possible MP for the university in 1658.[91]

Of the remainder, Thomas Arris, mentioned above as a justice, owed his medical qualifications to his being 'well affected' to Parliament in the 1650s; he was chosen for St Albans in 1661. Frederick and Herne, noted already as mayors, can be allocated to the mercantile interest.[92] Similar in type if not in character is the ruthless building entrepreneur and economist Nicholas Barbon (1637/40–1698/9), son of the London merchant and politician Praisegod Barbon (or Barebone), who began his career by qualifying in medicine in the Low Countries (MD Utrecht 1661). Barbon went on to play a key role in developing London after the Fire, and bought his seat in Parliament in 1690, probably to gain immunity from some forms of prosecution in the courts.[93] Representing the same locality (Bramber, in Sussex, 'a particularly venal borough') at the same period was the royal physician John Radcliffe (1650–1714, MD Oxford 1682), equally a strong personality, but more active both as practitioner and parliamentarian. Radcliffe, a Tory, also represented Buckingham in 1713, after buying estates in the county, and was a freeman of Bath.[94] In spite of his eminence, social aspirations, and (selective) attendance on royalty, Radcliffe, who was belittled for his middling birth and his bad temper, belongs among the hairy meritocrats rather than the smooth placemen.

Thirteen medical MPs, only six of them physicians, can be cited for the next century, but it is not possible here to deal with them individually. Certain themes can be identified. Medical MPs, and MPs with medical connections (even when as distant as a grandparent) continued to be twitted on their lowly origins. Continuity is also provided by royalist medical MPs (such as John Freind), and by medical MPs of a mercantile bent which often overlaps with stranger origins. Not new, but becoming more evident, and strengthened by the superiority of medical education in Enlightenment Scotland, are MPs with links to Scotland and Ireland. Other identities would be seen by most historians as characteristically eighteenth-century: the surgeon-adventurers, making somewhat dubious fortunes in India and the East Indies; the emergence of druggists and chemists among the metropolitan MPs; and the famous quacks or irregular practitioners who also became MPs, such as Joshua Ward and Thomas Dimsdale, who could be seen as primarily commercial, or as exercising an instinct for self-preservation, like Barbon.[95]

In spite of the influence of the public health movement, the situation with respect to medical MPs in the nineteenth century is not radically different. The well-known radical Joseph Hume (1777–1855), for example, qualifies as a

91   Rex, *University Representation*, p. 194.
92   On Frederick and Herne, see also Henning, *History of Parliament*, ii, pp. 363–5, 538–9.
93   *OxfordDNB*; D.W. Hayton et al., eds, *History of Parliament: The House of Commons 1690–1715* (5 vols, Cambridge, 2002), iii, pp. 131–3.
94   *OxfordDNB*; *DNB*; Hayton, *History of Parliament*, v, pp. 245–51, at p. 247. For other physicians made freemen 'by gift' (in Canterbury), see Mortimer, 'Medical assistance to the dying', ii, pp. 180, 202, 253, 268.
95   Chemists, etc. are excluded from the total of 13.

surgeon-nabob. Thomas Wakley (1795–1862), campaigning founder of *The Lancet* and radical MP for Finsbury, was also a surgeon. Bath continued to show a tendency to elect a physician as its MP. A number of MPs and peers illustrate points already made about medicine and the law. Sir James Mackintosh of Kyllachy (1765–1832, MD Edinburgh 1787), first returned to Parliament in 1818, took up medicine as a second-best, and reverted to the law, and to liberal politics, as soon as resources allowed. Another lifelong liberal, the 'reluctant peer' Henry Bickersteth (1783–1851), Baron Langdale, similarly began in medicine but entered Parliament as a lawyer. Robert Bannatyne Finlay (1842–1929), 1st Viscount Finlay, who became Lord Chancellor in 1916, practised medicine for only a few months after graduation from Edinburgh in 1858 and was called to the London Bar in 1867.[96]

As the discussion of justices of the peace has indicated, office-bearing by medical men in the nineteenth century becomes complicated with greater participation by the professional classes in general, and changes in the offices themselves. This is epitomized in the fact that Donald Dalrymple (1814–1873), active both as surgeon and MP, was also deputy lieutenant for the county of Norfolk, an incumbency hardly imaginable in earlier periods when lords lieutenant were personally responsible to the Crown for order in their shires.[97] Also significant, as indicated at the start of this essay, is the involvement in urban politics of public health reformers, like the surgeon and factory inspector Robert Baker (1803–1880), and the pioneer of industrial medicine George Calvert Holland (1801–1865, MD Edinburgh 1827).[98] However, the evidence so far suggests that while nineteenth-century medical men increasingly sought offices which were seen as honorific, and which were becoming more accessible to the middle class, their active engagement in political representation remained limited. Medicine gained in professional standing but this was accompanied by a stress on autonomy and scientific neutrality. An illustration of the social acceptability of such claims in the twentieth century is Lambert's depiction of the surgeon and medical officer of health John Simon as 'the open mind at work', celebrating the role of professional standards and scientific virtue in government administration rather than representative politics.[99] A twentieth-century medical MP could likewise reflect that 'doctors, in general, have not done outstandingly well in the House', and that, reciprocally, 'medicine, unlike the law, has never aroused great interest in the House of

---

96 For Mackintosh, Bickersteth, and Finlay, see *OxfordDNB*. Bickersteth's medical training was with his father, a Westmorland practitioner, and his uncle, a London accoucheur; he changed direction at Cambridge.

97 A. Batty Shaw, *Norfolk and Norwich Medicine: A Retrospect* (Norwich, 1992), p. 111; *idem, Norfolk and Norwich Hospital*, pp. 33–5.

98 See W.R. Lee, 'Robert Baker: the first doctor in the Factory Department. Part I. 1803–1858', *British Journal of Industrial Medicine*, 21 (1964), 86; *OxfordDNB*. Holland, the son of a wigmaker, became an alderman of his native city, Sheffield; he was an enthusiast first for phrenology and then homoeopathy.

99 Lambert, *Sir John Simon*.

Commons'.[100] Simon's politically active contemporaries in business or commerce could describe medical men as 'unpractical': this verdict recognizes the deliberate unworldliness of the aspiring professional, but it also suggests, for medicine, a surprising degree of detachment from the concerns of other men.[101]

Conclusions

It has not been feasible here to do more than suggest explanations for the tenuous links between medicine and politics in the British Isles, nor is it possible to explore the full range of consequences. However, I hope that a historical consideration of medicine and office-bearing has established both that the links are indeed tenuous and that there are long-term continuities involved. Glaser's pioneering study hypothesized that the *less* developed the profession, the *greater* the likelihood of political involvement, and ascribed modern medicine's detachment from politics to its success and its certainties.[102] In historical terms, we do find that certain marginalized groups either seek office or find it difficult to avoid, but for medicine, the case is different: detachment seems to be related to uncertainties, especially in terms of status. Moreover, Glaser's generalization leaves out of account the possible disadvantages of detachment, and it does not work for the other professions. At best, there is an early association between political disengagement and the self-image of physicians, who can be regarded as having had most influence on the development of the professional ethos in medicine. Crucially, however, this self-image was not yet recognized by the rest of society, and we also have to note significant exceptions in the shape of politically-active physicians of relatively assured status close to the Crown. Additionally, we have seen a marked disengagement of early modern physicians from urban life and the *cursus honorum*, which seems to be related to their hybrid character as belonging wholeheartedly neither to the town nor to the country. These disengagements were further associated with avoidance by physicians not only of the tax burdens involved in supporting civilian militias in the period before standing armies, but also of any form of military service. Whatever the advantages of this, as a strategy it had clear implications in terms of loss of masculine authority. Such authority was not defined by military service alone, but this source inevitably gains prominence for medical practitioners in the absence of other sources, such as 'ownership' of a

---

100   Henry Morris-Jones, *Doctor in the Whips' Room* (London, 1955), pp. 160, 164. See also the usefully detailed study by Roger Cooter: 'The rise and decline of the medical member: doctors and Parliament in Edwardian and interwar Britain', *Bulletin of the History of Medicine*, 78 (2004), 59–107. At the local level, see J.M. Lee, *Social Leaders and Public Persons: A Study of County Government in Cheshire since 1888* (Oxford, 1963).

101   E.P. Hennock, *Fit and Proper Persons: Ideal and Reality in Nineteenth-Century Urban Government* (London, 1973), p. 317.

102   Glaser, 'Doctors and politics', p. 234.

sacred text (as in the case of the clergy), or substantial property-holding (the lawyers, the upper clergy). The links between military service and political office-bearing are observable in other countries besides the British Isles, to a relatively late date.[103] Possibly even more pervasive are the consequences for office-bearing and public life of the limited overlap between medicine and law. Law, property, and power made an inextricable network, from which medicine was largely excluded.

It is arguably unsatisfactory to confine the discussion to the medical profession alone, but even if we do simplify in this way, we still have to give due importance to the differentials between the behaviour of physicians, and that of the more civic-minded surgeons and apothecaries. These differentials are enough in themselves to indicate that continuities in political disengagement are not adequately accounted for by practitioners' struggles to establish themselves, or by any ethos peculiar to medicine. At the same time, we have to take into account the blurring of medical identities, especially over the lifetime of a socially-mobile individual – as we have seen, a man might be known to posterity as a physician and yet have spent most of his working life as a surgeon – and the lingering effects of both civic and county family backgrounds. Further investigation is required. Nonetheless, that medicine, particularly as represented by physicians, is peculiar seems beyond doubt, and there is considerable fascination in exploring the consequences of its detachment, in the early modern period at least, from the structures of male authority, and the normal responsibilities of adult males in British society.

---

103   For example, in America: 'Doctors in government', pp. 362–4.

Chapter 6

A 'Sanative Contagion': Henry More on Faith Healing

Robert Crocker

The seventeenth century was a time of great religious expectation amongst Protestant Englishmen. The literature from this period is full of references to providential wonders and miraculous events suggestive of the close proximity to the world of men and women not only of the deity but of the world of spirits.[1] Millennial anxieties and providential concerns with spiritual safety, bodily health, and physical security in an uncertain, dangerous and rapidly changing world, undoubtedly added to this fascination. Collections of providential stories about prodigious natural events, witchcraft, and all kinds of other 'wonders' and 'signs' were popular, and the learned were much exercised in interpreting their meaning and significance.[2] But there was seldom unanimity in the way these extraordinary phenomena were to be interpreted. In the case of the briefly famous Martha Taylor, for example, the Derbyshire village girl's 'stupendous' maintenance of life without any apparent intake of food over several years was interpreted by some observers as an outstanding, even 'angelic', example of piety and by some as deliberately fraudulent. Others saw her as suffering an unusual but natural condition in her body, no more necessarily mysterious or mystical than several other unusual but known physical ailments.[3]

This divergence of opinion was naturally embedded in prior religious, philosophical and political commitments. What constituted a 'miracle' or merely a 'wonder', what was natural, preternatural or supernatural were questions that were usually cast within the larger sphere of Protestant providentialism, which had been

1   See William E. Burns, *An Age of Wonders: Prodigies, Politics and Providence in England, 1657–1727* (Manchester, 2002); Lorraine Daston, 'Marvellous facts and miraculous evidence in early modern Europe', in Peter G. Platt, ed., *Wonders, Marvels, and Monsters in Early Modern Culture* (London, 1999), pp. 76–104; Keith Thomas, *Religion and the Decline of Magic* (London, 1971); see also Alexandra Walsham, *Providence in Early Modern England* (Oxford, 1999), chaps 4–5.
2   See Burns, *Age of Wonders*, pp. 72ff.
3   Simon Schaffer, 'Piety, physic and prodigious abstinence', in O.P. Grell and A. Cunningham, eds, *Religio Medici: Religion and Medicine in Seventeenth Century England* (London, 1996), chap. 7: esp. pp. 180ff.

carefully constructed in opposition to the doctrines and 'false' miracles of the Roman Church and the religious sectarians. This meant that most Anglican theologians restricted the age of miracles to the apostolic age, and explained away more recent claims of miraculous events as probably natural rather than super-natural in origin.[4] Spiritual healing or 'faith healing' thus fell uneasily into a particularly ambiguous conceptual category: aside from the officially sponsored Anglican ceremonies of the 'royal touch' that Charles II exploited so successfully, most claims of 'miraculous' or divinely assisted healing in seventeenth-century England were interpreted by the Church authorities as 'natural' or magical and possibly even demonic in inspiration.[5]

The problem with this position, originally developed against both the various 'miraculous' cults of the Roman Church and the legitimizing claims of the radical sectarians, was that it depended upon a critique of false miracles that was contra-dicted by the example of the healing king himself, and on occasion by the appearance of a handful of notable but sincere faith healers, who could not easily be depicted as witches, 'cunning-men', or enthusiasts.[6] It was the contradictory, contested nature of this terrain, and the widely held official response that the age of miracles had passed, that led an increasing number of intellectuals to favour 'natural' explanations for these typically extraordinary examples of healing or recovery, but at the same time to frame this within a pious providentialism, in which God was held to be worthy of praise, even if not taken to be directly involved in producing the event under discussion.[7]

Accordingly, it was suggested that natural events, such as sickness or accidents affecting the believer's health or fortunes, were providential, and thus 'signs' of moral and spiritual states and processes, which could not always be immediately read or understood – hence the fundamental requirement of faith to be patient and accepting.[8] While a general providential view of sickness as 'a trial or punishment' sent by God was common in the period, some adopted an overtly spiritualistic view of this account of the body and its ailments, in which physical illness and suffering were to be read as a more specific providential sign of

---

4 See Walsham, *Providence*, pp. 226ff.; and esp. David Harley, 'Spiritual physic, Providence and English medicine, 1560–1640', in O.P. Grell and A. Cunningham, eds, *Medicine and the Reformation* (London, 1993), chap. 5.

5 See Thomas, *Decline of Magic*, pp. 148–51, 235ff.

6 *Ibid.*, and Walsham, *Providence*, pp. 228–30. See also Charles Webster, 'Paracelsus confronts the saints: miracles, healing and the secularisation of magic', *Social History of Medicine*, 8 (1995), 403–42.

7 See Thomas, *Decline of Magic*, pp. 238–41, and R.M. Burns, *The Great Debate on Miracles: from Joseph Glanvill to David Hume* (East Brunswick, NJ, 1981), chap. 3, and below.

8 See Harley, 'Spiritual physic, Providence and English medicine'.

spiritual status, and also, perhaps, as an incitement to greater faith, resignation and self-denial.[9]

Wonders, signs and spiritual gifts: Henry More's psychology of illumination

The writings and letters of Henry More, the Cambridge Platonist (1614–1687), provide many examples of this 'spiritualistic' providentialism. This can be seen developed first in his early cycle of Platonic poems on the 'life of the soul', *Psychodia Platonica, or a platonical song of the soul* (1642). Born into a family of well-to-do Lincolnshire gentry, More was brought up a Calvinist, but like many of his generation reacted against Calvinism's strictures while still a student at Cambridge.[10] His subsequent discovery of Platonism and the writings of the 'mystical divines' led him to adopt a perfectionist, illuminist theology that laid considerable emphasis on the close relationship between the moral and spiritual status of the soul and that of the body. In his view an active, intelligent and immaterial soul, inspired by a divine 'seed' planted in it by God in the beginning, was progressively united to three material 'vehicles' in its 'descent' into this 'out-world': a 'terrestrial' vehicle (the living physical body), an 'aerial' vehicle (a more subtle body also inhabited by the souls of the dead, and most other 'fallen' spirits), and the immortal 'aetherial' vehicle or body of light that was united to the soul at its creation, and promised to the saints and the faithful in heaven.[11]

For More a Plotinian psychology provided the framework for the soul's 'return' to this primordial spiritual perfection, through a lengthy process of

9   Gary K. Waite, 'Demonic affliction or divine chastisement? Conceptions of illness and healing among spiritualists and Mennonites in Holland, c.1530–c.1630', in M. Gijswijt-Hofstra et al., eds, *Illness and Healing Alternatives in Western Europe* (London and New York, 1997), chap. 3, esp. pp. 61ff.

10 For a biography of More, see *DNB*, and also my 'Henry More: a biographical essay', in Sarah Hutton, ed., *Henry More (1614–1687): Tercentenary Studies* (Dordrecht, 1990), pp. 1–18; 'The role of illuminism in the thought of Henry More', in G.A.J. Rogers et al., eds, *The Cambridge Platonists in Philosophical Context* (Dordrecht, 1997), chap. 9; and *Henry More, 1614–87: A Biography of the Cambridge Platonist* (Dordrecht, 2003).

11 See my 'Role of illuminism', pp. 129–32. The earliest outline of this psychology occurs in *Psychathanasia*, book I, canto ii in More, *Psychodia Platonica: Or a Platonical Song of the Soul...* (Cambridge, 1642), and also in *Philosophical Poems* (Cambridge, 1647), and More, *The Immortality of the Soul* (London, 1659), book II, chapter xiv; and More, *An Explanation of the Grand Mystery of Godliness* (London, 1660), book II, chapter xi. For convenience I have referred here to the book, chapter or canto and section or stanza numbers rather than page numbers for More's works because each of his major works was produced in several editions. All further references to More's poems will be to the *Philosophical Poems* (1647, henceforth *Poems*) which contains the second edition of the original four poems contained in the *Psychodia Platonica*, plus additional poems, annotations and glossary.

purification that he likened to a 'pilgrimage' or journey in his first major poem, *Psychozoia*.[12] This 'return' was triggered, first, by the Christian's faith in the power of Christ to perfect the believer in his image, and secondly, by a 'perfect' self-denial, which for More was a deliberate and conscious withdrawal from all bodily and egoistic concerns. He distinguished this sharply from the tainted illuminism of the religious sectarians or 'enthusiasts', with which he feared his own rather austere spiritualistic Christian Platonism would be associated. To counter this danger, he laid considerable emphasis on the sectarians' egoism, attachment to body, and resulting psychosomatic impurity, an impurity that resulted from their following a constitutionally dependent 'false light', rather than the true 'inner light' of Christ they claimed to follow.[13] More's later and better-known writings against enthusiasm took up this theme and expanded on it in some detail: the enthusiasts' 'false' perception of the 'inner light' was based upon their imagination's reflection of a psychosomatic impurity, derived ultimately from a failure to engage fully in the self-denial, repentance and faith in the power of Christ's spirit that for More were the hallmarks of the path to true illumination or 'deification'.[14] As this implies, More's concept of enthusiasm – rational and intellectualist as it has always been made to seem – was constructed against a central spiritualist notion of what 'true enthusiasm' or illumination involved: for More, a 'divine life' of true Christian devotion that he believed could lead to spiritual perfection.[15]

Although More's better-known controversial writings tend not to detail this devotional stance, his poems, early sermons and letters confirm that the original context of his definitions and criticisms of the 'false light' of the enthusiasts was his own strong central notion of what 'true' enthusiasm or illumination involved.[16]

12   *Psychozoia*, canto ii. This was the first poem included in his *Psychodia Platonica* (1642).

13   See More's additional verses describing the position of his own illuminism in relation to the dominant positions around him: *Psychozoia*, only in *Poems*, canto ii, 57–125. His distinction between 'true' and 'false' light derives from *Theologia Germanica*, ed. Dr Franz Pfeiffer, trans. S. Winkworth (London, 1854), chap. xl. See *Psychozoia*, canto ii, 112–16, and More, *Enthusiasmus Triumphatus* (London, 1656), sig. A5; and *Mystery of Godliness* (1660), II, xi ('On the divine life'). See also my 'Mysticism and enthusiasm in Henry More', in Hutton, *Henry More*, pp. 137–56: pp. 143–4.

14   More, *Cupid's Conflict*, in *Poems*, pp. 299–312: pp. 302–3; *Discourses on Several Texts of Scripture* (London, 1692), p. 54; *Divine Dialogues* (2nd edn, 2 vols in 1, London, 1713), pp. 303–6; Richard Ward, *The Life of Henry More Parts 1 and 2*, ed. S. Hutton et al. (Dordrecht, 2000), pp. 33–8; and More, *Mystery of Godliness*, VIII, xii ('Of the light within us').

15   See *Enthusiasmus Triumphatus*, p. 2, for More's definition of 'Enthusiasm' as a 'false' perception of divine inspiration, and also *Mystery of Godliness*, II, xii ('Of the divine life'), and references in note 14 above. See also Michael Heyd, 'The reaction to enthusiasm in the seventeenth century', *Journal of Modern History*, 53 (1981), 258–80.

16   This notion of a deluding 'false light' was adapted from the *Theologia Germanica*, chap. xl. See my 'Role of illuminism', pp. 131–5.

Referring to Plotinus's own experience of illumination, he declared in the explanatory notes attached to his poems, for instance, that 'our endeavour must be not onely to be without sin, but to become God, that is impassible, immaterial, quit of all sympathy with the body, drawn up wholly into the intellect'.[17] Probably influenced by his former tutor at Christ's College, Robert Gell, to take up first this 'way of purgation and illumination', described best for More in the works of the 'Platonists and mystical divines', More's vigorous early criticisms of Calvinist pessimism and predestinarianism are closely aligned to a spiritual perfectionism similar to that found in the works of Calvin's influential opponent, Sebastian Castellio, also one of Gell's favourite authors.[18]

The creation and maintenance of the 'divine life' was thus for More the main aim of Christian devotion, and was founded upon a belief in the power of Christ's spirit to purify and perfect the soul in its image.[19] In More's view, there was a certain 'temper' in the body engendered by this process of purification and spiritual devotion, a 'divine body' that developed alongside this 'divine life' of the regenerate Christian's experience.[20] According to Richard Ward, at one time More's amanuensis and later his biographer, More laid as great an emphasis on this notion of a 'divine body' as upon:

17 *Poems*, p. 371; Plotinus, *The Enneads*, ed. and trans. Stephen McKenna (5 vols, London, 1921), iii, pp. 143–4 (IV, viii, 1). See also C.A. Patrides, *The Cambridge Platonists* (Cambridge, 1969), pp. 16–18, on the crucial significance of Plotinus to More and the Platonists.

18 On Gell, see John Peile, *Biographical Register of Christ's College Cambridge* (2 vols, Cambridge, 1910), i, p. 301, and Gell, *Remaines*, ed. N. Bacon (2 vols, London, 1676). Comments on his 'perfectionism', interest in Jacob Boehme, and alleged 'familism' can be found in John Etherington, *A Brief Description of...Familisme* (London, 1645), p. 10; Richard Baxter, *Reliquiae Baxterianae*, ed. M. Sylvester (2 vols, London, 1696), i, p. 78; and in a letter from Jeremy Taylor to John Evelyn, cited in Marjorie Nicolson, *The Conway Letters*, ed. S. Hutton (Oxford, 1992) p. 155, note 3. See also Castellio, *Of Obedience, and his modes apology and defence of himself* (London, 1679), and *A Conference on Faith* (London, 1679); Castellio, *On Heretics*, ed. R. Bainton (New York, 1935), pp. 10ff. On Castellio's perfectionism in Gell, see Gell, *Remaines*, i, pp. 148, 155–80. See also D.W. Dockrill, 'The heritage of patristic Platonism in seventeenth-century English philosophical thought', in Rogers et al., *The Cambridge Platonists in Philosophical Context*, pp. 55–77.

19 See for instance More, *Mystery of Godliness*, II, xii.

20 He seems to have attributed this to Boehme, even if he felt that Boehme had been misled by the 'chymists', and Paracelsus in particular. See Sarah Hutton, 'More and Jacob Boehme', in Hutton, *Henry More*, pp. 157–68; More, *Philosophiae Teutonica Censura*, Quaestio 2, sections 7 and 9, in More, *H. Mori Cantabrigiensis Opera Omnia* (3 vols, London, 1675–9), ii (1679), pp. 541–2, and see also More to Anne Conway, in Nicolson, *Conway Letters*, p. 306. See also More, *Divine Dialogues*, p. 467.

the Divine Life itself; and upon the former because of the latter. For he supposes that it always dwells in it, and is no where fixable out of it, and of how much any Person partakes of more of Righteousness and Virtue, he hath also a greater Measure of this Divine Body or Celestial Matter, within himself.[21]

This 'divine body', associated for More with an awareness of the soul's original 'aetherial vehicle' or 'body of light', gave a practical, psychosomatic dimension to his discussion of purification, illumination and the spiritual life. Indeed, he was convinced, from his own experience:

> that there is a holy Art of Living, or certain sacred Method of attaining unto great and Experimental Praegustations of the Highest Happiness that our Nature is capable of: And that the degrees of Happiness and Perfection in the Soul arise, or ascend, according to the degree of Purity and Perfection in that Body or Matter she is united with: So that we are to endeavour a Regress from the Baser Affections of the Earthy Body; to make our Blood and Spirits of a more refined Consistency; and to replenish our Inward Man with so much larger Draughts of Aetherial or Coelestial Matter.[22]

Henry More, Anne Conway, and Matthew Coker, spiritual healer and prophet

As this strong, underlying current of illuminism in More's writings suggests, his interest in spiritual healing or 'faith healing' needs to be placed in the context of his understanding of the intimate relationship between spirit and body in the sincere believer: the body, he considered, reflected the life of the spirit, and this manifested itself through the animal spirits and the individual's constitution. Claims of sanctity, of spiritual visions and experiences, and also examples of spiritual healing, were thus of considerable interest to More, as testamentary evidence for his spiritual beliefs.[23] And what gave this interest in spiritual healing in particular an additional personal dimension was his close, lifelong friendship with Anne, Viscountess Conway.[24]

Anne Conway was an invalid for most of her adult life, suffering from a mysterious and steadily worsening crippling illness, involving periodic bouts of prostrating headaches. As Sarah Hutton has pointed out, Anne Conway was wealthy and apparently patient enough to suffer almost every possible type of cure then available, many of them first recommended, and sometimes even tested

---

21   Ward, *Life*, p. 33. See also More, *Divine Dialogues*, pp. 293–5; and *Enchiridion Ethicum* (1667), III, v, 10.

22   Ward, *Life*, pp. 33–5.

23   See my 'Mysticism and illuminism', pp. 139–41.

24   See *DNB*, and Sarah Hutton, 'Of physic and philosophy. Anne Conway, Francis Mercury van Helmont and seventeenth-century medicine', in Cunningham and Grell, *Religio Medici*, chap. 9.

personally, by her devoted friend and philosophical mentor, Henry More.[25] More's compassionate reaction to her terrible suffering, and his advice, provide a rich source for his own understanding of the body and its relationship with the spiritual and moral life. More had taught Anne's half-brother, John Finch, at Christ's, and was introduced to Anne and her family, and then the Conways, through him.[26] While still a young girl, Anne had fallen seriously ill with a dangerous fever, and from this time onwards had suffered from recurring bouts of a debilitating illness, involving increasingly protracted and destructive bouts of severe headache. Some of England's foremost physicians, including her own relative William Harvey, attempted to treat her terrible affliction, but without success.[27]

More's letters to her are of special interest because they reveal his own and her view of the close relationship between the parallel spheres of spiritual and medical advice and treatment, with More frequently recommending specific readings and meditations to assist her to find a spiritual value in her suffering, in addition, of course, to finding an effective cure.[28] As Sarah Hutton has shown, their letters also reveal much about the kind of medical treatments available to her, including three prolonged administrations of mercury (via 'salivation') – a frightful treatment reserved, as custom would have it, for the worst diseases, such as syphilis and its associated symptoms.[29] At one time, even more seriously, Anne Conway was advised to undergo a 'trepan', an extreme surgical intervention during which a hole was bored through the front of the skull, supposedly to relieve the pressure that was thought to cause the headaches – an extreme cure, that she fortunately never consented to, apparently on the advice of her Platonist friend.[30] Alongside these

25   See Hutton, in Nicolson, *Conway Letters*, p. viii, and below; Hutton, 'Of physic and philosophy', pp. 230–1.
26   On Finch, see *DNB*, and Archibald Malloch, *Finch and Baines: A Seventeenth-Century Friendship* (Cambridge, 1917).
27   On Conway's illness and medical treatments, see Hutton, 'Of physic and philosophy', and *idem*, in Nicolson, *Conway Letters*, pp. vii–ix. See also Allison Coudert and Taylor Corse, *Anne Conway, Principles of the most Ancient and Modern Philosophy* (Cambridge, 1996), Introduction.
28   See More to Anne Conway on his developing spiritual and moral interpretation of her illness and suffering, in Nicolson, *Conway Letters*, pp. 104, 130–2, 153–4, 168–9, 181–2, 280–1. See also Harley, 'Spiritual physic, providence and English medicine', pp. 102–5; and Waite, 'Demonic affliction or divine chastisement?', pp. 61 ff. See also David Harley, 'The theology of affliction and the experience of sickness in the godly family, 1650–1714: the Henrys and the Newcomes', in Cunningham and Grell, *Religio Medici*, chap. 11.
29   Nicolson, *Conway Letters*, pp. 91, 107, 113.
30   Proposed by Harvey for Anne Conway, *ibid.*, pp. 106, 116. For the general context, see also Lucinda Beier, *Sufferers and Healers: the Experience of Illness in Seventeenth-Century England* (London, 1987). See also Hutton, 'Of physic and philosophy', pp. 232–3.

many medical failures, and at least one case of medical dishonesty,[31] More also encouraged his friend to try other, more unconventional, spiritual methods of healing, including 'stroking' by the now obscure faith healer and self-styled prophet, Matthew Coker.[32]

What we know of Matthew Coker derives largely from four small pamphlets he published between April and July, 1654.[33] He appears to have been a lawyer, an educated man, from Lincoln's Inn, and we know that for some time he attended the sermons of More's former tutor and friend, Dr Robert Gell, at this time Rector of St Mary Aldermary in London.[34] Coker, while personally unknown to Gell until he published his pamphlets, was briefly a member of Gell's congregation, and judging by his pamphlets was greatly influenced by the writings of Jacob Boehme, whom Gell seems to have admired.[35] Interestingly, Coker published his first, 'prophetical' pamphlet in Latin (now lost) and dedicated it to the Protector, to whom he apparently presented it in person, but the only surviving copy of this is a translation he issued some months later as *A Prophetical Revelation given from GOD himself unto Matthew Coker of Lincoln's Inne* (1654). In the preface to this English pamphlet Coker included a description of his original moment of illumination, or 'awakening', during which he had received the twin gifts of prophecy and

31   On Frederick Clodius, Dutch chymist and son-in-law of Samuel Hartlib, see Nicolson, *Conway Letters*, pp. 94ff. More's outraged anger at Clodius's behaviour is spread over several letters, starting in May 1654, pp. 97–8. See also Hutton, 'Of physic and philosophy', p. 233.

32   See Nicolson, *Conway Letters*, pp. 98ff, and Matthew Coker, *A Short and Plain Narrative of Matthew Coker... In reference to His Gift of Healing* (London, 1654).

33   It appears he first published a 'prophecy' in Latin, which was then translated as the second of the tracts below, *A Short and Plain Narrative* (the signature is dated 17 March 1653); *A Prophetical Revelation given from God himself unto Matthew Coker... declaring things shortly to come to pass thorowout all Christendom* (1654) – signature of Epistle dated 24 April 1654, text dated 'Munday the 9th of January'; and *A Whip of Small Cords to scourge Antichrist...out of the Temple of God* (1654), dated 25 May 1654, which includes *A Knot at the End of the Whip* (dated 25 June 1654); and *The Sheerer sheer'd, and casheer'd; the Shaver shav'd, and the Grinder ground* (26 June 1654). In the last two pamphlets, as well as adopting a more stridently apocalyptic style in which Antichrist is depicted as the leader of his more troublesome enemies in London, he signs himself 'Matthew Coker, the Apostolical Prophet and Prophetical Apostle'.

34   For Gell's letter to Anne Conway about Coker, see Nicolson, *Conway Letters*, pp. 98–9.

35   See especially, Coker, *A Whip of Small Cords*, which provides questions and answers on the crucial question of whether 'miracles had ceased' as the Church of England maintained – like Gell, Coker declared them 'much abated' but not ceased (pp. 2–3) – and also makes a distinction between miracles (resulting in immediate cures) and healings by touch where cures were more gradual (p. 4), but it is clear that he regarded the self-same Holy Spirit as responsible for both, a view that Gell's letter, above, indicates he shared.

healing.[36] It appears from this preface that his moment of illumination came over him suddenly, and he describes how he could not open his eyes for some time afterwards, so powerful did this experience appear to him. Showing the influence of Boehme's writings or of Gell's preaching, the resulting prophetical message was a mystical and irenical vision of the coming millennium, where all Christians, including Catholics, would be known by no other name than 'Christian' and be united in peace.[37]

Coker's second pamphlet and his first to be published in English was *A Short and Plain Narrative of Matthew Coker, Touching Some Mistakes and Mis-Recitals in a Pamphlet this day...In reference to His Gift of Healing* (May, 1654), produced some two months after his (now lost) Latin *Prophetical Revelation*. This described some of Coker's healing experiences, beginning with his first apparently successful case, the cure of a leprous beggar named Henry Flemming. This is an interesting incident, and is reminiscent of some of the healing encounters between the Quaker leader, George Fox, and certain 'poor madmen' that followed him also in expectation of a cure.[38] After Flemming had called upon him in a loud voice several times, apparently expecting something remarkable from Coker, Coker questioned him closely as to his history and state of health, but only before witnesses did he then proceed to try out his new gift. Flemming, he says:

> satisfied us that his Father was a Leper and Lame, and that he was and had been lame about three years, not able to go without Crutches; besides, weak even in every part of his body, and having a sore in his thigh. We found clearly that he was not able to stand off from a Wall or Leaning place without help; and his posture was much bowed. Then I came to him, and with my hands straightened his body, and laying my hand on his back and also on his knee and leg, he was presently able to stand upright, and go a step or two without Crutches, upon my saying to him, *Stand up and Walk*. After that, I applied an Ivy-leaf to his sore, and he bound it up, and then he walked somewhat better, saying, he hoped to run by to morrow: but I said, *Nay sooner then you think for*: and a few hours after, he was able to run: and since, I have found him to walk as well as any one.[39]

Coker then went on to describe many other notable instances of the operation of his gift, including an exorcism – a 'casting out' of the 'evil spirit' which had struck a child dumb for a week – a type of spiritual healing also fairly typical amongst the leading radical sectarians at the time.[40] In this he emphasized, against

36 *A Prophetical Revelation*, sig. A2–A2v.
37 *A Prophetical Revelation*, sig. A2–A2v. For More's view see Nicolson, *Conway Letters*, p. 101.
38 Coker, *Short and Plain Narrative*, p. 4; for George Fox, see Michael MacDonald, *Mystical Bedlam: Madness, Anxiety and Healing in Seventeenth-Century England* (Cambridge, 1981), p. 228.
39 Coker, *Short and Plain Narrative*, p. 4.
40 *Ibid.*, pp. 5–6; and see MacDonald, *Mystical Bedlam*, chap. 5; Thomas, *Decline of Magic*, pp. 227–51; and also David Harley, 'Mental illness, magical medicine and the

his unknown conservative critic (whose pamphlet is not extant), that he did not take anything in exchange for his service, 'lest the gift *freely received*, should not be *freely given*'.[41]

Anne Conway must have heard of the claims concerning Coker's abilities while in London, and immediately made enquiries of Gell, whom she knew through More. In his surviving reply to her letter, dated 26 May 1654, Gell describes meeting Coker and observing his method of curing.[42] He concluded that Coker had a genuine gift of healing, having himself witnessed several cures performed by him, although he emphasised his own belief that these cures were indeed miraculous, demonstrations that God 'alone doth wonderous things', and pointedly criticizing the then orthodox Anglican view that 'miracles had ceased', a standpoint that clearly undermined his own perfectionism.[43] It appears from a letter More wrote to Anne Conway on Coker's alleged gifts, shortly after this time (7 June 1656), that Anne Conway had already approached Coker for assistance, but that perhaps because of the demands put upon him by the crowds of sick people who sought him out, he had put her off, at least for a time.[44] From his letter to Anne Conway it is clear that More had made a detailed study of Coker's pamphlets and the available evidence for his gift. After denying that Coker could be just another 'enthusiast' or 'impostor', because of the evidence of his sincere beliefs and genuine abilities, More went on to speculate about how the healing took place, along lines very different to those proposed by his former tutor and friend, Robert Gell:[45]

> And I must confess what he does I do not at all suspect to be by the power of the Devil, but by a power partly natural and partly devotional, and that it does not at all amount to a miracle, as I conceive, properly so called, which methinks the manner of his healing does intimate. For they recover their strength by degrees, as in the taking of a medicine, as I observe in all these stories. Wherefore I have this odd conceit concerning this matter, that the blood and spirits of this party is become sanative and healing, by long temperance and devotion, as I suppose, nature being so hugely advanced and perfectly concocted, that his blood and spirits are a true elixir, and therefore he laying his hands upon diseased persons, his spirits run out of his own body into the party diseased, and actuate and purify the blood and spirits of the diseased party, which I conceive they do with more efficacy, if he add devotion to his laying on of hands, for that sets his spirits afloat more copiously and animates them more strongly, and they being no spirits of a melancholy man but thus refined and sublimated, they are the more fierce and

Devil in northern England, 1650–1700', in Roger French and Andrew Wear, eds, *The Medical Revolution of the Seventeenth Century* (Cambridge, 1989), chap. 4.

41   Coker, *Short and Plain Narrative*, p. 5.
42   Gell, in Nicolson, *Conway Letters*, pp. 98–9.
43   Gell, in *ibid.*, p. 99. It is significant that Gell saw this orthodox denial of post-apostolic miracles as closely associated with Calvinist pessimism. See my 'Role of illuminism', pp. 131–2, and Walsham, *Providence*, pp. 226–34.
44   More, in Nicolson, *Conway Letters*, pp. 100–2.
45   More, in *ibid.*, p. 101.

strong in their motions, and more effectual for the kindling of life and spirit in such dead and diseased limbs as he is said to have healed... I could wish, if he could be persuaded to it, that he would continue his hand upon the Temples of your head or your forehead, or if he could come to the place where your pain most resides, to let it rest there a good while, when you are in a fit, for I conceive the virtue will be then perceptible.

For More, Coker's body was 'infectiously healthful', and his healing 'natural', but greatly augmented by the effect on his body of his notable piety and devotion – a providential effect of the evident purity of his 'divine body'. As to his prophecy of the future unity of all Christians, More denied that a prophetical gift was necessary to recognize a promise made in the Bible, and one that, he considered, all 'regenerate' Christians should believe.[46] Interestingly, More earnestly entreated Anne Conway not to reveal his explanations to Coker himself, in case a 'rational consideration' of his gifts might 'weaken' his present facility, which he suspected might not last for very long, for which reason also he urged her to make use of Coker while she could.[47] This naturalistic, psychosomatic understanding of Coker's gift is significant, since it echoes More's understanding of the development of the 'divine life' as something involving a spiritual or devotional augmentation of the normal bodily state or 'constitution', in this way producing a 'divine body' that spontaneously exhibited signs of greater refinement, spiritual energy, 'healthful' effects or 'effluvia', and thus a demonstrable degree of spiritual 'perfection'.[48]

A few days later (18 June), More replied to Anne Conway's suggestion that Coker might really be performing miracles – an argument that took up Gell's suggestion, and which was in her view strengthened by Coker's claim to have also cured some children and others merely by his word and his prayers. More's response is again typically cautious, even sceptical, favouring a naturalistic and material explanation for what appeared to her to have no obvious 'natural' explanation:

As for Mr Coker curing the absent, and children by mere speaking unto them, it is to be enquired, whether they are immediately cured, at the very hour he first prays for them, or speaks to them, or in some compass of time and then whether all or but some though most. For if there be any considerable space of time required, and beside that, he does not cure universally, it seemes to me to be a fallacy, or a mistake of his. For lett any man pray for or speak to all the sicke persons of any one town, his prayers or speaking will seeme oftener to take effect then to be frustrate, because there is no man can dye more then once but he may and usually has severall fitts of sickness, before he dyes. Wherefore whosoever prayes for, or speakes to by way of cure, all the sick persons of a town, he oftener seeing his endeavours take place then be frustrate, he may deceive himself and others too, as if it were done by the vertues of his Devotion or Words, and not by the strength of

46 *Ibid.*
47 *Ibid.*
48 More, in Ward, *Life*, p. 33.

Nature. Which Imposture is also upon the Physicions though not so fully. For I think they very seldome cure, but where nature by ordinary country meanes and abstinence would cure itself.[49]

As is apparent from Coker's last pamphlets, *A Whip of Small Cords, to scourge Antichrist* and *The Sheerer sheer'd, and casheer'd; the Shaver shav'd and the Grinder Ground* (both late June, 1654), his prophetic pretensions had grown greatly along with the feverishly prophetic spirit of the times, and so, apparently, had his orthodox enemies.[50] Now styling himself 'the Apostolical Prophet and Prophetical Apostle', it was not long before poor Coker was taken to Bedlam, according to a report relayed to More.[51]

Henry More and Valentine Greatrakes: the spiritual healer's 'sanative' touch

More considered that the great spiritual devotion and 'purity' of the faith healer had so refined his 'animal spirits' that they had become 'sanative' in their effects, and were able to pass through his hands to influence the 'animal spirits', and thus the bodily health of his patients.[52] The apparently 'miraculous' performance that resulted was viewed sceptically by More, as mainly the result of popular ignorance, and the occult but natural processes involved in its material cause. This did not require any special medical or expert knowledge, but rather called upon what might be regarded as a common fund of rapidly expanding natural and medical knowledge shared by More with the majority of his educated readers, although it is clear that for More its purpose was 'evidential', underpinning his broader Platonic metaphysic and psychology.[53]

When over ten years later (in 1666), his friend Edward Conway invited the Anglo-Irish farmer, Valentine Greatrakes, to come to England to attempt to cure his invalid wife, More offered a similar interpretation of this second, more famous healer's 'sanative virtue'. He was similarly enthusiastic about the possibility that

49   More, in Nicolson, *Conway Letters*, p. 103.
50   It is difficult to determine who exactly opposed him, but it is likely that clerical and medical opposition would have been aroused by his activities.
51   As More reports to Anne Conway, 31 July [1654], in Nicolson, *Conway Letters*, p. 104.
52   More, in Nicolson, *Conway Letters*, p. 101, where he mentions the 'Great Elixir they [the chymists] talk of'. On the increasing popularity of Helmontianism from the late 1640s, see Ole Peter Grell, 'Plague, prayer and physic: Helmontian medicine in Restoration England', in Cunningham and Grell, *Religio Medici*, chap. 8, and Charles Webster, *The Great Instauration: Science, Medicine and Reform 1626–1660* (London, 1975), pp. 276ff. More seemed to think that a similar process, part-spiritual and part-natural, explained how the witch could make her victim ill. See my *Henry More*, chap. 9.
53   See Daston, 'Marvellous facts and miraculous evidence', pp. 93–4.

his invalid friend might be assisted by being 'stroked' by this healer.[54] Unfortunately, nothing came of Greatrakes's more widely publicized attempts to cure Anne Conway, despite his remarkable successes with the other sick people whom he attracted to him at her home in Warwickshire and later in London. His visit, certainly, was the occasion of much public discussion, and a number of educated observers, including More, Ralph Cudworth, Benjamin Whichcote, George Rust, Jeremy Taylor and Robert Boyle, witnessed the proceedings and tried various experiments to test the extent and reliability of his powers.[55]

It is interesting to note that in the surviving testimonies attached to Greatrakes's printed apologia, and in the pamphlets accepting and explaining Greatrakes's cures, More's theory of a 'sanative virtue', 'contagion' or 'effluvia' – a natural energy that passed through the healer's hands to his patients – became effectively the orthodox moderate Anglican explanation for what was happening.[56] For instance, when Lord Conway wrote to his brother-in-law, Sir Heneage Finch, as early as the end of August, 1665, before Greatrakes could be induced to come to England, he also considered the healer's cures not to be miraculous but the result of 'a sanative virtue' or a 'natural efficiency', explicitly citing More's concept.[57] Similarly, More's former pupil, George Rust, then Dean of Connor, described Greatrakes's activities in a letter to Joseph Glanvill in terms of a similar 'sanative contagion'. After noting the 'talk in the coffee houses' about Greatrakes, and that 'some take him to be a Conjuror, and some an Impostor, but others again adore him as an Apostle', Rust then described meeting the healer at Ragley with the Conways, and seeing him touch over a thousand persons, sometimes with remarkable success. Echoing More's early views of Coker, he then described his method

54 The Greatrakes visit and subsequent publicity have been repeatedly discussed and documented, starting with Nicolson, in *Conway Letters*, chap. 5; see esp. Eamon Duffy, 'Valentine Greatrakes, the Irish stroker: miracle, science and orthodoxy in Restoration England', in Keith Robbins, ed., *Religion and Humanism*, Studies in Church History, XVII (Oxford, 1981), pp. 251–73; and Nicholas Steneck, 'Greatrakes the stroker: the interpretations of the historians', *Isis*, 73 (1982), 161–77.

55 See the testimonies of John Wilkins, Benjamin Whichcote, Ralph Cudworth, George Rust and Simon Patrick, appended to Greatrakes's *A Brief Account of Mr Val. Greaterak's* (London, 1666), pp. 56–63. This was addressed to Boyle. On Boyle's view, see next note.

56 See Boyle's letter to Henry Stubbe (9 March 1666), rejecting his controversial interpretation of Greatrakes's cures as similar to those of Jesus and his followers, in Thomas Birch, *The Life of the Honourable Robert Boyle*, in Birch, ed., *The Works of the Honourable Robert Boyle* (6 vols, London, 1778), i, pp. lxxvi–lxxxv, esp. p. lxxvii on Boyle's own, typically qualified version of More's 'sanative contagion': 'Mr Greatraks's touch may work not only as a cordial or strengthener of nature, but as a proper remedy of qualities opposite to those of the causes of the diseases he cures. For I do not see, why it may not be possible for the sanative, and perhaps anodyne steams of his body to be of such a texture, that they may both invigorate the spirits, and by appropriated qualities oppose and subdue the morbific matter or ferment'.

57 Conway in Nicolson, *Conway Letters*, p. 268.

of healing and its remarkable but rather mixed results:

> But yet I have many reasons to perswade me, that nothing of all this is miraculous. He pretends not to give Testimony to any Doctrine, the manner of his Operation speaks it to be natural, the Cure seldom succeeds without reiterated touches, his Patients often relapse, he fails frequently, he can do nothing when there is any Decay in Nature, and many Distempers are not at all obedient to his Touch: so that I confess, I refer all his vertue to his particular Temper and Complexion, and I take his Spirits to be a kind of Elixir, and universal Ferment, and that he cures (as Dr M[ore] expresseth it) by a sanative contagion.[58]

But the controversies surrounding Greatrakes's visit were considerably amplified by their circumstances, and cannot readily be compared with the brief publicity given to Coker's healing activities ten years earlier. As several scholars have noted, in the religious and political terms of the Restoration Church, Greatrakes's activities needed to be clearly distinguished from the 'miraculous' cures claimed by the Catholic Church for its saints and relics, from the similarly legitimizing claims of the radical sectarian leaders, from the orthodox ceremonies of royal thaumaturgy performed by King Charles II and now sponsored by the Anglican Church, and also from the magical, possibly demonic cures of the 'cunning-men' and wise women or witches.[59] These were precisely the politically charged negative associations deliberately emphasised by the Anglican minister, David Lloyd, in his pamphlet attacking Greatrakes, a pamphlet that provoked a most interesting apologetic response from Greatrakes himself.[60] For this reason too the Platonist, Benjamin Whichcote, who had himself received an extraordinary cure from the healer, attempted, in his brief testimony supporting Greatrakes, to distinguish his method from that of the cunning-men or magicians: 'I have very diligently observed him, but did never perceive him to use any form of words, nor saw him do any thing (in my judgment) liable to any suspicion of any ill art or device'.[61]

To Lloyd, and presumably many orthodox churchmen, Greatrakes and his enthusiastic popular reception seemed to present a direct challenge to the authority of the Church. Greatrakes therefore, he tried to assert, must either have been cheating or using illicit natural magic. Lloyd also emphasised Greatrakes's discredited former sympathies with the Independents, his 'Latitudinarianism' (predictably implying, for Lloyd, 'no religion' or 'any'), his Quaker-like subjection to 'imagination' and 'impulses', and, through his pretension to heal scrofula or 'the King's Evil', his implicit attack on, and attempt to 'level' the popular royal ceremony of

---

58   Rust in *ibid.*, p. 274.
59   See Duffy, 'Valentine Greatrakes, the Irish stroker', pp. 263–6; and Thomas, *Decline of Magic*, pp. 227ff (on healing by touch) and 239–42 (on Greatrakes).
60   [David Lloyd], *Wonders no Miracles: or Mr Valentine Greatrates Gift of Healing Examined, Upon occasion of a Sad Effect of his Stroaking* (London, 1666), pp. 13–14.
61   Whichcote, in Greatrakes, *A Brief Account of Mr Val. Greaterak's*, p. 58.

healing.[62] Indeed, one gets the impression from this rather scurrilous attack that not only is the age of miracles past, but only those miracles approved by the Church could be allowed.[63] Apparently recognizing the broad acceptance of More's interpretation as an alternative, naturalistic view, Lloyd goes on explicitly to attack 'Dr More's theory' regarding the healer's sanative 'crasis or complexion' – an interpretation Lloyd then tries to muddy with 'the Atheists obsolete cavil against Christ's miracles', that they too were all 'natural', an association More was of course at pains to deny.[64]

As can be seen from Lloyd's pamphlet, it was More's naturalistic, psychosomatic notion of a 'sanative contagion', passing through the healer's hands to the body and spirits of the patient, that seems to have crept into nearly all the remaining positive accounts of Greatrakes's powers, including, unfortunately for More and also Boyle, that more notorious appraisal published by the physician and former Independent and anti-clerical pamphleteer, Henry Stubbe.[65] In a similar but more overtly medical manner, Stubbe, who was one of those who witnessed Greatrakes's performances at Ragley, attributed Greatrakes's powers to 'effluvia' or to his 'temperament', which was able to change the constitution, blood and spirits of his patients.[66] While this was broadly acceptable to, and not entirely dissimilar to the rather hesitant conclusions of Boyle, and quite close to More's theory, Stubbe subverted their carefully circumscribed naturalism by directly comparing Greatrakes's abilities with those of the apostles and Christ himself.[67] By implication this suggested the dangerous 'atheistic' corollary proposed by Lloyd, that Greatrakes's

---

62 See above. According to Lloyd, *Wonders no Miracles*, his cures were 'lying wonders' (p. 2) and Greatrakes himself a 'Latitude-man, that is, one that being of no Religion himself, is indifferent what Religion others should be of', and a man troubled by 'Fancies and Imaginations', in other words an 'enthusiast' (p. 10). His touching for the King's Evil was a direct attack on the King, 'levelling his Gift... and Office' (p. 14).

63 See his 'Rules to discern true miracles from false', *Wonders no Miracles*, pp. 36–7. According to the *DNB*, Lloyd, as 'William Foulis', had recently published a similarly vituperative attack on nonconformity as political rebellion: *Cabala; or the History of Conventicles unvail'd* (London, 1664).

64 *Wonders no Miracles*, pp. 26–8.

65 *The Miraculous Conformist: or an account of severall Marvellous Cures performed by a Stroking of the Hands of Mr Valentine Greatarick; with a Physical Discourse thereupon, in a letter to the Honourable Robert Boyle Esq* (Oxford, 1666). On Stubbe and his pamphlet, see *DNB*; Christopher Hill, *The Experience of Defeat: Milton and some Contemporaries* (London, 1984), pp. 252–77; James R. Jacob, *Henry Stubbe: Radical Protestantism and the Early Enlightenment in England* (Cambridge, 1983); and Duffy, 'Valentine Greatrakes, the Irish stroker', pp. 265–8.

66 Stubbe, *Miraculous Conformist*, p. 10, quoted below, note 68.

67 *Ibid.*, p. 10, on the peculiar 'effluvia' and their effects (see below, next note), and also pp. 25–7, for Stubbe's comparison of Greatrakes's cures to those of Christ. For Boyle's detailed refutation of this comparison, see his letter to Greatrakes (9 March 1666), in Birch, *Life*, in Birch, *Works of the Honourable Robert Boyle*, i, pp. lxxvi–lxxviii, and also note 56, above.

activities, if they were to be accepted as real but not miraculous, could be con-
strued to demonstrate that the biblical miracles were also natural, a corollary that
both Boyle and More had taken pains to deny.[68] Stubbe's pamphlet, dedicated to
Boyle without his prior knowledge or consent, naturally embarrassed and angered
him and provoked an outcry.[69]

The naturalism embodied in 'Dr More's theory', in tune with, even if not
strictly aligned to, the emerging 'philosophical' account of the nature of disease
and health propounded by Boyle and his fellow virtuosi, and adjusted here to suit
the modest, rational theological exigencies of the Platonists and Latitudinarians, is
evidenced even in Greatrakes's own final apologia for his gifts and activities. This
was written, probably under Boyle's guidance, in response to the outcry provoked
by Stubbe's ill-timed pamphlet, and also the orthodox clerical backlash embodied
in Lloyd's *Wonders no Miracles*.[70] This influence can be surmised because
Greatrakes's published account does not coincide entirely with the recollections of
the views of his powers he had apparently expressed when he had been in Ireland.[71]

In this final account, after telling his own story and the appearance of his
special gift of healing, and detailing several of his cures – modestly laying no claim
to any special spiritual or moral attainment – Greatrakes went on to provide three
related and modestly rational theological reasons for his role as a healer, which
certainly could have been suggested to him by Boyle or by More – 'to convince
this Age of Atheism' of God's existence and power, to reveal the 'goodness of
God, out of compassion to poor destressed man', and, by using an unworthy
Protestant such as himself, to 'abate the pride of the Papists (that make Miracles
the undeniable Manifesto of the truth of their Church)'[72] – certainly a telling
argument for a Protestant Irish planter. But then in response to the typical questions
raised about his operation of his gift, questions that were perhaps suggested to him

68   Rust, in Nicolson, *Conway Letters*, p. 274, is clearly indicative of More's judgment;
      no letter from More on this subject survives. On Stubbe's physical understanding of
      Greatrakes's cures, see *Miraculous Conformist*, p. 10: 'God had bestowed upon Mr
      Greatarick a peculiar temperament, or composed his Body of some particular
      Ferments, the Effluvia whereof, being introduced sometimes by a light, sometimes by
      a violent friction, should restore the Temperament of the Debilitated parts,
      reinvigorate the Bloud, and dissipate all heterogeneous Ferments out of the Bodies of
      the Diseased'. Boyle's own views on whether there was something miraculous in
      Greatrakes's performances, characteristically, were never entirely resolved, although it
      is clear that he sympathized most with the naturalistic explanation put forward by
      More and his friends. See Duffy, 'Valentine Greatrakes the Irish stroker', p. 268, on
      Boyle's typically scrupulous, lengthy manuscript queries on Greatrakes's complexion,
      religion, etc.
69   Stubbe, *Miraculous Conformist*, pp. 2–3, 26–8.
70   Greatrakes, *A Brief Account of Mr Val. Greaterak's*.
71   Michael Boyle, Archbishop of Dublin, on first interviewing Greatrakes, found his
      ideas disturbing, for not dissimilar reasons to Lloyd. See Michael Boyle to Lord
      Conway, 29 July 1665, in Nicolson, *Conway Letters*, pp. 262–3.
72   *A Brief Account of Mr Val. Greaterak's*, pp. 30–31.

by Boyle, his account finished with an answer to the question, 'whether this operation of my Hand proceeds from the Temperature of my Body, or from a Divine Gift, or from both?' While Greatrakes typically preferred to think of his special ability as an 'extraordinary Gift from God', he now was apparently willing to accept the possibility that 'an extraordinary Gift may be exercised by natural means':

> I suppose no man will question but that an extraordinary Gift may be exercised by natural means, or that God may confer in an extraordinary manner such a Temper of Body upon a person as may by a natural efficacy produce these effects; Only by the way I shall suggest to you an Experiment made at the House of that excellent Person, your Sister, the Lady Ranelaghs where I tried (to satisfie the curiosity of some there) with a Napkin which I rubbed my breast withal, and with my Shirt which I had pulled off, being very hot; whether that would remove the pains of a Woman, which was in strange fits there (as my glove, being tried, did often times) and it would not.[73]

While not directly appropriating More's notion of a 'sanative contagion', even Greatrakes himself had clearly moved some way towards More's part-spiritual, part-naturalistic psychosomatic explanation of his own gift and powers, as a divine 'gift' exercised by 'natural means'.

73   *Ibid.*, p. 34.

Chapter 7

William Petty and Anne Greene: Medical and Political Reform in Commonwealth Oxford

Scott Mandelbrote

On 16 December 1650, William Petty (1623–87) wrote from Oxford to his friend and supporter, Samuel Hartlib.[1] In this letter, Petty gave an account of two incidents involving members of 'the club' of experimenters that was then meeting in his lodgings in Buckley Hall (107 High Street), which was also the house of John Clarke, who had been William Harvey's apothecary.[2] The first of these consisted of the replication of an experiment initiated by Captain Bulmer, which involved raising weights by blowing into bladders that had been placed beneath them, with the intention of being able 'to blow a Boy or a Boate over London-bridge'. The second was altogether more unusual, although it also related to the

I should like to thank the following individuals for their willingness to discuss Anne Greene with me over the years: Jonathan Barry, Douglas Chambers, Cliff Davies, Mark Goldie, David Harley, Mark Jenner, Bent Juel-Jensen, Lauren Kassell, Margaret Pelling, Joad Raymond, Richard Smith, Keith Thomas, Paul Weindling. I am also grateful for comments from the audiences at seminars that were held in the Oxford Wellcome Unit and at the Department of History and Philosophy of Science in Cambridge. The ideas generated by the student members of a 'Research Challenge' class for the M.Phil. in Early Modern History at Cambridge, held in November 2003, have proved particularly fruitful.

1   New Haven, Connecticut, Yale University, Beinecke Rare Book and Manuscript Library, James Marshall and Marie-Louise Osborn Collection, OSB MSS File 16797; a copy of the letter may be found at Sheffield University Library, MSS Hartlib Papers, 8/23/1A–2A.

2   For the meetings of this group, see Charles Webster, *The Great Instauration: Science, Medicine and Reform 1626–1660* (2nd edn, Oxford, 2002), pp. 154–9; Lindsay Gerard Sharp, 'Sir William Petty and some aspects of seventeenth-century natural philosophy', unpublished Oxford University D.Phil. thesis (1976), pp. 60–106; Robert G. Frank, Jr., *Harvey and the Oxford Physiologists* (Berkeley, 1980), pp. 51–7; Penelope Gouk, 'Performance practice: music, medicine and natural philosophy in Interregnum Oxford', *British Journal for the History of Science*, 29 (1996), 257–88.

power of human respiration. It involved a young Oxfordshire woman who had been discovered concealing the lifeless remains of her new-born child. Although the birth was later presented as having been very premature, she was convicted of infanticide and executed, apparently according to due process of law. Her body was then taken to Petty's lodgings to be dissected, but before the anatomists could get to work the young woman showed signs of life. They revived her and when she recovered, she was pardoned for her crime. An outburst of comment, beginning with Petty's letter, followed on the event. This essay will consider what was said and by whom. It will then seek to uncover the debates and disagreements that lay behind a particular moment of medical and political reform. In the process, it will reveal the opportunities and the costs of a very peculiar experiment.

Petty's description of the event was as follows:

> Here hath happened lately a very miracle. Viz. A Maid was condemned to bee hanged for killing her owne new borne Infant w[hi]ch [she] tooke upon her death had never life not being a span long and shee not bee much aboue halfe gone w[i]th Child and alledging divers other circumstances whereby I am fully perswaded shee was innocent as to the Murther. But notw[i]thstanding all this shee was hanged neare halfe an houre beaten on the breast w[i]th many violent stroakes w[i]th the Butt end of a Musket then Cut downe and laid in a coffin w[hi]ch I had sent for her being to dissect her, when shee was brought to the place shee rattled in the throate but a friend of hers thinking to dispatch her stamped w[i]th his feet upon her three times. Soone after this I and one or two more came in to have opened her I found her then to rattle againe where-upon wee fell to worke w[i]th her, let her blood and vsed many other various remedies, which you shall know hereafter and now to the great admiration of all shee is almost recovered beyond all danger of her life where upon wee have gotten her repreive and made faire way for her pardon collected her monies to defray the charge of Medicines in her cure and hope to right her in refference of the persons that wronged her: Thousands of people come from all parts to admire the great and powerfull hand of God; in this businesse I shall further adde, that shee cannot remember how shee came out of Prison, how shee was hanged what shee said on [th]e Gallows (although shee spake liberally) but all things done before very perfectly.

Stories after the event

The account that Petty sent to Hartlib was the first of several retellings of the events that had taken place on 14 December 1650 and the ensuing days. Almost immediately, the weekly Parliamentarian newsbook, Marchamont Nedham's *Mercurius Politicus* carried a version of the story, in a letter dated 18 December. This gave far more circumstantial detail about the 'remarkable act of providence, that much amazeth the ordinary sort, and much affects the most discreet and reasonable men'. It revealed the identity of the woman ('One *Anne Green*, a servant in Sir *Thomas Roads* house at *Ounstu* in *Oxfordshire*'); that she had been made pregnant by the grandson of her master, and that she had given birth in 'the house of Office' as a result of straining herself through overwork when she was 'near the fourth moneth of her time'.[3] It provided more information about Anne Greene's state of health, about her trial, and about the execution that had taken place in the yard of Oxford Castle. It also explained that Greene was to be dissected 'before the company of Physitians, and other ingenuous Gentlemen, who have a weekly meeting at Mr. *Clarks* the Apothecary, about naturall enquiries and experiments'. Moreover, it identified the doctors who had treated Greene: 'one Dr. *Petty*, lately come from *London* to the Anatomy Reader in this University... with Mr. *Clerk* of *Magdalen* Colledg, and Mr. *Willis* of *Christ Church*', and gave further details of their actions in recovering her. Finally, it noted that Greene had now been reprieved by the Governor of the garrison at Oxford, remarked (as Petty had done) on the 'thousands of people' who had come to see Greene, and concluded with an assertion of her innocence: "'tis apprehended to be such a contrary verdict from heaven that may strike terror to the consciences of those who have been any way faulty in this businesse'.

Nedham later returned to the case of Anne Greene, picking up her story by printing another letter that had been sent from Oxford on 6 January 1651 and that reached him on 9 January. The main thrust of this letter was to describe what Greene remembered of her ordeal. It suggested that Petty had tried to stop the women who had attended Greene from suggesting 'unto her to relate of strange Visions and apparitions to have been seen by her in that time wherein she seem'd Dead (which they had begun to doe)' and that he had taken care over a number of days to test her memory. It revealed that she could not recall any part of the ceremony that attended her execution, nor of the speech that she had made on the gallows, and it drew attention to her piety and patience.[4] Given the speed with which Nedham had obtained information about Anne Greene, and the similarity of his descriptions to those given in the earlier letter to Hartlib, it is tempting to suppose that Petty himself was the anonymous author of the letters that were printed in *Mercurius Politicus*. Certainly, when Petty wrote up a more detailed account of his treatment of Anne Greene, he drew attention to several of the points that Nedham also developed.[5] By the time that Nedham published the second letter from Oxford, however, a competitor had entered the marketplace of cheap print.

3   *Mercurius Politicus*, 28 (12 December to 19 December 1650), 468–9. There are several misprints or mishearings in the passage quoted: the name of Greene's master was Sir Thomas Read and his house was at Duns Tew. See also Joad Raymond, ed., *Making the News* (Moreton-in-Marsh, 1993), pp. 182–3.

4   *Mercurius Politicus*, 32 (9 January to 16 January 1651), 520–1; cf. Raymond, *Making the News*, pp. 183–4.

5   Petty's detailed account of the incident and of his treatment of Greene is preserved in London, British Library, MS. Add. 72892, H75. Its title, 'History of the Magdalen', appears to me to be a later addition. The manuscript is printed (with several errors and omissions) in Marquis of Lansdowne, ed., *The Petty Papers* (2 vols, London, 1927), ii, pp. 157–67. For evidence of the date of its composition, see footnote 22 below.

This was a brief pamphlet, purporting to be a letter from Oxford written by 'W. Burdet' on 13 January 1651. A copy of the pamphlet, *A Wonder of Wonders*, reached the London stationer and collector of tracts, George Thomason, by 15 January 1651.[6]

A Wonder of Wonders claimed to be '*Witnessed by Dr. Petty, and Licensed according to Order*', although it is only known in a copy that lacks an imprint. Certainly, it heaped praise on 'the great pains of honest and faithful Dr. Petty'.[7] Despite this, the pamphlet presented a rather different view of events from that set out by Petty himself and by Nedham. It strengthened the emphasis on the role of divine providence in Greene's survival, to which both Petty and Nedham had alluded.[8] The title-page of the pamphlet bore a woodcut illustration in two parts, showing on the right-hand side an execution scene similar to that described in accounts of Anne Greene, and, on the left-hand side, a coffin and two female figures in a bed, recalling one of the details of Petty's treatment of Greene, in which 'Wee persuaded a Woman to goe into bed with her, and to keepe rubbing her lower parts gently'.[9] In this woodcut, a bubble of speech emerged from the mouth of one of the female figures, proclaiming 'Behold Gods providence'. According to the title-page of *A Wonder of Wonders*, when Anne Greene awoke 'the first words she spake were these; *Behold Gods Providence! Behold his miraculous and loving kindness!*' Elsewhere, Burdet suggested that she had said:

> Behold Gods providence, and his wonder of wonders, which indeed, is a deliverance so remarkable, since the ceasing of Miracles, that it cannot be parallel'd in all Ages, for the space of 300 years, And withall, it may remain upon record, for a president to all Magistrates, and Courts of Judicature, to take a special care in denounsing of sentence, without a due and legal process, according to the known Laws of the Land, by an impartiall and uncorrupted Jury, either of men or women, &c.[10]

Moreover, Burdet argued that it was only through the intervention of 'some honest Souldiers' that 'a great man' was dissuaded from taking Greene from her sick bed

6   W. Burdet, *A Wonder of Wonders* ([London], 1651), p. 6. The sole surviving copy of this tract (London, British Library, Thomason Tracts E621 (11)) bears Thomason's date of acquisition. Unfortunately, the second digit of the date has been altered and then smudged: Thomason's note could read 'Jan: 10. 1650' (according to ESTC), or 'Jan: 14. 1650' (according to Falconer Madan, *Oxford Books* (3 vols, Oxford, 1895– 1931), iii (1931), p. 2) or, conceivably, 'Jan: 15. 1650'.

7   Burdet, *A Wonder of Wonders*, title-page and p. 6.

8   On providentialism in pamphlet literature and related publications, see Alexandra Walsham, *Providence in Early Modern England* (Oxford, 1999), esp. pp. 32–224; Peter Lake, 'Deeds against nature: cheap print, Protestantism and murder in early seventeenth-century England', in *Culture and Politics in Early Stuart England*, ed. Kevin Sharpe and Peter Lake (Basingstoke, 1994), pp. 257–83, 361–7.

9   London, British Library, MS. Add. 72892, H75, fol. 4v.

10 Burdet, *A Wonder of Wonders*, p. 5.

to be hanged again for her crime. These sentiments were very different from Petty's own reticent account of Anne Greene's words on her recovery:

> Before Wee lett her blood, having putt all [th]e Company out of [th]e roome saving myselfe & 3 men of our faculty Wee asked what she could remember of all that had beene done to her, Shee answerd that, since shee had putt off her bod[ice] w[hi]ch cost her 5s. and gave w[i]th One of her coates to her Mother w[hi]ch was betimes in the Morning and that she had heard some say that Old Townesend was... to putt her to death, shee remembred... Neither how shee was came out of [th]e prison, went up the ladder &c nor what shee had spoken... Another thing is observable that her first speeches after shee came to herselfe were Much like those shee had used immediately before her execution with often sighes &c.[11]

Unlike Petty, Burdet also gave a detailed version of the words that Anne Greene had uttered at her execution, supposedly spoken on the ladder before the hangman turned her off to die. Despite suggesting that Greene had rebuked her 'false accusers' and referred to herself 'as an innocent woman to be in a moment cut off in the prime of her years', this text echoed many of the conventions of speeches from the scaffold that had already been established over decades in the publication in cheap print of accounts of criminals and their fates.[12] Although, according to Burdet, Anne Greene might seem to approach her death in a fashion that presaged the self-confidence with which criminals of the eighteenth century would be portrayed as going to the gallows, she in fact appeared to remain penitent and alert to divine retribution once she addressed her fate.[13] This was certainly the tone of the petition for a pardon that Greene presented after her recovery, which it seems reasonable to suppose that Petty helped to draft.[14] Nevertheless, Burdet's account differed from that published by Nedham and those written by Petty both in the extent of its providentialism and in its reflections on the social order.

Some time after the publication of *A Wonder of Wonders*, the London book-seller John Clowes issued another pamphlet, entitled *A Declaration from Oxford, of Anne Green*. Its title-page bore the same woodcut illustration that had decorated the front of *A Wonder of Wonders* and its contents overlapped considerably with those of the earlier work.[15] There were, however, some additions to Burdet's version of

11   London, British Library, MS. Add. 72892, H75, fol. 6r. The text has been damaged in places, making the sense obscure. These have been indicated with ellipses in this transcription.

12   Burdet, *A Wonder of Wonders*, p. 3; cf. J.A. Sharpe, '"Last Dying Speeches": religion, ideology and public execution in seventeenth-century England', *Past and Present*, no. 107 (1985), 144–67.

13   Cf. Andrea McKenzie, 'Martyrs in low life? Dying "game" in Augustan England', *Journal of British Studies*, 42 (2003), 167–205.

14   London, British Library, MS. Add. 72892, H75, fol. 8r.

15   There are other similarities, for example the decorative headpiece that is found on p. 1 of both pamphlets. Madan, *Oxford Books*, iii, pp. 2–3, is almost certainly correct to assert that they must have been issued from the same press.

the story. In particular, *A Declaration from Oxford* included an account of what Greene, who had now completed her recovery, had seen 'during her Trance'. The details provided by the author of *A Declaration from Oxford* were of precisely the kind that Nedham had suggested that Petty had tried to protect Greene from, or to prevent her from supplying. According to *A Declaration from Oxford*, Greene had thought herself 'in a Garden of Paradice' and had seen '4. little boyes with wings, being four Angels, saying, *Woe unto them that decree unrighteous Decrees, and take away the right from the Judges, that the innocent may be their prey*'. The pamphlet also included a long prayer, which it claimed that Greene now used, and which was 'fit to be read in all Families, throughout *England, Ireland, Scotland, and Wales*'. This likened Greene explicitly to Mary Magdalen, with whom she wished to '*testifie the love and thankfulness of my heart with abounding tears*!' A sense of the prayer's tone, as well as its relevance to the contemporary state of the four kingdoms of the British Isles, racked by nearly a decade of civil war, can be gained from the following lines: '*My sins deserved punishment, and thou hast corrupted me; but hast not given me over unto death*'.[16] As a whole, *A Declaration from Oxford* displayed even more of the features of providentialist cheap print than were apparent in *A Wonder of Wonders*. It concluded by juxtaposing the experience of Anne Greene with a story about the discovery in Derbyshire of a living child in the grave of a woman who had died in childbirth.[17]

That Petty and his Oxford allies disapproved of the presentation of Anne Greene's recovery set out in the two pamphlets that appeared early in 1651 is clear from a further publication that was rushed through the presses of Henry Hall and Leonard Lichfield later that year. Thomason acquired his copy of *Newes from the Dead. Or a True and Exact Narration of the Miraculous Deliverance of Anne Greene* on 6 March 1651.[18] The book consisted of 14 pages of verses, with 32 poems in Latin, English, and French, composed by a wide range of authors, many of whom had matriculated in the university within the previous two years. The poetry was followed by ten pages of prose, which set out in a tone that differentiated it at once from the pamphlets that had preceded it:

> There happened lately in this Citty a very rare and remarkeable accident, which
> being variously and falsely reported amongst the vulgar (as in such cases it is

16   *A Declaration from Oxford, of Anne Green* (London, 1651), quotations from the title-page and pp. 4–5.

17   *A Declaration from Oxford, of Anne Green*, p. 6; on the content and form of godly pamphlets, see Tessa Watt, *Cheap Print and Popular Piety 1550–1640* (Cambridge, 1991), pp. 296–320; Jerome Friedman, *Miracles and the Pulp Press during the English Revolution* (London, 1993); Ian Green, *Print and Protestantism in Early Modern England* (Oxford, 2000), pp. 445–502.

18   Thomason noted the date of acquisition on the title-page of his copy, now London, British Library, Thomason Tracts E625 (14); for evidence that the printing of the work was divided between the shops of Hall and Lichfield, see Madan, *Oxford Books*, iii, p. 5.

usuall) to the end that none may be deceived, and that so signall an act of Gods mercy and providence may never be forgotten, I have here faithfully recorded it, according to the Information I have received from those that were the chiefe Instruments in bringing this great worke to perfection.[19]

Newes from the Dead gave a detailed account of the events surrounding Anne Greene's trial, execution, and recovery. It amended the stories that had circulated previously, both in points of detail and in a more substantial manner. For example, it provided a full and accurate identification of Greene's master, her place of employment, and the circumstances of her pregnancy, thus correcting the information given in *Mercurius Politicus*. It described the regime of treatment that Petty and his colleagues provided for Greene. This description was based directly on the full version of events that Petty himself had composed, following its day-by-day assessment of Greene's condition and behaviour, and summarizing its narrative of the actions and prescriptions of the physicians attending her.[20] Moreover, *Newes from the Dead* echoed Petty's careful and restrained use of providentialist claims and language. When its author reviewed the case against Greene, he set out the arguments for believing that her child must have been stillborn that Petty had used in composing the petition for his patient's pardon. He suggested that, when 'the Governour and the rest of the Justices of Peace' were considering whether to reprieve Greene, 'they readily apprehended the hand of God in her preservation, and [were] willing rather to co-operate with divine providence in saving her, then to overstraine justice by condemning her to double shame & sufferings'. Describing the death of Greene's master and chief accuser, Sir Thomas Read, three days after the hanging, the author of *Newes from the Dead* limited himself to the observation that 'because he was an old man...such Events are not too rashly to be commented on'. Accounts of 'what visions this maid saw in the other world; what coelestiall musicke, or hellish howling she heard; what spirits she conversed with; and what Revelations she brought backe with her' were explicitly left to the imagination of the poets of the first part of *Newes from the Dead*, rather than

19 [Richard Watkins], *Newes from the Dead* (Oxford, 1651), second pagination, p. 1. For information about the authors of the poetry in this work, see Joseph Foster, *Alumni Oxonienses 1500–1714* (4 vols, Oxford, 1891–2); James Sutherland, 'Anne Greene and the Oxford poets', in *The Augustan Milieu*, ed. Henry Knight Miller, Eric Rothstein, and G.S. Rousseau (Oxford, 1970), pp. 1–17. For the attribution of the prose to Watkins, see Anthony Wood, *Athenae Oxonienses*, ed. Philip Bliss (4 vols, 3rd edn, London, 1813–20), iv [*Fasti Oxonienses*, vol. ii], p. 103, and Wood's note in his copy of the 2nd impression of *Newes from the Dead* (Oxford, 1651), now Oxford, Bodleian Library, Wood 515 (12).

20 This can be seen by comparing [Watkins], *Newes from the Dead*, esp. second pagination, pp. 4–9, with London, British Library, MS. Add. 72892, H75, esp. fols 4v–8v.

concerning the pen of the historian who composed its prose section.[21] Finally, *Newes from the Dead* presented an interpretation of the legal and social context of Greene's case that bolstered the contemporary hierarchy, however uncertain its claim to legitimacy. Thus, Greene's survival and pardon was a product of 'the generous attempt of those Gentlemen that freely undertooke, and have soe happily performed the Cure'; the Governor of Oxford was 'a Gentleman as much to be belov'd for his Courtesie, as he is honour'd for his Prudence', and he and others of 'the better sort' had been allowed access to the convalescing Greene through making a payment 'for their Curiosity' when 'multitudes' had been kept out.[22]

Newes from the Dead was reprinted twice in 1651, with additions and corrections, mainly to its verses.[23] In the long run, it succeeded in defining the story of Anne Greene, and in confirming William Petty's role as her saviour. The limits of its achievement as a work of publicity, however, can be gauged by a brief consideration of the continuing currency of Greene's experiences after 1651. Four contemporary historians of mid-seventeenth-century English affairs mention the recovery of Anne Greene. The author of *Britannia triumphalis* (London, 1654) based his account largely on the letters in *Mercurius Politicus*, repeating the errors of detail to be found there.[24] His conviction that the reviving of Greene was a special providence and that '[h]erein did the hand of God wonderfully appear, in detecting the unadvised actings of men, and in shewing us the danger we are in, when we are sway'd either by passion or prejudice against the meanest of his Creatures', however, seemed to owe more to *A Wonder of Wonders* than to Petty's version of events.[25] James Heath was similarly indebted to *Mercurius Politicus* for his description of Anne Greene, again repeating its errors of detail, and was apparently unacquainted with any of the other versions of the story.[26] Thomas

---

21   [Watkins], *Newes from the Dead*, at pp. 4, 9, and 10. In practice, none of the poems did in fact engage with the theme of Greene's experiences (imagined or otherwise) during the period immediately before she was revived, although several compared her fate with the classical myth of Eurydice, whom Orpheus tried to rescue from the underworld by the power of his playing on the lyre.

22   [Watkins], *Newes from the Dead*, at pp. 10, 7–8. The funds that were raised by exhibiting Anne Greene were used to pay her apothecary's bill, her board and lodging, legal expenses, and, eventually, to provide for her after her recovery. These details are not recorded in Petty's manuscript account (London, British Library, MS. Add. 72892, H75), which must therefore have been composed in late December 1650, before the outcome of Greene's petition was certain.

23   The second impression seems to have appeared in April 1650: see Andrew Clark, ed., *The Life and Times of Anthony Wood* (5 vols, Oxford, 1891–1900), i, pp. 169–70.

24   These errors were corrected in manuscript by the Oxford antiquary, Anthony Wood, on p. 82 of his copy, now Oxford, Bodleian Library, Wood 190: see Nicolas K. Kiessling, *The Library of Anthony Wood* (Oxford, 2002), p. 102.

25   *Britannia triumphalis; a Brief History of the Warres and other State-Affairs of Great Britain* (London, 1654), pp. 82–4, at p. 84.

26   James Heath, *A Brief Chronicle of the Late Intestine War in the Three Kingdoms of England, Scotland & Ireland* (London, 1663), pp. 512–13.

Fuller's short notice of Anne Greene as a 'memorable person' in Oxfordshire, however, indicated knowledge of the poetry of *Newes from the Dead*, as well as revealing that Greene was 'married, and liveth in this County in good reputation'.[27] The English continuator of Denis Petau's *History of the World* (London, 1659) told the tale of Anne Greene with some unique elements of his own. He claimed that the father of Greene's child was a servant or friend of Sir Thomas Read, rather than his grandson, and suggested that Read had died from choking on his food when he heard of Greene's recovery.[28]

The chemist and natural philosopher, Robert Plot, later repeated some of these details from Petau's *History* when he considered Anne Greene. However, Plot must also have had access either to gossip about Greene, or to oral tradition, or to some other branch of what Daniel Woolf has called 'history by almanac, ballad, and chapbook'. He alone named '*Mason* a *Tayler*' and 'one *Orum* a Soldier' ('as some say') as the onlookers at Greene's execution who tried charitably to ensure that she was dead before she was placed in her coffin. He similarly revealed that Greene had 'retired into the *Country* to her *friends* at *Steeple-Barton*' and that her marriage had produced three children before her death in 1659.[29] At least one of Plot's readers was disturbed by his ignorance of *Newes from the Dead* and by his embellishment of the suggestion, originally made in cheap print, that Greene had had a vision of paradise ('*she* said, *she* had been in a fine *green meddow*, having a *River* running round it, and that all things there glittered like *silver* and *gold*').[30] In his 'Adversaria Physica', the Wiltshire natural philosopher, John Aubrey, remarked that any vision that Greene had had must have been caused by 'the nerves constringed' in her neck. He later communicated this view to Plot. In February 1680, Aubrey composed a life of Petty in which he referred directly to the narrative printed in *Newes from the Dead*.[31] Anthony Wood, who was a contributor of verses to the second impression of *Newes from the Dead*, perhaps unsurprisingly preferred

27 Thomas Fuller, *The History of the Worthies of England* (London, 1662), p. 341 (sig. 3X2r).

28 Denis Petau, *The History of the World: Or an Account of Time...Continued by Others to the Year of Our Lord, 1659* (London, 1659), p. 502.

29 Robert Plot, *The Natural History of Oxfordshire* (Oxford, 1677), pp. 197–9; cf. Daniel Woolf, *The Social Circulation of the Past. English Historical Culture 1500–1730* (Oxford, 2003), pp. 259–391, esp. p. 320. Writing in September 1703, John Evelyn believed that Anne Greene had still been alive in 1665: see London, British Library, MS. Add. 4229, fol. 56v; Michael Hunter, ed., *Robert Boyle by Himself and his Friends* (London, 1994), p. 94.

30 Plot, *Natural History of Oxfordshire*, p. 199.

31 Oxford, Bodleian Library, MS. Hearne's Diaries 158–9, second pagination, p. 214X; Andrew Clark, ed., *'Brief Lives', Chiefly of Contemporaries, Set Down by John Aubrey, between the Years 1669 & 1696* (2 vols, Oxford, 1898), ii, pp. 141, 148; Michael Hunter, *John Aubrey and the Realm of Learning* (London, 1975), pp. 80, 130, 237–8.

its version of Anne Greene's story to that given by Plot.[32] Watkins's account also influenced the natural theologian William Derham's choice of Anne Greene to illustrate the providence of God in the design of the respiratory system. In his Boyle lectures of 1711–12, Derham wondered whether Greene's survival might have been due to the extraordinary strength of the human windpipe.[33]

Contexts for an event: medical and political reform in Commonwealth Oxford

The story of Anne Greene's survival with the accounts that were woven around it poses many interesting problems of evidence and interpretation. It has been worth telling it at some length in part because the difficulties posed by the relationships between the various texts describing Anne Greene have never been fully tackled.[34] The real reason, however, for rehearsing it has been to provide the necessary background for a more important set of questions. Given that Greene was not the first person to survive being hanged, what was special about the way in which she recovered and for what reasons did Petty and others present her survival in the manner in which they did? The answers to these questions will help us to understand what happened to Anne Greene, but they will also allow us to trace the practice of reform at Oxford in the years around 1650.

There is one aspect of the appearance of Anne Greene in the literature of cheap print that can be considered directly in the light of the comparison of the chapbook accounts of her death with those presented in other sources. This is the possibility that the story of Anne Greene was in large measure a fiction, drawing on a number of formulaic elements commonly to be found in godly pamphlets aimed at a popular audience. A different kind of homage to literary tradition was certainly paid by the authors of the verses that accompanied *Newes from the Dead*. More-

32   Clark, *Life and Times of Wood*, i, pp. 165–6; cf. p. 251. For a judicious assessment of the argument that one of Wood's brothers might have been the author of the poem printed at p. 21 of [Watkins], *Newes from the Dead* (2nd impression, Oxford, 1651), see Kiessling, *Library of Anthony Wood*, p. 603.

33   William Derham, *Physico-Theology* (3rd edn, London, 1714), p. 157. Derham believed that *Newes from the Dead* was largely the work of Petty's collaborator, Ralph Bathurst. This opinion was rebutted by Thomas Warton, *The Life and Literary Remains of Ralph Bathurst, M.D.* (London, 1761), pp. xv, 43, 295–6. There have been a number of more recent medical commentators on Anne Greene's survival: see Bent Juel-Jensen, 'News from the dead: the remarkable history of Anne Green', *Oxford Medical School Gazette*, 14 (1962), 135–40; J. Trevor Hughes, 'Miraculous deliverance of Anne Green: an Oxford case of resuscitation in the seventeenth century', *British Medical Journal*, 285 (1982), 1792–3; S.G. Braye and G. Guy, 'Miraculous deliverance of Anne Green', *British Medical Journal*, 286 (1983), 556.

34   Cf. Joad Raymond, *Pamphlets and Pamphleteering in Early Modern Britain* (Cambridge, 2003), pp. 113–15. Two novels have attempted to make sense of Anne Greene's experiences: Douglas Angus, *The Green and the Burning* (London, 1958) and Iain Pears, *An Instance of the Fingerpost* (London, 1997).

over, the legend of Anne Greene lived on in the tradition of cheap print until well after it must have lost any particular or personal significance that it might once have had.[35] Elements of the story were strongly reminiscent of those to be found elsewhere in the religious ballads and chapbooks that represented nearly a third of the market for cheap print in the 1650s. Some of these were cautionary tales in which punishment for sin or preparation for death and divine judgement played an important role. Others were stories of strange and unusual events that were intended as much to entertain as to edify. Although they did not all repeat the explicitly providentialist language of the pamphlets that described Anne Greene, many echoed the fascination with the wondrous and marvellous that also marked the accounts of her execution and recovery.[36]

Infanticide was a common theme in chapbook and pamphlet literature.[37] Another aspect of Anne Greene's experience that interested the purveyors of cheap print was the display of unexpected signs of life. For example, a ballad of 1661 told about Lawrence Cawthorn, a London butcher, who had been declared dead prematurely and then buried alive.[38] The repentant criminal, Thomas Savage, who was hanged twice for the same murder, was the subject of numerous pamphlets after his execution in 1668. Several of these noted the remarkable fact that Savage had revived when his body was laid out in a public house after the first hanging.[39] There were also many later accounts of similar survivors of hanging, at least one of which contained a number of details found in descriptions of Anne Greene, although most of these abandoned the literary traditions of the godly pamphlet for

---

35   *A Full and True Relation of Anne Green who was Hanged at Oxford 14th December 1650* (Norwich, 1741); the Hackney merchant and moral reformer, Nehemiah Lyde, recorded a vague memory of Anne Greene's story in *A Narrative of the Life of Mr. Richard Lyde of Hereford* (London, 1731), p. 50.

36   See Margaret Spufford, *Small Books and Pleasant Histories* (London, 1981), pp. 194–218; cf. Green, *Print and Protestantism*, esp. pp. 472–502. For secular developments in the literature of marvels and wonders, see Lorraine Daston and Katharine Park, *Wonders and the Order of Nature* (New York, 1998), esp. pp. 215–53.

37   See Frances E. Dolan, *Dangerous Familiars. Representations of Domestic Crime in England, 1550–1700* (Ithaca, 1994), pp. 121–70; Christopher Durston, *The Family in the English Revolution* (Oxford, 1989), pp. 153–4.

38   *Misery to bee Lamented* (London, [1661]).

39   Robert Franklin, Thomas Vincent, Thomas Doolittle et al., *A Murderer Punished and Pardoned* (London, 1668), p. 43; *God's Justice against Murther* (London, [1668]), pp. 10–11; *The Murtherer Turned True Penitent* (London, [1668]), p. 21; *The Wicked Life and Penitent Death of Tho. Savage* (London, [1668]), p. 18. On Savage, see Lincoln B. Faller, *Turned to Account* (Cambridge, 1987), pp. 28–31; Green, *Print and Protestantism*, pp. 488–9; Peter Lake, 'Popular form, puritan content? Two puritan appropriations of the murder pamphlet from mid-seventeenth-century London', in *Religion, Culture and Society in Early Modern Britain*, ed. Anthony Fletcher and Peter Roberts (Cambridge, 1994), pp. 313–34; John J. Richetti, *Popular Fiction before Richardson: Narrative Patterns 1700–1739* (Oxford, 1969), pp. 53–5; Sharpe, '"Last Dying Speeches"', pp. 151–5.

the factitious ones of journalism.[40] More important than such later examples might be a comic ghost story recounted in 1617 by John Taylor. This related the liberation from the gallows of a German robber, who had been left to hang in a thunderstorm. The robber proceeded to make off with a horse that belonged to the farmer who had cut him down, but was eventually recaptured and lynched by his victim. This in turn caused wonder and foreboding among those who had noticed the disappearance of the criminal's body from the gallows and who now remarked on its strange reappearance.[41] A French tract that appeared in two editions at Douai in 1589, however, provides the most tantalizing evidence for the role of a literary tradition in shaping accounts of Anne Greene. Together with a similar story published in Rennes in 1588, this *occasionnel* was produced in the context of the resurgence of interest in the miracles of the Virgin that accompanied the success of the Catholic League. It described the execution of a young woman who had been unjustly accused of infanticide. She was hanged, but prayed to Our Lady of Liesse, and so survived. In due course, she was rescued, recovered, and reprieved. The French pamphlet reveals a tradition of miracles associated with the intervention of the Virgin to save innocent women from hanging. Stories from this tradition were still being reprinted in France in the 1630s.[42] Despite many similarities in the circumstances that they recount, it nevertheless seems unlikely that these examples of Catholic piety and propaganda provided a direct model for any of the accounts of the experience of Anne Greene. Although Anne Greene's story was quickly assimilated to the traditions of cheap print, both in form and content, its details did not always sit easily with the ideas of providence and the miraculous, or with the aims of entertainment, that characterized that genre. Moreover, the appearance of

40   For examples, see *The Gentleman's Magazine*, 1 (1731), 172; 6 (1736), 422; 10 (1740), 570; 37 (1767), 90; Arthur Griffiths, *The Chronicles of Newgate* (2 vols, London, 1884), i, pp. 280–1; [James Guthrie], *The Ordinary of Newgate, His Account of the Behaviour, Confession, and Dying Words, of the Malefactors, who were Executed at Tyburn, on Monday the 24th of November* (London, 1740), esp. pp. 6–8, 18–19; Alfred Marks, *Tyburn Tree: Its History and Annals* (London, [1908]), pp. 221–3, 226; J.L. Mayner and G.T. Crook, eds, *The Complete Newgate Calendar* (5 vols, London, 1926), ii, pp. 4–8; iii, pp. 44–6, 110. Guthrie mentions Anne Greene and also describes the recovery and pardon of Margaret Dixon of Musselburgh, who was hanged for infanticide in 1728. The currency of Anne Greene's story in the 1740s (see footnote 35 above) may have been partly due to him.

41   John Taylor, *Three Weekes, Three Daies, and Three Houres Observations and Travel from London to Hamburgh in Germanie* (London, 1617), sigs C3v-D1r. The story was reprinted in *All the Workes of Iohn Taylor* (London, 1630), sigs 3G6v-3H1r. See also Bernard Capp, *The World of John Taylor the Water-Poet 1578–1653* (Oxford, 1994), pp. 18–19. Taylor was rediscovered by Robert Southey, whose poem ('Roprecht the Robber') based on this story can be found in *The Poetical Works* (10 vols, London, 1837–8), vi, pp. 241–59.

42   See Roger Chartier, 'The hanged woman miraculously saved: an *occasionnel*', in *The Culture of Print*, ed. Roger Chartier, trans. Lydia G. Cochrane (Cambridge, 1989), pp. 59–91, and plates II-III. This also provides translations of the original publications.

Anne Greene in the literature of cheap print was more contentious than most godly pamphleteering.

In an English context, one of the oddest things about Anne Greene's story was that it had a happy ending. By contrast, on 22 April 1658, Elizabeth Russell was brought before the Sessions of the Peace in Oxford 'for murthering a Bastard female infant borne of hir bodie was for the same arraigned & found guiltie & had judgment to bee hanged'. Hers was one of 36 cases heard that day, four of which related to bastardy.[43] On 4 May, Russell was hanged:

> After shee was cut downe and taken away to be anatomiz'd, [William] Coniers a physitian of S. John's Coll and other yong physitians, did in short time bring life into her. But the bayllives of the towne hearing of it, they went between 12 and one of the clock at night to the house where she laid, and putting her into a coffin carried her into Broken hayes, and by a halter about her neck drew her out of it, and hung her on a tree there.[44]

According to Anthony Wood, who was highly critical of the Oxford magistrates and of city government at the time, Russell was alert and prayed before she was executed for the second time. Wood claimed that the women of Oxford responded to the bailiffs' actions with abuse and by cutting down the tree from which Russell had been hanged. Wood also attributed the later bankruptcy of one of the bailiffs, Henry Mallory, to divine judgement on his role in this affair. The details of Elizabeth Russell's case were remarkably similar to those of Anne Greene. Russell was also a servant, and, like Anne Greene, she had sought to conceal her dead child in a privy. Furthermore, Conyers's treatment of Russell, which involved bleeding and putting her to bed with another young woman, was reminiscent of Petty's actions in December 1650.[45] In spite of Wood's disapproval, however, the Oxford authorities acted according to the letter of the law in their treatment of Russell. As Petty's care in obtaining a pardon for Anne Greene indicated, to survive the procedure of hanging did not acquit a convict of the penalty of execution.

The experiences of both Anne Greene and Elizabeth Russell also indicate the unusual nature of the crime of infanticide in mid-seventeenth-century England. Anne Greene's case in particular suggested some of the special difficulties that confronted female servants in resisting sexual pressure applied by their masters or by other figures of authority in the household. By contrast, sexual availability could be a high-risk strategy for young women eager to win a better life for themselves through a form of entrapment, although Anne Greene's uncertainties about her pregnancy, as well as her youth, perhaps reveal that this was not the

---

43   Oxfordshire Record Office, City Archive, MS. O.5.11, fols 11v–13r, at fol. 12v (Sessions Roll, 1656–76).

44   Clark, *Life and Times of Wood*, i, pp. 250–1.

45   *Ibid*. See also Plot, *Natural History of Oxfordshire*, pp. 199–200.

course that she had been following.[46] Instead, Greene's experience provided a reminder of the emotional and personal challenges faced by young women, working away from home, in assessing and responding to changes in their own bodies and in interpreting the evidence of pregnancy, particularly when the child was stillborn.[47] Supporting the petition for Anne Greene's pardon, Petty cast doubt on her condition and redefined the birth of her child as a miscarriage. He denied that the circumstances of the birth indicated a desire to conceal the pregnancy or gave substance to the accusation of infanticide: they were also evidence of the unwitting behaviour of Greene, who 'might not at that tyme certainly know shee was with child Or that she had beene delivered thereof'. Petty's claims were buttressed by reference to the opinion of the midwife who had examined the birth, the views of women that he had consulted in Oxford, and the gossip of Anne Greene's fellow servants.[48] Greene's petition and its supporting documents were carefully contrived to exploit the room for negotiation that existed in the case of a woman accused of infanticide.

Trials for infanticide were carried out under the terms of a statute of 1624, which sought to deal with the obstacles raised against successful prosecution in cases where the birth and subsequent death of a child had been concealed. Under the normal terms of common law, absence of proof that a child had been born alive had rendered many efforts to prosecute for infanticide fruitless. The Parliament of 1624 was dominated by discussions of the disastrous turn in European affairs that seemed to threaten the extinction of Protestantism.[49] Despite this, more than thirty public Acts were passed between February and May 1624. Most of these had already been debated as bills in the Parliament of 1621 that James VI and I had cut short. Several of them related to legal reforms, for example to the power of JPs, the jurisdiction of local courts and of the prerogative courts, the corruption of judges, and the inadequacy of jurors. A number reflected contemporary concern about the diminution of trade and the effects of a depression in land values. Uniquely among the public bills, that concerning infanticide had not been introduced in 1621.[50] The

---

46   Cf. Tim Meldrum, 'London domestic servants from depositional evidence, 1660–
      1750: servant-employer sexuality in the patriarchal household', in *Chronicling
      Poverty. The Voices and Strategies of the English Poor, 1640–1840*, ed. Tim
      Hitchcock, Peter King, and Pamela Sharpe (Basingstoke, 1997), pp. 47–69; Tim
      Meldrum, *Domestic Service and Gender 1660–1750* (Harlow, 2000), pp. 100–27;
      Laura Gowing, *Common Bodies. Women, Touch, and Power in Seventeenth-Century
      England* (New Haven, 2003), pp. 59–65.
47   See Laura Gowing, 'Secret births and infanticide in seventeenth-century England',
      Past and Present, no. 156 (1997), 87–115; Gowing, *Common Bodies*, pp. 17–51, 111–
      48.
48   London, British Library, MS. Add. 72892, H75, fols 8v–9r.
49   Thomas Cogswell, *The Blessed Revolution* (Cambridge, 1989).
50   See Conrad Russell, *Parliaments and English Politics 1621–1629* (Oxford, 1979), pp.
      190–4; Stephen D. White, *Sir Edward Coke and the Grievances of the Commonwealth*
      (Manchester, 1979), pp. 46–85.

infanticide statute of 1624 was passed in the context of the desire to control moral behaviour, in particular illicit sexual activity, and to limit the costs to parish ratepayers of relief of the poverty of unmarried women and bastard children. It was supposed to encourage women to reveal the identity of the fathers of their living children, by introducing the presumption that concealment of a child that was found to be dead after its birth would lead to the conviction of the mother for infanticide.[51]

This was the presumption under which both Anne Greene and Elizabeth Russell were convicted, since neither could produce the single witness to the birth that the law required. The statute of 1624 had the effect of increasing substantially the number of women who were convicted of homicide or its equivalent. Its consequences were particularly severe in the case of female servants, especially those who had been sexually involved with their masters, since these women were likely to lose their jobs and thus their livelihoods if they revealed the circumstances of their pregnancies. Before the extension of benefit of clergy to women in 1691, those who were convicted of infanticide were also very likely to be executed.[52] As Garthine Walker has noted, however, the apparent harshness of the law on infanticide paradoxically meant that the courts were more willing to explore circumstances that might mitigate the crime than they were in other cases of violence by women. In the first place, evidence was required that concealment was deliberate. Secondly, proof was needed that death had occurred after birth, for example from the evidence of a midwife who had examined the corpse of the baby. Finally, judges showed a willingness to recommend for pardon women who had been convicted of infanticide that they did not extend to other female murderers.[53]

The actions of Anne Greene's friends in December 1650 exploited the full range of mitigating circumstances that were available in cases of alleged infanticide. They asserted that Greene had confessed to fornication before the time of the birth; that the birth had been so premature that Greene might reasonably have been unsure whether or not she was pregnant; that Greene had not concealed the birth, but had miscarried naturally, perhaps as an unwitting result of performing too much physical labour; that the midwife and the other women who had examined the birth after it had been discovered 'did not thinke it ever to have life' and 'that [th]e whole rather seemed a lump of flesh, then a Mature and Onely

---

51   Steve Hindle, *The State and Social Change in Early Modern England, c. 1550–1640* (Basingstoke, 2000), pp. 153–62; Martin Ingram, *Church Courts, Sex and Marriage in England, 1570–1640* (Cambridge, 1987); Mark Jackson, *New-Born Child Murder* (Manchester, 1996), esp. pp. 30–6.

52   See J.M. Beattie, *Crime and the Courts in England 1660–1800* (Oxford, 1986), pp. 113–24; Keith Wrightson, 'Infanticide in earlier seventeenth-century England', *Local Population Studies*, 15 (1975), 10–22. Many examples of the working of the statute of 1624 can be found in the Proceedings of the Old Bailey, London (1674 to 1834), now available at www.oldbaileyonline.org.

53   Garthine Walker, *Crime, Gender and Social Order in Early Modern England* (Cambridge, 2003), pp. 148–58.

formed child'. Finally, they suggested that the sentence that Anne Greene had received was a product of 'the desires and good intentions of her Judges to discover and punish Wickednes as also their excusable Unacquaintance with [th]e physicall part of these cases... [rather] than any cleere demonstrations of her guiltines of a crime deserving so severe a punishment'.[54] In some ways, this was a remarkable conclusion, since it is hard to see how, if what Petty and others said was true, Anne Greene could ever have been found guilty, even under the terms of the infanticide statute of 1624.

The suspicion that some sort of foul play might indeed have occurred in the prosecution of Anne Greene, as the cheap print accounts of her ordeal suggested, may gain a little substance when the local circumstances of the village in which the alleged crime took place are considered. The manor in the parish of Duns Tew was held by the Read family, whose main property was in Berkshire, but who also owned land in Oxfordshire, Northamptonshire, Hertfordshire, and Cambridgeshire. Sir Thomas Read (1575–1650) is said to have settled the estate at Duns Tew in 1639 on his eldest surviving son, John (1617–94). Sir Thomas Read had been knighted in 1619. He served in a variety of local offices over a period of more than forty years. He had been an opponent of ship money, but was active on the Royalist side in the first civil war. Nevertheless, he made his peace with the King's opponents quickly, and was placed on the Committee for the County of Oxford in 1646. He was buried at Duns Tew on 20 December 1650. That there may have been generational conflict within the Read family was apparent in the accounts of the treatment of Anne Greene. Furthermore, another of Read's sons, Geoffrey, was estranged from his father and was one of several members of the family not to be mentioned in his will. Another Geoffrey Read (baptized 20 April 1634), the fifth son of the eldest of Sir Thomas Read's sons to reach adulthood (also Thomas, 1606–34), was mentioned in the will but was unusual among Read's grandchildren in receiving nothing by it. This younger Geoffrey Read was the grandchild of Sir Thomas Read by whom Anne Greene became pregnant in late summer 1650. Greene herself was not quite a local girl, having been born in the neighbouring parish of Steeple Barton. The Reads were not on particularly good terms with the other significant landowners in Duns Tew, who seem to have mounted successful opposition to an enclosure scheme of theirs in 1652. The Reads' tight management of their estate contributed to a remarkable increase in levels of poverty in the parish during the middle years of the seventeenth century and a growing polarization of wealth. The limited funds available in Duns Tew for poor relief and charity thus grew more and more stretched, exacerbating the tensions within households and between neighbours, and reducing tolerance for illicit adolescent sexual behaviour. At the level of the village, therefore, there were a number of factors that were likely both to promote belief in Anne Greene's guilt and to encourage a willingness

54   London, British Library, MS. Add. 72892, H75, fols 8r–9v. A similar, if less developed case, was also made in *Mercurius Politicus*, 28 (12 December to 19 December 1650), 468–9.

to interpret the evidence of her crime in the harshest possible terms. Conversely, there would have been many people in Duns Tew and its neighbourhood who would not have been unhappy with the damage done to the reputation of the Read family by some of the comments that appeared in the pamphlet literature about the recovery of Anne Greene.[55]

Although the petition of Anne Greene was careful to avoid suggesting that any injustice had been done, the issue of the punishment of infanticide nevertheless resonated strongly with contemporary political debates about morality and the legal system. For this reason, it was not surprising that Anne Greene's case generated the highly charged comments concerning justice that were contained in both *A Wonder of Wonders* and *A Declaration from Oxford*. These were unlike the positions taken up by Petty and his allies in a number of ways. Firstly, both *A Wonder of Wonders* and *A Declaration from Oxford* began with a description of the birth of Anne Greene's child that contradicted the details given in her petition. Although pointing out that the child was 'abortive', they agreed that Greene had 'laid it in a Corner…and covered it with dust and rubbish'. A dialogue between Greene and a fellow servant, 'Mary', which both pamphlets presented, revealed that Greene had kept secret both her pregnancy and the illicit sexual activity that had preceded it. These points sensationalized the story, but complicated, without invalidating, the claim that Greene was innocent of infanticide. Such complexity was, however, in part a reflection of a second difference between the pamphlet accounts and those with which Petty was involved. In *A Wonder of Wonders* and *A Declaration from Oxford*, the suggestion was made that Greene's crime and her punishment were in some sense a product of unjust laws made for an unjust society, to be contrasted with her own natural innocence and piety. Both pamphlets drew attention to the social status of the father of Greene's child ('a Gentleman of good birth and kinsman to a justice of Peace'). They both emphasized the speed with which her case was heard and stressed the importance of due process in all trials. Finally, they gave Anne Greene a voice with which to denounce her tormentors.[56]

Concern with the speed of trials, with due process in common law, and with the impartiality of juries was a widely noted feature of the campaign for legal reform that represented one part of the demands of the Leveller movement at the end of the 1640s. Capitalizing on grievances within the Parliamentary army, spokesmen associated with the Levellers presented a broad programme of social and political reform, particularly between March 1647 and May 1649. Following the imprisonment of several Leveller leaders in London in spring 1649, Leveller women presented petitions that stressed the threat to the unity and probity of the

55   See A. Tomkinson and C.J. Day, 'Duns Tew', in *The Victoria History of the County of Oxford. Volume XI: Wootton Hundred (Northern Part)*, ed. Alan Crossley (London, 1983), pp. 209–22; for information on the Reads, see Compton Reade, *A Record of the Redes* (Hereford, 1899), pp. 18–47.

56   Quotation from Burdet, *A Wonder of Wonders*, p. 2; cf. *A Declaration from Oxford, of Anne Green*, p. 2, which is identical except for capitalization. See also the references given in footnotes 10 and 16 above.

household posed by the actions of the Army grandees and defended themselves and their husbands against slanderous imputations of sexual misconduct. Leveller literature contrasted the honest and natural morality of the free household with the licentiousness and immorality that derived from placing a privileged oligarchy above the law.[57]

It is not straightforward to suggest the influence of Leveller writing on the presentation of Anne Greene in *A Wonder of Wonders* and *A Declaration from Oxford*. For one thing, the Leveller movement had largely been suppressed a year and a half before the publication of these pamphlets. In any case, the Leveller belief that politics was best conducted by individuals who were not only born free, but who were also free to act independently, implied limitations on the expression of female opinion and largely excluded servants from any discussion of reform.[58] Nothing is known of 'W. Burdet', the supposed author of *A Wonder of Wonders*. John Clowes, the printer of the anonymous *A Declaration from Oxford*, did publish some works associated with expressions of grievance in the army in 1648, but was not connected with any of the more prominent Leveller writings.[59] What may be more important, however, is not whether *A Wonder of Wonders* and *A Declaration from Oxford* really did derive any of their content from Leveller thought, but whether their readers would have believed that they might have done so. In this context, the similarities between the two pamphlets and a text that would certainly have resonated in Oxford remain striking.

On the night of 17 May 1649, Sir Thomas Fairfax and Oliver Cromwell lodged at All Souls College, Oxford, fresh from the bloody suppression at Burford of an army mutiny that had broken out at Banbury on 6 May, in support of the imprisoned Leveller leaders. The manifesto of the mutineers, *Englands Standard Advanced*, complained about the subversion of trial by jury and the establishment of oligarchy. It attacked summary justice and appealed to divine and natural law. The mutineers aimed 'to set the unjustly imprisoned free, to relieve the poor, and settle this Commonwealth, upon the grounds of Common Right, Freedome, and Safety'.[60] It does not seem implausible to link memories of the aims and fate of the Burford mutineers with the presentation in cheap print of the execution and

---

57   See Donald Veall, *The Popular Movement for Law Reform 1640–1660* (Oxford, 1970), esp. pp. 98–106, 128–38, 152–9; G.E. Aylmer, ed., *The Levellers in the English Revolution* (London, 1975), pp. 22–49; Ann Hughes, 'Gender and politics in Leveller literature', in *Political Culture and Cultural Politics in Early Modern England*, ed. Susan D. Amussen and Mark A. Kishlansky (Manchester, 1995), pp. 162–88; William Haller and Godfrey Davies, eds, *The Leveller Tracts 1647–1653* (New York, 1944), esp. pp. 152, 158–9, 219.

58   Keith Thomas, 'The Levellers and the franchise', in *The Interregnum: The Quest for Settlement 1646–1660*, ed. G.E. Aylmer (London, 1972), pp. 57–78, 219–22.

59   For example, *The Copies of Two Petitions from the Officers and Souldiers of Col. Charles Fleftwoods Regiment* (London, 1648).

60   [Clement Walker], *The Compleat History of Independency* (4 pts, London, [1660]), ii, pp. 168–73, quotation at p. 170.

recovery of Anne Greene, and in particular to the claim made, according to *A Wonder of Wonders*, by 'some honest Souldiers', that 'it was contrary to all right and reason, that any further punishment shuld be inflicted upon her'.[61]

Although Marchamont Nedham, who published the first account of Anne Greene, was a public critic of Leveller ideas, his own brand of republicanism was not so distant from theirs.[62] In December 1650, however, when Cromwell's forces were triumphing in Scotland, it was difficult for Nedham to criticize the Republic. The journal that Nedham had started six months before, *Mercurius Politicus*, took the side of the Rump for reasons that perhaps owed more to the prospect of personal and financial reward than they did to conviction. Having been bankrupted as a result of an earlier change of horses that led him to support the Royalist cause from 1647 until 1649, Nedham was ready to support the rule of the Commonwealth because it offered stability, order, and protection and thus deserved to command the obedience of the people.[63] By the late autumn of 1650, the threat that had been posed to the Commonwealth regime by the alliance of the Royalists with the Scottish Presbyterians was receding. In its place, however, political efforts to conciliate English Presbyterians, whom Nedham detested, seemed to be gathering pace. Such a shift threatened to destabilize Nedham's newly found confidence in the regime. One aspect of the change that attracted the open opposition of Henry Marten and others in Parliament whom Nedham supported may also have helped to interest him in Anne Greene. On 10 May 1650, Parliament passed the Adultery Act, which returned to the secular authority the right to make judgements in matters of moral behaviour that had previously been reserved to the ecclesiastical courts. The Adultery Act made incest and adultery into felonies, for which execution was the penalty, and established imprisonment for three months as the punishment for fornication. Thanks to the efforts of Marten and his allies, however, the teeth of the Adultery Act were drawn by the exclusion of certain categories of offence and by the imposition of higher standards of evidence than had originally been intended. Nevertheless, this was an opportune time for Nedham to publicize the case of Anne Greene and to present her as a victim of the excesses of zeal that might occur if the power of the secular courts were to be turned to consider moral offences, or if members of the same household were to be encouraged to bear witness against one another's sexual behaviour.[64]

61   Burdet, *A Wonder of Wonders*, p. 6.
62   See Jonathan Scott, *Commonwealth Principles. Republican Writing of the English Revolution* (Cambridge, 2004), pp. 82–4.
63   Marchamont Nedham, *The Case of the Common-Wealth of England, Stated* (London, 1650); Blair Worden, 'Marchamont Nedham and the beginnings of English republicanism, 1649–1656', in *Republicanism, Liberty, and Commercial Society, 1649–1776*, ed. David Wootton (Stanford, 1994), pp. 45–81; David Norbrook, *Writing the English Republic* (Cambridge, 1999), pp. 221–5.
64   See Keith Thomas, 'The puritans and adultery: the act of 1650 reconsidered', and C.M. Williams, 'The anatomy of a radical gentleman: Henry Marten', both in *Puritans and Revolutionaries*, ed. Donald Pennington and Keith Thomas (Oxford, 1978), pp.

During the autumn and winter of 1650–1, Nedham's friends in Parliament won recognition for those who had secured the execution of Charles I and promoted policies, through the newly established Council of Trade, which they had advocated, to encourage English trade and shipping. Several members of the circle around Samuel Hartlib took part in these new developments. Benjamin Worsley, for example, who had been involved in Hartlib's schemes from the mid-1640s, was appointed as secretary to the Council of Trade in August 1650. Another one of its members was Sir Cheney Culpeper, whose support for Hartlib went back to the heady days of 1641. Culpeper had complained to Hartlib about his fears of 'the Presbiterian Popery, (I meane that persecutinge Spirite which they haue pulled downe in others that themselues myght get in the saddle)' in January 1648.[65] Anxiety about the intentions of the Presbyterians and fears about the establishment of a divisive form of prelacy underlay the attitudes of many reformers in 1650 and helped to explain their willingness to bind themselves to the Rump by taking the Engagement, an oath of loyalty to the Republic. One of those who advocated doing so, thus earning the opprobrium of the Presbyterian controversialist, William Prynne, was Hartlib's long-term collaborator, John Dury.[66]

The Royalist journalist and rival of Marchamont Nedham, Sir John Birkenhead, asked in summer 1651 'whether the Mayd at *Oxford* that was hanged and reviv'd, had subscrib'd the *Ingagement?*'[67] Like most of the jokes traded by pamphleteers at this time, Birkenhead's facetious question hit on a serious political point. The Parliamentary visitors who eventually descended on the University of Oxford following the defeat of Charles I in the first civil war expelled approximately 50 per cent of the fellows of the colleges. The leading figures in this visitation were prominent Presbyterians, and the men whom they appointed to the places that were left vacant after 1648 could be expected to be sympathetic to their

257–82 and 118–38 respectively; Blair Worden, 'Milton and Marchamont Nedham', in *Milton and Republicanism*, ed. David Armitage, Armand Himy, and Quentin Skinner (Cambridge, 1995), pp. 156–80; Worden, '"Wit in a Roundhead": the dilemma of Marchamont Nedham', in *Political Culture and Cultural Politics*, ed. Amussen and Kishlansky, pp. 301–37.

65   Charles Webster, 'Benjamin Worsley: engineering for universal reform from the Invisible College to the Navigation Act', in *Samuel Hartlib and Universal Reformation*, ed. Mark Greengrass, Michael Leslie, and Timothy Raylor (Cambridge, 1994), pp. 213–35; M.J. Braddick and Mark Greengrass, eds, 'The letters of Sir Cheney Culpeper (1641–1657)', *Camden Miscellany* 33, Camden 5th Series, 7 (1996), pp. 105–402, quotation at p. 317.

66   John Dury, *Considerations Concerning the Present Engagement* (London, 1650); cf. William Prynne, *The Time-Serving Proteus, and Ambidexter Divine* ([London], 1650). See also John M. Wallace, *Destiny His Choice* (Cambridge, 1968), pp. 43–68, which notes that many Presbyterians themselves took the oath.

67   [Sir John Birkenhead], *Paul's Church-Yard. Libri theologici, politici, historici, nundinis Paulinis (unà cum Templo) prostant venales* ([London, 1651]). Thomason acquired his copy of this pamphlet (London, British Library, Thomason Tracts E637 (15)) on 24 July 1651.

views.[68] The rising power of the Independents, however, especially after the imposition of the Engagement, led to the prospect of further intervention. Several important places did indeed change hands: for example, Cromwell's chaplain, John Owen, was appointed as Dean of Christ Church, and Jonathan Goddard, the physician to the Cromwellian army, became Warden of Merton, and later played a significant part in the activities of the Oxford experimentalists. The acceptance of *de facto* authority implied by the Engagement oath also allowed a number of Royalists to retain or advance their positions in Oxford. These included Ralph Bathurst, who participated in the Oxford experimental club and was one of the first witnesses to the recovery of Anne Greene.[69] Thomas Willis (1621–75), who assisted Petty in treating Anne Greene, had fought in the Royalist army during the civil war and initially played a role in resisting the visitors by allowing services according to the rites of the Church of England to take place in his rooms at Christ Church. Although Willis later moved into the city to practise as a physician, his continued malignancy does not seem to have bothered the Independents.[70] One of those who eventually owed his position to the Parliamentary visitors, who had deprived ten of the 17 fellows of his college (nine of whom did indeed leave Oxford) in 1648, was William Petty of Brasenose.[71] Petty's approach to the changing circumstances in the university in 1650 was straightforward. In August, he wrote to John Dury, looking forward to benefits that he might derive from the 'new evacuation of the University about the Engagement'.[72] By December, he had been appointed as Tomlins reader in anatomy, a post that required him to assist the Professor of Physic at an annual salary of £15.

Throughout the late 1640s and early 1650s, Petty seems to have regarded the practice of reform in science and medicine, and the promotion of practical and useful knowledge in general, as a route to advancement of his own career. In this respect, his interests appear more self-seeking than those of Samuel Hartlib and some other members of his circle. The difference may have been as much circumstantial as temperamental. Petty, who was the son of a Hampshire clothier, was young and ambitious, and had benefited from a period of education at the Jesuit college in Caen and from extensive foreign travel in the early 1640s that

68   Ian Roy and Dietrich Reinhart, 'Oxford and the civil wars', in *The History of the University of Oxford. Volume IV: Seventeenth-Century Oxford*, ed. Nicholas Tyacke (Oxford, 1997), pp. 687–731, esp. pp. 723–31.

69   Blair Worden, 'Cromwellian Oxford', in *Seventeenth-Century Oxford*, ed. Tyacke, pp. 733–72, esp. pp. 734–9.

70   Robert G. Frank, Jr., 'Thomas Willis and his circle: brain and mind in seventeenth-century medicine', in *The Languages of Psyche*, ed. G.S. Rousseau (Berkeley, 1990), pp. 107–46, esp. pp. 112–13; Kenneth Dewhurst, ed., *Willis's Oxford Casebook (1650–52)* (Oxford, 1981), pp. 5–21.

71   Roy and Reinhart, 'Oxford and the civil wars', p. 730.

72   James Marshall and Marie-Louise Osborn Collection, OSB MSS File 16809; cf. Webster, *Great Instauration*, pp. 154–5.

introduced him to many of the leading intellectual figures in Europe.[73] The characters of several of the older members of the Hartlib circle, by contrast, had been formed largely by their experience of exile and of the destructive European warfare of the 1620s and 1630s, which tempered their personal hopes even if it did not dampen their confidence in prospects for the renewal of society. The confidence in the working of providence that they sometimes displayed also seemed relatively alien to Petty. Once he had been introduced to the Hartlib circle, perhaps through the mathematician John Pell, however, Petty rapidly embraced the interests of its members in improvement through the advancement of learning and in institutional reform.[74] On 16 November 1647, Hartlib described Petty as 'not altogether a very dear *Worsley*, but a perfect Frenchman, and good linguist in other vulgar languages besides Latin and Greek, a most rare and exact anatomist, and excelling in all mathematical and mechanical learning; of a sweet natural disposition and moral comportment. As for solid judgment and industry altogether masculine'. Even at this stage, however, Hartlib noted the expense and ambition of Petty's projects.[75]

Among Petty's schemes from the late 1640s were plans for establishing new educational and medical institutions, and for the reform of Gresham College in London.[76] By July 1649, Hartlib was trying to assist Petty in using these proposals as a springboard to a position at Gresham College.[77] At the same time, Petty was completing his medical education at Oxford. On 25 June 1650, he was elected a candidate and admitted to the London College of Physicians, partly on the strength of the Oxford doctorate of medicine that he had recently obtained.[78] The background provided by Petty's search for patronage via his contacts with Hartlib and through him with Robert Boyle and his sister, Lady Ranelagh, is essential for understanding his response to the recovery of Anne Greene in December 1650.

In the winter of 1650–1, Petty was eager to capitalize on the opportunities that political change might provide to speed up his material and professional advancement. He was associated with a group of individuals who were broadly supportive of the new regime and eager to prevent it from degenerating into a revived form of clerical tyranny. At Oxford, he was already demonstrating his anatomical skill, his interest in experimental learning, and his dedication to the performance of his duties.[79] He was thus in an excellent position to benefit from helping to create the

---

73   For an outline of Petty's career, see E. Strauss, *Sir William Petty* (London, 1954).
74   Pell certainly provided Petty with an introduction to Thomas Hobbes in 1645 and also recommended him to Sir Charles Cavendish: see Noel Malcolm and Jacqueline Stedall, *John Pell (1611–1685) and his Correspondence with Sir Charles Cavendish* (Oxford, 2005), pp. 434, 441.
75   Michael Hunter, Antonio Clericuzio, and Lawrence M. Principe, eds, *The Correspondence of Robert Boyle* (6 vols, London, 2001), i, pp. 63–4.
76   William Petty, *The Advice of W.P. to Mr. Samuel Hartlib* (London, 1648); Webster, *Great Instauration*, pp. 548–51.
77   Hunter, Clericuzio, and Principe, *Correspondence of Boyle*, i, pp. 78–9.
78   London, Royal College of Physicians, MS. 2290, pp. 25–7.
79   Frank, *Harvey and the Oxford Physiologists*, pp. 101–3.

remarkable story of Anne Greene's recovery and pardon, when the chance came his way. Petty shaped the publicity about Anne Greene in ways that would profit him, not least by managing to counter more providentialist readings of her experiences with the history and verses printed in *Newes from the Dead*. That collaborative publication had the additional advantage of cementing Petty's place within a community of young Oxford natural philosophers, many of whom were either the direct beneficiaries of the effects of recent political change on the university or, like Bathurst, had resigned themselves to them.[80] Anne Greene did not subscribe to the Engagement, but several of her supporters did, and in doing so they committed themselves to a *de facto* form of politics that ruled out some of the most extravagant interpretations of her recovery. This need not have involved any abandonment of a commitment to justice, however imperative to Petty's personal hopes it might have been that his skill should succeed in preserving Greene's life as well as in recovering it. For example, it seems likely that his acquaintance with the commander of the Oxford garrison, Colonel Kelsey, proved as important in obtaining Anne Greene's pardon in 1650 as it had been in providing testimonials towards Petty's doctorate a year earlier.[81] What was nevertheless remarkable was that Petty, although stage-managing the presentation of Anne Greene's recovery in order to highlight his role as her saviour and to play down the politically, religiously, and socially disturbing elements of her case, seems to have prevented his name from appearing in public as the author of any statements about Anne Greene. The one possible exception to this was his implicit authorship of the testimony of Anne Greene's physicians that was attached to her petition for a pardon. That apart, Petty seemed content to let others appear to do the talking, provided that they stuck to his brief.

When Petty wrote to Hartlib on 16 December 1650 to give the first account of Anne Greene's survival, he asked him to 'Communicate these things to whome you thinke fitt', suggesting that Lady Ranelagh might be a potential recipient of the information. He also noted happily that 'my endeavours in this businesse haue bettered my reputation'.[82] Throughout the rest of his career, Petty seems to have regarded the recovery of Anne Greene as a decisive turning point in his own fortunes. Thus John Evelyn, who dined at Petty's house on 22 March 1675, thought it worth recording that '[he] was growne famous as for his Learning, so for his recovering a poore wench that had ben hanged for felonie'.[83] At the start of 1650, Petty had savings amounting to less than £30; by September 1652 he could call on £480 that he held in cash. In 1651, Petty became Vice-Principal of Brasenose, succeeded in obtaining a grant to buy instruments for his anatomical lectures, and was appointed to the professorship of music at Gresham College. His various

80   See footnote 19 above.
81   Robert G. Frank, Jr., 'Medicine', in *Seventeenth-Century Oxford*, ed. Tyacke, pp. 505–58, at p. 544; Plot, *Natural History of Oxfordshire*, p. 198.
82   See footnote 1 above.
83   E.S. de Beer, ed., *The Diary of John Evelyn* (6 vols, Oxford, 1955), iv, pp. 56–7.

positions there and at Oxford now gave him an annual income of £120.[84] This was a good beginning, but it paled into insignificance beside the rewards that Petty was able to heap up following his appointment to succeed Goddard as physician to the army in Ireland in September 1652. Contacts in Ireland, perhaps including members of Lady Ranelagh's network of acquaintances, as well as Petty's recently acquired fame may have helped to secure him this post. In April 1651, however, Petty had already been given permission to leave Oxford for two years from the following March.[85]

Despite the brevity of the period during which Petty held an active appointment in Oxford, his presence there played a crucial role in reinvigorating the local community of natural philosophers and physicians. In addition to the success of his anatomical lectures, particularly those delivered in 1651, Petty helped to create and sustain a group of experimentalists with an interest in mechanical and chemical philosophy. More importantly, given the development of natural philosophy at Oxford in the later 1650s and in the 1660s, Petty's own interests represented the bringing together of two contemporary bodies of work. These were the anatomical and physiological concerns of William Harvey and the physicians who had worked in Royalist Oxford before 1646, and the traditions of atomism and chemistry that Petty had encountered in the Parisian circle of Marin Mersenne and that excited a number of Hartlib's other correspondents.[86] When he first wrote to Hartlib about the resuscitation of Anne Greene, Petty coupled his account of her with one of the replication of Captain Bulmer's experiments with the inflation of bladders. The explanation for this apparently nonsensical juxtaposition might be haste or chance. But it is also possible to argue that Petty thought that both reports gave information about a common object of enquiry: the strength and capacity of the human respiratory system. The anatomy and physiology of breathing was one of the topics that fascinated Harvey's disciples, in particular Ralph Bathurst. Thomas Willis also later used Bulmer's experiment to suggest how vital spirits communicated from the brain by the nerves might cause the muscles to expand and contract, generating movement.[87]

Petty's record of the treatment that he and Willis employed to recover Anne Greene hinted at an awareness of many of the questions that predominated in subjects for research and experiment in the Oxonian natural philosophy of the following decade and a half. In lectures that he gave in the early 1660s, Willis

---

84 Strauss, *Sir William Petty*, p. 32; Marquis of Lansdowne, ed., *The Petty-Southwell Correspondence 1676–1687* (London, 1928), p. 222; Frank, 'Medicine', p. 545; John Ward, *The Lives of the Professors of Gresham College* (London, 1740), p. 218.

85 Montagu Burrows, ed., *The Register of the Visitors of the University of Oxford, from A.D. 1647 to A.D. 1658*, Camden Society N.S. 29 (London, 1881), p. 335.

86 For these bodies of work, see Frank, *Harvey and the Oxford Physiologists*; Antonio Clericuzio, *Elements, Principles and Corpuscles* (Dordrecht, 2000).

87 Kenneth Dewhurst, ed., *Thomas Willis's Oxford Lectures* (Oxford, 1980), p. 55; a full account of a similar experiment can be found in Thomas Birch, *The History of the Royal Society of London* (4 vols, London, 1756–7), i, p. 36.

argued that 'Our life, therefore, is very similar to that of a burning lamp, and a man lives as long as his blood is being burnt in his heart'. He went on to describe the role of the blood and of vital spirits in sleep, coma, and lethargy. The treatments that Petty and Willis used to recover Anne Greene were predominantly aimed at restoring the free flow of blood of good quality and the promotion and control of sensation. They employed the same kinds of recipes that Willis used in his normal practice. Although these did not include examples of the chemical remedies whose function Willis and Petty certainly discussed together around 1650, they were nevertheless responses to symptoms that could also be found in disorders that the physicians were used to treating and whose physiology they were attempting to elucidate by the application of ideas drawn from chemical medicine. They were thus similar to the suggestions that Willis later made for the combating of lethargy and other maladies that he likened to sleep. The observation that Petty made concerning Anne Greene's interrupted memory of the events at her execution was echoed in Willis's descriptions of the powers of recall of lethargic patients.[88]

The recovery of Anne Greene was therefore part of the development of a reformed understanding of physiology. Experimentation was important in the formation of this new interpretation of the body and the resuscitation of Anne Greene was also presented in that context. The reform of medicine and science did not take place without regard to personal circumstance, however, and for both the main protagonists the events of 14 December 1650 had unexpected consequences that changed their lives. This process of change drew both William Petty and Anne Greene into the public world of political and social debate, where Petty at least was committed to a position that supported contemporary *de facto* authority in both law and politics. In that arena, Petty functioned as a puppet-master, and, to some extent, Anne Greene became his puppet. The result was that an unusual, but by no means unique, event became, as Petty put it to Hartlib, 'a very miracle', or, in words that one would still like to think belonged to Anne Greene, a 'wonder of wonders'.

---

88   Dewhurst, *Willis's Oxford Lectures*, pp. 53, 60, 100–11; Dewhurst, *Willis's Oxford Casebook*, esp. pp. 23–40.

Chapter 8

Between Anatomy and Politics: John Finch and Italy, 1649–1671

Stefano Villani

In the chapel of Christ's College at Cambridge, one may visit the burial monument of John Finch and Thomas Baines. Two medallions with the sculpted portraits of two friends, their eyes peering at the observer, are posed on two tablets, on which runs a single, long Latin inscription celebrating the knot of friendship which in life and death linked the two for more than thirty years, permitting them to share 'interests, fortunes, counsels'.[1]

Finch and Baines met each other, in their twenties, in that college in the 1640s. Finch came to Christ's in 1648, having completed part of his studies at Oxford, and there he met Baines, who was introduced to him by Henry More, their common tutor. From that moment onwards, and for the rest of their lives, the two men became inseparable from one another.

John Finch and Thomas Baines

Born in 1626, Finch was about four years younger than Baines and came from one of the most illustrious families in England: his father, Heneage Finch, who died in 1631, had been Speaker of the House of Commons and both his uncle Thomas and, later, his cousin Heneage were earls of Winchilsea.[2] We know very little about the years that Finch and Baines spent together in Cambridge. What is sure is that, after their initial acquaintance, the two men embarked upon a deep and lasting friendship that made them virtually indissoluble in the minds of their contemporaries and

I would like to express my thanks to Sandra Cerrai, Sara Bonechi, Mario Caricchio, Maria Pia Donato, Giuseppina Petroccia, Adriano Prosperi, and Mario Rosa for their help.

1   Alan Bray, *The Friend* (Chicago, 2003). Just a few weeks before his death in 2001, I corresponded with Alan Bray and he very kindly sent to me the chapter from his forthcoming book dealing with the friendship of Finch and Baines.
2   See Arthur Collins, *Peerage of England*, ed. Sir Egerton Brydges (9 vols, London, 1812), iii, pp. 378–9.

of posterity. It was a friendship that Finch, in a poem written after the death of his friend, described as *Animorum Connubium* and that, as a matter of fact, resembled in every respect a marriage. From 1649, Baines, who came from a modest family, followed Finch like a shadow in all his travels and stays abroad, and the two figures seemed as one.

The two friends, after having completed their MA degrees in 1649 – the fatal year in which Charles I was beheaded – decided to leave their country, now in the hands of people who seemed to them to be the enemies of friendship, and set off for Italy.[3]

John Finch at Padua

> I left England in that unhappy time when honesty was reputed a crime, religion superstition, loyalty treason; when subjects were governors, servants masters, and no gentleman assured of any thing he possessed.... This posture of affairs so changed the face of home, that to live there appeared worse than banishment; which caused most of our youth (especially such whose families had adhered to the late king) to travel; amongst others myself.[4]

These were the reasons that, Sir John Reresby declared, with some emphasis, had induced him in 1654 to abandon England and to travel on the continent. And these were certainly the reasons that also persuaded Finch – who came from a royalist family and had perhaps served in the army of Charles I – to leave his country and to go to Padua to study medicine.[5]

In autumn 1651 Finch, with his already inseparable friend Baines, set off for a new life on the continent. The two spent the winter of 1651 in Paris and in April 1652 reached Geneva, where they stayed for some months.[6] Then they started their journey to Padua, where they arrived in October of that year.[7]

---

3   Thomas Archibald Malloch, *Finch and Baines, A Seventeenth-Century Friendship* (Cambridge, 1917). For the supposed enmity of Cromwell's soldiers to friendship see G. Cozzi, *Venezia barocca. Conflitti di uomini e idee nella crisi del Seicento veneziano* (Venice, 1995), p. 405.

4   Albert Ivatt, ed., *The Memoirs and Travels of Sir John Reresby* (London, 1904), p. 1.

5   For the possibility that Finch participated in the civil war see Malloch, *Finch and Baines*, pp. 2–3.

6   See the letters by John Finch to Anne Conway, Paris 10/20 November 1651, Paris 1/11 December 1651, Geneva 27 April/7 May 1652, Geneva 1/10 August 1652, in Marjorie Hope Nicolson, ed., *Conway Letters* (New York, 1930), pp. 55, 58–61, 62–4, 64–7.

7   Horatio F. Brown, 'Inglesi e scozzesi all'Università di Padova 1618–1775', in *Contributo del R. Istituto Veneto di scienze, lettere ed arti alla Celebrazione del VII Centenario della Università di Padova* (Venice, 1921), pp. 140–213. See letters by John Finch to Anne Conway, Venice 10/20 February 1653, Venice 9 N. S. April 1653,

The University of Padua was then organized into the two student corporations of the *Universitas Iuristarum*, for those who studied law, and of the *Universitas Artistarum*, for those who studied philosophy, medicine and arts. Both of these universities were structured by 'Nations' which designated representatives who formed the university council, headed by a syndic and pro-rector, who was elected annually at the beginning of August. Because the English nation was not present as an organized body in the *Universitas Artistarum*, Finch and Baines, who intended to study medicine (as indeed did almost all the Englishmen who studied at Padua), instead matriculated amongst the jurists.[8] Their professor of anatomy was Antonio Molinetti, author of important studies on the sense organs, who had succeeded Johann Wesling in the chair after his death.[9] On 1 August 1656 John Finch was nominated pro-rector and syndic of the jurists and, at the end of his year in government, in autumn 1657, he graduated. With him, naturally, graduated also his inseparable friend, Baines.[10]

Eight years had already passed since the two friends left their own country. We do not know if Finch wanted to return to England, but almost certainly he preferred not to come back to his country when Cromwell was still in power and at the height of his influence on both the English and international scenes. Possibly, in the months after they had taken their degrees, he and Baines travelled in Italy.[11] In any case, in spring 1659, the two relocated to Tuscany.

The first period of John Finch as lecturer at the University of Pisa

In 1659 the Grand Duchy of Tuscany was certainly the place in Italy where the finest resources to pursue their researches were offered to scholars of the anatomical and biological sciences. Moreover, it afforded the best opportunities for scholarly discussion and for interrogating the results obtained by other researchers.

Padua 6 November N. S. 1653, Padua 9/19 November 1653, Padua 30 November/10 December 1653, in Nicolson, ed., *Conway Letters*, pp. 73–4, 77–9, 86–90.

8   The matriculation roll of Englishmen has been published by Gian Luigi Andrich, *De Natione Anglica et Scota Iuristarum Universitatis Patavinae ab a.* MCCXII *p. ch. n. usque ad a.* MDCCXXXVIII (Padua, 1892). For the English students at Padua see Lucia Rossetti, 'Membri del "Royal College of Physicians" di Londra laureati nell'Università di Padova', *Atti e Memorie della Accademia Patavina di Scienze, Lettere ed Arti*, 75 (1962–3), 175–201; for the Tudor years see Jonathan Woolfson, *Padua and the Tudors* (Cambridge, 1998), p. 28.

9   On Molinetti see Andrea Bosatra, 'L'organo dell'udito negli studi di Antonio Molinetti anatomico padovano del '600', *Minerva otorinolaringologica*, 4 (1954), 99–102.

10   In the same year (1656) Baines was elected counsellor for the English nation. See Lucia Rossetti, ed., *Gli stemmi dello studio di Padova* (Trieste 1983), numbers 328, 2339, 2795, 2810–2810bis. For Baines see numbers 1095, 2812.

11   See London, British Library, MS. Add. 23, 214, fols 32, 38.

Both Ferdinand II, Grand Duke of Tuscany from 1620, and his brother Prince Leopold, a sort of 'minister of culture' of the grand dukedom, showed great personal interest in the new Galilean science. After Galileo's condemnation they tried to find a point of equilibrium between the will to further scientific research – which bestowed enormous prestige upon the Medici dynasty and which afforded a real intellectual pleasure both to the Grand Duke and, especially, to his brother Leopold – and the pressing necessity to avoid incurring any further ecclesiastical censure that would inevitably have brought about an end to these kind of researches. The strategy that had been adopted was to promote and finance biological and meteorological studies especially, letting the scholars involved in such researches clearly understand that it was necessary to avoid drawing any consequences of a general order about the structure of the universe or of the physical world. Thanks to Leopold's wishes, from 1657 research activity structured itself into an academy that came to be known by the name *Cimento*. In order to pursue the strategy that we have described, intellectuals with different philosophical and methodological orientations were called to be its members: there was a conservative group which included Carlo Rinaldini and, especially, the acknowledged Aristotelian Alessandro Marsili; there was the group of moderate Galileans which included Vincenzo Viviani, Francesco Redi and Lorenzo Magalotti; and, eventually, a group of innovators which included Giovanni Alfonso Borelli and Antonio Oliva.[12]

Finch was not the only British intellectual to find an appointment in Tuscany in these years. One year before his arrival in Pisa, the Scotsman Thomas Forbes, who had been at the University of Padua in the same years as Finch, was appointed Extraordinary Professor of Philosophy and then, after one year, took the chair of Theoretical Medicine, a chair that he kept for three academic years until 1662, the year in which he decided to return to his own country.[13] The Catholic Hellenist John Price lived in Florence between 1651 and 1658, being maintained by the Grand Duke and by Prince Leopold.[14] The Catholic priest Peter Fitton, who was for

12   On the Academy of the Cimento see W.E. Knowles Middleton, *The Experimenters. A Study of the Accademia del Cimento* (Baltimore, 1971); Paolo Galluzzi, 'L'accademia del Cimento: "Gusti" del Principe, filosofia e ideologia dell'esperimento', *Quaderni Storici*, 16 (1981), 788–844; Ugo Baldini, 'Un libertino accademico del Cimento Antonio Oliva', *Supplemento agli Annali dell'Istituto e Museo di Storia della Scienza*, 1 (1977), 33–5; Galluzzi, ed., *Scienziati a Corte. L'arte della sperimentazione nell' Accademia Galileiana del Cimento (1657–1667)* (Livorno, 2001).

13   Forbes matriculated in February 1650 and in August of that year he was elected counsellor for the Scotch nation. On John Forbes see Alistair Tayler and Henrietta Tayler, *The House of Forbes* (Aberdeen, 1937), pp. 300, 472. See *Storia dell' Università di Pisa* (Pisa, 2000), vol. I*, p. 310; see Brown, 'Inglesi e scozzesi all'Università di Padova', number 433c, p. 157; Andrich, *De Natione Anglica et Scota*, pp. 112, 176.

14   Edward Chaney, *The Grand Tour and the Great Rebellion. Richard Lassels and 'The Voyage of Italy' in the Seventeenth Century* (Geneva, 1985), pp. 263, 274–5, 290; Giovanni Targioni Tozzetti, *Notizie degli aggrandimenti delle scienze fisiche accaduti in Toscana nel corso di anni LX del sec. XVII* (3 vols, Florence, 1780), i, p. 489; see

a long time in Italy, took care of the Medicean collection of medals until his death in October 1656.[15]

So there is some truth to Redi's description of the court of Florence as 'a court to which from all the parts of the world' were welcomed 'great men, who with their pilgrimages' were 'searching and bringing goods of virtue' ('*merci di virtude*').[16]

Finch was appointed lecturer in anatomy at the University of Pisa and at Florence at the beginning of May 1659. For the pleasure of Prince Leopold, Finch and Baines performed a first anatomical demonstration which was received with general admiration.[17]

In the long-lasting conflict between the moderate group of the majority of the academicians of Cimento and the more radical Borelli, Finch lined up without question alongside the former. They were closer to him from both a personal and from a scientific point of view. We know for example that in a discussion with Oliva regarding the vacuum, Finch and Baines denied its existence strongly.[18] In the space of a few months, the initial curiosity that Borelli had shown towards the two English anatomists (the 'notomisti inglesi') transformed rapidly and progressively into an open and explicit hostility, of which we can find many traces in his numerous letters to Malpighi from this period.[19]

In April 1660, with the end of the academic year approaching, Finch asked for and obtained permission to come to England and to stay there for a while, until the end of the vacation. The English political situation had been completely transformed in just a few months: Cromwell died in September 1658 and, in a tumultuous run of events, preparations were now being made for Charles II's restoration.[20]

also Laura Giovannini, ed., *Carteggio d'artisti dell'Archivio di Stato di Firenze x Lettere di Ottavio Falconieri a Leopoldo de' Medici* (Florence, 1984), pp. 21, 166–7. There are many letters written by Price to Redi in the Biblioteca Laurenziana, Florence, MSS Redi 222, fols 91–129, and from Price to Prince Leopold in the Biblioteca Nazionale Centrale, Florence (hereafter BNCF), MS. Lettere Aut. Palat. 75.

15   On Fitton, properly Biddulph, see Chaney, *The Grand Tour*, p. 261.

16   Francesco Redi, *Esperienze intorno a diverse cose naturali...*, in Redi, *Opere* (5 vols, Venice, 1712), ii, pp. 2–3.

17   *Storia dell'Università di Pisa*, vol. I**, pp. 519, 559; Targioni Tozzetti, *Notizie degli aggrandimenti*, ii, p. 599.

18   Borelli to Malpighi, Pisa 7 November 1659, printed in Howard B. Adelmann, ed., *The Correspondence of Marcello Malpighi* (Ithaca, 1975) (hereafter, *Malpighi Correspondence*), p. 22; see also Baldini, 'Un libertino accademico del Cimento Antonio Oliva', p. 35.

19   *Malpighi Correspondence, passim*. For the scientific activity of Finch in this period see BNCF, MS. Baldovinetti 258 III.19 and *Report on Finch Papers*, ii, pp. 500–1 (Targioni Tozzetti, *Notizie degli aggrandimenti*, i, p. 269).

20   BNCF, MS. Gal. 276, fols 27ʳ–28ᵛ; Finch to Leopold. See Anna Maria Crinò, 'Inediti su alcuni contatti Tosco-Britannici nel Seicento', *English Miscellany*, 12 (1961), 147–209.

And so the two friends left for London, reaching the city a few weeks after the arrival of Charles Stuart.[21]

An important English intermezzo (1660–2)

As is well known, the king did not forget the people who had remained loyal during the difficult years of his exile, and, among those who had proof of the affection and gratitude of the sovereign, there were many members of Finch's family. In June 1660 John's elder brother Heneage Finch was appointed solicitor-general and made a baronet and his cousin, also a Heneage Finch, already the governor of Dover castle, was created a baron.

Finch and Baines evidently appreciated the new political climate of their country and, contrary to what they had initially envisioned, stayed on in England till the end of 1662, well after the date of December 1660, when they had originally expected to return to Italy.

The year 1661 was really an *annus mirabilis* for the two Englishmen: on 26 February 1661 both were elected extraordinary members of the College of Physicians; in March, Baines was appointed Professor of Music at Gresham College; and finally, in June, Finch was knighted. In a couple of weeks both he and Baines were awarded the degree of doctor of physic by the University of Cambridge.

During these two and a half years spent in England, Finch wrote with some regularity to Prince Leopold, each time offering apologies and excuses for the impossibility of his returning to Florence because of his duties and the important affairs of his family ('affari importanti di casa') which kept him in his homeland. Apart from excuses and compliments, his letters generally dealt with the English political situation, giving notice of the successes of Charles II's domestic and foreign policy.[22] The tone of the letters makes it clear that Finch wanted to return to his chair of anatomy in Tuscany, but nevertheless what emerges is a progressive dimming of his general medical-naturalistic interests for, significantly, in the majority of his letters there is not any trace of discussion of scientific problems. In

21   See Finch to ?, in Archivio di Stato, Florence (hereafter ASF); MS. Misc. Medicea 62/2, fols 543–4; see letter by Oldenburg to Boyle, October 1661, in *The Correspondence of Henry Oldenburg*, edited and translated by A. Rupert Hall and Marie Boas Hall (13 vols, Madison and Milwaukee, London, Philadelphia, 1965–1986) (hereafter *Oldenburg Correspondence*), i, pp. 440–2; Michael Hunter, Antonio Clericuzio, and Lawrence M. Principe, eds, *The Correspondence of Robert Boyle* (6 vols, London, 2001), i, p. 466.

22   In the *fondo galileiano* of the BNCF are kept these letters by Finch to Leopold: 12/22 October 1660 (MS. Gal. 281, number 148, fols 181^r–183^r); 30 November 1660 (*ibid.*, number 26, fols 32^r–33^r); 12/22 April 1661 (MS. Gal. 280, number 39, fols 77^r–78^r). All of them have been transcribed thanks to the Progetto Galileo and it is possible to access the digitized version of the letters and their transcripts at this web address: <http://www.bnseefirenze.sbn.it/cgi-galileo/makeQuery.cgi>.

this respect the first letter (dated 17 August 1660), in which Finch recounts at length both a meeting he had in Rotterdam with the anatomist Lodewijk Bils and an encounter with a blind man of Maastricht allegedly capable of distinguishing colours by touch, is an exception.[23]

On 28 November 1660 the little group of philosophers and scientists who for a long time met at Gresham College to discuss issues in experimental philosophy and natural science decided to create a more organized structure, and the following week they produced an ample petition to the king to obtain an official sanction that was signed also by John Finch.[24] On 18 January 1661 Finch hastened to let Prince Leopold know that in London – thanks to a 'royal command' – an experimental Academy ('per far delle esperienze') had been born, similar to the Florentine Accademia del Cimento, and that he, knowing the attitude ('il genio') of the prince, had proposed to some 'virtuosi' the idea of starting a correspondence with Tuscany.[25] Having received from Leopold some encouragement to start this correspondence, Finch, in June of that year, advised that the experimental Academy (the future Royal Society) instructed him to thank the prince formally for his goodwill.[26]

The absence of its lecturer in anatomy, however, was starting to create problems for the University of Pisa, where – as noted with malevolent satisfaction by Borelli – the students were starting to complain about Finch's absence ('per l'assenza dello Sfinchio'). These complaints were provoked by the fact that Tilman Trutwin, the Flemish anatomist who since the time of Aubry (Finch's predecessor as professor of anatomy) had collaborated with a reputedly extraordinary dexterity on the dissections of the professors of anatomy, was now able only to cut but not to

---

23 BNCF, MS. Gal. 280, number 40, fols 79^r–82^r (a manuscript copy is in the Istituzione 'Biblioteca Città di Arezzo', MS. 188, fol. 124). See Angelo Fabroni, *Lettere inedite di uomini illustri* (2 vols, Florence, 1773–5), i, pp. 261–5; Targioni Tozzetti, *Notizie degli aggrandimenti*, i, pp. 272–3. Boyle spoke of the blind in *Experiments and Considerations Touching Colours* (London, 1664): see Michael Hunter and Edward B. Davis, eds, *The Works of Robert Boyle* (14 vols, London, 1999–2000), iv, pp. 40–5; see also, Hunter, Clericuzio and Principe, *Correspondence of Robert Boyle*, ii, pp. 373, 552.

24 Thomas Birch, *The History of the Royal Society of London for improving of Natural Knowledge from its first rise* (4 vols, reprinted New York, 1968), i, pp. 3–4.

25 Finch to Leopold, in BNCF, MS. Gal. 276, number 2, fols 2^r–3^r.

26 Finch to Leopold, 9 June 1661, in BNCF, MS. Gal. 276, number 67, fol. 130^{r-v}. Finch, with some courtly flattery, said that the Academy was born to make some experiments ('per far delle esperienze') following the model of the Florentine one. See also an undated answer by Leopold (*ibid.*, fol. 217). See W.E. Knowles Middleton, 'Some Italian visitors to the early Royal Society', *Notes and Records of the Royal Historical Society of London*, 33 (1979), 157–73, at p. 157; Knowles Middleton, *The Experimenters*, p. 288.

speak.[27] Yet, for the second consecutive academic year, the chair remained deserted and it was only on 25 October 1662 that Finch and Baines left England to come back to Italy.[28]

For the second time in Italy: Florence (1663–4) and Padua (1664–5)

As soon as Finch arrived in Pisa in January 1663, he was immediately engaged in an anatomical demonstration,[29] and over the following months he continued apace with his academic activity. In autumn 1663 Finch and Baines went to Naples. Their Neapolitan stay was very short, but useful: there they had very detailed news ('particolarissima notitia') of Tommaso Cornelio – 'Cartesian and a great defender of new things' ('cartesiano et molto difensore delle cose nuove') – and were able to purchase part of Severino's library. In Rome, on their way back to Tuscany, they met Michelangelo Ricci, a sort of ambassador of the Medici court for scientific affairs in the Roman curia.[30]

27 Borelli to Malpighi, 13 January 1662, in *Malpighi Correspondence*, p. 112 (see also the letter of 29 December 1661, at p. 93). See ASF, MS. Misc. Med 87/6, fol. 6ʳ. In September 1661 Finch apparently wanted to come back to Pisa and both he and Baines asked for and obtained permission from the College of Physicians to leave England, but then they postponed their departure; see John Ward, *The Lives of the Professors of Gresham College* (London, 1740), p. 229.

28 *Calendar of State Papers, Domestic Series of the Reign of Charles II, 1661–2* (London, 1861), pp. 463, 513. See letter by Thomas Bankes to Viviani, 6 December 1662, in BNCF, MS. Gal. 162, fol. 34.

29 See Bruto Annibale Molara to Viviani, Pisa 22 January 1662, in BNCF, MS. Gal. 161, fol. 352ʳ; cf. ASF, MS. Misc. Med. 87/6. For some of Borelli's malevolent comments see his letters to Malpighi of 2 February 1663, and of 24 January 1663, in *Malpighi Correspondence*, pp. 144, 146. Both Finch and Baines were called to be members of the Academy of the *apatisti*, as can be seen from BNCF, MS. Marucelliano A. 36, fol. 64ᵛ. This dates the inscription of Thomas Baines ('D. Tommaso Fana inglese') to the year 1661 and that of John Finch ('cav. Gio. Finchio') to the year 1662: see Alessandro Lazzeri, *Intellettuali e consenso nella Toscana del 600: l'accademia degli apatisti* (Milan, 1983), pp. 93–4 (but the two Englishmen were surely called to be members of the Academy in 1663). See also *Calendar of State Papers, Domestic Series of the Reign of Charles II, 1663–4* (London, 1862), p. 226.

30 Leopold to Ricci, 16 October 1663, in BNCF, MS. Gal. 282, number 60, fol. 78ʳ⁻ᵛ. For this letter see also Fabroni, *Lettere inedite di uomini illustri*, p. 533 and Targioni Tozzetti, *Notizie degli aggrandimenti*, i, p. 274; Ricci to Leopold, 12 November 1663 and 29 November 1663, in BNCF, MS. Gal. 276, fols 223ʳ (number 139); 229ʳ (number 143); Finch to Leopold, 10 Dec. 1663, BNCF, MS. Gal. 276, fols 230ʳ–231ʳ (transcript in *Lettere di Uomini Illustri* (Florence, 1773), pp. 268–70 and see also Malloch, *Finch and Baines*, p. 42); Ricci to Leopold, Rome 10 December 1663, BNCF, MS. Gal. 276, number 145, fol. 232ʳ. Regarding the purchase by Finch of part of Marco Aurelio Severino's library, see Max H. Fisch, 'The Academy of the Investigators', in E.A. Underwood, ed., *Science, Medicine and History. Essays on the Evolu-*

With the beginning of the new academic year, in December 1663, Finch started again his work as an anatomist in Pisa and the following months were passed making anatomical demonstrations on animals and conducting experiments in the presence of the prince.[31] At the beginning of the holidays, in May 1664, Finch and Baines took their leave of Leopold, with the intention of returning to England. But before setting off for their native land, the two wanted to stop at Padua, probably to see the novelties undertaken in that university in the previous years; and, perhaps, under direction from Leopold, to see which among the professors of Padua could be recruited by the University of Pisa. The two friends stayed in Padua for almost one year, at least until the middle of April 1665, and Finch was afforded the opportunity to improve his experience of dissecting human bodies, both adults and children, since, unlike in Pisa, there were more than enough of these provided ('provisti soverchiamente').[32] From Padua, Finch wrote with a certain regularity to Prince Leopold, recommending as a possible professor at Pisa his onetime teacher Molinetti as well as a young Greek student named Alessandro Maurocordato.[33]

At the beginning of April, Finch and Baines moved to Venice, with the intention of setting off from there to England in a short time. But, presumably while the two friends were preparing for the journey, Finch received the appointment as English resident to the Grand Duke of Tuscany, Ferdinand II.[34]

And so the two friends came back to Tuscany, this time not as anatomists but as diplomatic representatives of the English monarchy. Finch made his official entry into Florence on 6 July 1665 and Borelli let Malpighi know that the two English *signori* had become residents of the King of England along with the most

tion of Scientific Thought and Medical Practice Written in Honour of Charles Singer (2 vols, Oxford, 1953), i, pp. 521–63. On the role of Ricci at Rome see P. Galluzzi, 'Nel "teatro" dell'Accademia', in Galluzzi, *Scienziati a Corte*, pp. 12–25, at p. 14.

31   See Targioni Tozzetti, *Notizie degli aggrandimenti*, i, p. 274. See letters by Borelli to Malpighi of 21 March 1664 and of 11 April 1664 in *Malpighi Correspondence*, pp. 204, 208; see also *Report on Finch Papers*, ii, pp. 500–1.

32   Padua 14 November 1664, BNCF, MS. Gal. 277, number 30, fol. 39^{r-v}.

33   Finch stayed at Padua from July 1664 to February 1665; see his letters in BNCF, MS. Gal. 277, fol. 51^{r-v} (Padua, 16 July 1664); fol. 23 (Padua 6 February 1665); number 67, fol. 99^{r-v} (Padua 14 November 1664); number 30, fol. 39^{r-v} (Padua 12 March 1665); MS. Gal. 281, number 55, fols 66^{r}–67^{r} (a seventeenth-century copy of this letter is in Istituzione 'Biblioteca Città di Arezzo', MS. 188, fols 128^{r}–129^{v}). BNCF, MS. Gal. 282, number 74, fol. 91^{r-v} (Leopold to Finch, 21 March 1664). See also Targioni Tozzetti, *Notizie degli aggrandimenti*, i, pp. 274–5.

34   Finch received the news of his appointment on 15 May: see Finch to Arlington, 15 May 1665, The National Archives (PRO), London, MS. SP 99/46, fol. 47 (see fols 50 and 52) and Finch to Leopold, 16 May 1665, BNCF, MS. Gal. 281, number 59, fols 71^{r}–72^{r}; *Calendar of State Papers, Domestic Series of the Reign of Charles II, 1664–5* (London, 1863), p. 286; Knowles Middleton, *The Experimenters*, p. 287. For the diplomatic instructions given to Finch, see The National Archives, London, MSS SP 98/5 (12 April 1665); SP 104/174B, pp. 61–4. For his diplomatic correspondence, see MS. SP 98/5–13.

superb pomp and solemnity ('con una pompa, e fasto superbissimo'). But he
wanted to inform him as well that neither he nor his friends went to visit Finch or
to watch the spectacle of his entry.[35] In the two previous years the concealed hostility that, from the beginning, Borelli had felt towards the two Englishmen, had
been transformed into an irreparable and open rupture. The Englishmen's Tuscan
stay of 1663–4 was in fact studded with continuous polemics and quarrels with
Borelli and his school. In spring 1663 the two Englishmen disputed with Lorenzo
Bellini about the existence of salivary ducts.[36] In December 1663 they debated with
Carlo Fracassati about the acid juice or ferment of the stomach that – according to
Finch, erroneously – was a 'residue of food' ('reliquia dei cibi precedenti').[37] In the
following months they quarrelled with Antonio Oliva about the origin of the idea
of colouring with a red pigment the rock salt of Volterra to distinguish it from
common salt, as a measure that might put an end to the active contraband trade in
this commodity that had always been practised.[38] Also in this period there was an
animated discussion that saw a neat and sharp break between Aristotelians and
Atomists, in which Finch in fact took sides with the traditional party.[39] In January
1664 the controversies developed into a veritable war when, faced with Malpighi's
discoveries about the structures of the optical nerves of swordfish, at first Finch
and Baines denied the validity of Malpighi's findings and then affirmed that they
were already well known.[40] Borelli, who evidently wanted to settle accounts with
the English, addressed an ample memoir to the Grand Duke Ferdinand in which he
ascribed these discoveries to Malpighi and commented with irony on the attitude of
people who wanted to deprive 'the inventors of new things' of their merit while
offering as proof nothing more than 'a single word incidentally uttered as an enigma' ('una sola parola incidentalmente detta modo di enigma').[41]

35   See letter from Borelli to Malpighi, 10 July 1665, printed in *Malpighi Correspon-
      dence*, p. 266. Finch's successor to the chair of anatomy was called Carlo Fracassati,
      who announced to Malpighi that he got the place of 'sig. Finchio che hora qui sta in
      posto di Cavallerizzo ed è residente del re d'Inghilterra': Fracassati to Malpighi, 15
      August 1665, in *Malpighi Correspondence*, p. 278. See Finch to Leopold, Padua 6
      February 1665, in BNCF, MS. Gal. 277, number 67, fol. 99^{r-v}.
36   See letters from Borelli to Malpighi, 22 March 1663, 15 February 1663, 30 March
      1663, in *Malpighi Correspondence*, pp. 148, 153, 156. See Howard B. Adelmann,
      Marcello Malpighi and the Evolution of Embryology (5 vols, Ithaca, 1966), i, p. 216.
37   Carlo Fracassati to Malpighi, 22 January 1664, in *Malpighi Correspondence*, p. 195.
38   For Ferdinand II's decree of November 1664, see Angelo Fabroni, *Historiae
      Academiae Pisanae* (3 vols, Pisa, 1791–5; reprinted Bologna, 1971), iii, pp. 614–15;
      Baldini, 'Un libertino accademico del Cimento Antonio Oliva', pp. 33, 34, 35;
      Vincenzo Antinori, *Scritti editi e inediti* (Florence, 1868), p. 195.
39   Galluzzi, 'L'accademia del Cimento', pp. 808, 819–23. On Marsili and Rinaldini see
      Galluzzi, 'Nel "teatro" dell'Accademia', pp. 22–3.
40   Carlo Fracassati to Malpighi, 22 January 1664, in *Malpighi Correspondence*, p. 195
      (cf. p. 133); Baldini, 'Un libertino accademico del Cimento Antonio Oliva', pp. 33–5;
      Fabroni, *Historiae Academiae Pisanae*, iii, pp. 466–7 .
41   *Malpighi Correspondence*, pp. 215–16, 217; see Adelmann, *Embryology*, i, p. 233;

Significantly the Grand Duke, after having read the memoir, ordered that an end be put to this controversy as soon as possible for several political reasons ('per diverse ragioni politiche') and, first of all, 'not to disgust the queen and the king of England, to whom this subject [i.e. Finch] has been appointed physician and knight' ('per non dar disgusto alla regina d'Inghilterra, et al re dei quali questo soggetto è dichiarato medico, e cavaliere').[42] One year later, as we have seen, the 'medico e cavaliere' Finch was also appointed resident. And of course Borelli's memoir was published only in 1698 – when all the protagonists of the conflict were already dead.[43]

John Finch as English resident in Tuscany (1665–71)

Contrary to the Grand Duke's expectations, and considering the extent of their acquaintance, Finch always had a very pugnacious attitude towards the Tuscan authorities, and the years in which he was resident in Tuscany (staying usually in Florence and in the first months of the year, in Livorno) were characterized by frequent and harsh conflicts. Between 1665 and 1671 about forty memorials were given to the grand-ducal authorities in Italian complaining about more or less serious wrongs experienced by the rich and numerous English community of Livorno.

One of the questions that for a long time poisoned the relationship between the English and Tuscans in those years was the attempt made by the British Factory of Livorno to obtain permission to celebrate Protestant religious services for its members. Finch tried in every way formally to obtain freedom of worship for the English of Livorno and initiated a sharp diplomatic battle, the only result being the issuing of humiliating exclusion orders for the Protestant preachers who went to Livorno in September 1666, December 1668, and January 1671.[44]

Luigi Guerrini, 'Medicina e scienze naturali nell'attività dell'Accademia del Cimento', in Galluzzi, *Scienziati a Corte*, pp. 48–51; Baldini, 'Un libertino accademico del Cimento Antonio Oliva', p. 34. Finch obviously had these polemics in mind when he spoke of the *Cerebri anatomie nervorumque descriptio et usus* by Thomas Willis in a letter of 26 December 1664: BNCF, MS. Gal. 277, fol. 70^{r-v}.

42 Borelli to Malpighi, 10 January 1664, in *Malpighi Correspondence*, p. 193. Later, when Maurocordato attacked Malpighi, Oliva thought that he acted on behalf of the two Englishmen.

43 The memoir was published with the posthumous works of Malpighi edited by Pierre Regis in 1698.

44 For the relationship between Finch and the Medicean authorities see ASF, MSS Mediceo del Principato 4244, 1828; F.J. Routledge, ed., *Calendar of the Clarendon State Papers* (5 vols, Oxford, 1869–1963), v, *passim*. For the attempt of the British Factory of Livorno to be allowed a Protestant preacher, see Stefano Villani, '"Cum scandalo catholicorum...". La presenza a Livorno di predicatori protestanti inglesi tra il 1644 e il 1670', *Nuovi Studi Livornesi*, 7 (1999), 9–58.

Both formal and personal relationships between Finch and the officials of the Tuscan court became more and more tense and one may suppose that it was a genuine relief for Finch to be recalled from his appointment in 1671 to undertake the more prestigious role of ambassador to Constantinople. Finch stayed in Turkey for almost ten years. In September 1681 his beloved companion Baines died and, a few months later, Finch came back to England where he died in November 1682.[45]

If relationships between Finch and the authorities in the years in which he was resident in Tuscany were characterized by tensions and disagreements, relationships between Finch and his former colleagues at the University of Pisa were almost non-existent.

In the history of the Royal Society that he published in 1667, Thomas Sprat wrote that Tuscany had the 'excellent priviledge' of having one of the Society's Fellows as resident for the king of England, whose presence allowed a continuous and valuable intellectual exchange with the 'most Noble wits' of Italy, and chiefly with Prince Leopold, 'the Patron of all Inquisitive Philosophers of Florence'.[46] Sprat here clearly speaks of Finch who when he was lecturer of anatomy in Pisa, had been appointed Fellow of the Royal Society.[47] But, contrary to what Sprat might lead one to believe, during the years in which Finch had a diplomatic function, he did not do very much himself to promote Anglo-Italian cultural exchanges. That he no longer wanted to deal with either anatomy or arts ('[né] di notomia né di lettere') because he was completely concerned with affairs of state ('negozi di stato') was immediately clear to Borelli who gave news of Finch and Baines to Malpighi on 14 August 1665.[48] That Finch did not want to become engaged substantially with scientific matters was however very less clear to the Royal Society. One of the major aims of the Society was to build up a network of international collaboration, especially for the circulation of scientific information, and its members intended to rely on Finch to establish a productive link with the Academy of Prince Leopold, which was considered by those in England as being more structured than it actually was.

Already on 7 December 1665 therefore, the indefatigable secretary of the Royal Society, Henry Oldenburg, had written to John Finch asking that he be informed about everything that might go on at the philosophical theatre in Florence

45   See G.F. Abbott, *Under the Turk in Constantinople. A Record of John Finch's Embassy 1674–1681* (London, 1920).

46   Thomas Sprat, *The History of the Royal Society of London for the Improving of Natural Knowledge* (London, 1667), p. 126; Knowles Middleton, *The Experimenters*, p. 290.

47   Finch was elected FRS on 20 May 1663: see Birch, *History*, i, pp. 239–40; Knowles Middleton, *The Experimenters*, p. 291; Michael Hunter, *The Royal Society and its Fellows 1660–1670. The Morphology of an early Scientific Institution* (2nd edn, Oxford, 1994), pp. 102, 103, 116, 249 n. 8, 261 n. 1, 262 nn. 5, 13, 265 n. 12, 269 n. 27.

48   Borelli to Malpighi, 14 August 1665, in *Malpighi Correspondence*, p. 276.

and in other Italian academies.[49] Finch did not answer and so, on 10 April 1666, Oldenburg wrote another letter to him urging him again to keep the Royal Society informed about everything that from time to time was being done by the 'Excellent Virtuosi of Italy'.[50] The months passed without any reply from Finch.

This situation was starting to become embarrassing and irritating, not least because in the meantime the Royal Society had promoted – with clear propagandistic and celebrative intentions – the publication of its history by Sprat, and it would now be necessary to present a copy of it to Prince Leopold. Thus on 26 November 1667 Oldenburg wrote for the third time to Finch. Enclosed with the letter were a copy of the *History of the Royal Society* for presentation to Prince Leopold and a long covering letter addressed to him.[51]

Only on 14 July 1668 did Finch finally respond to the letter sent to him more than seven months before (and that he claimed that he had just received). He said that he had already let Leopold, now a cardinal, have a copy of the book through Dr Baines.[52]

It has been suggested that one of the reasons that could explain the silence of Finch in response to the many questions posed to him by Oldenburg about the Academy of Cimento, could have been his embarrassment at having to explain that the Academy had already ceased its activity a few years before.[53] But it is much more probable that his silence was determined instead by the reasons that – with typical malevolence, but not falsehood – Borelli had pointed out when Finch was appointed to the office of resident: that 'negozi di Stato' were the only things that were now of interest to him.

Although it is true that in 1668 the Academy had already ceased to meet, as a matter of fact it is also true that, on the Tuscan side, in those years there was a very strong desire to construct cultural and scientific relationships with England. The growing economic, political and cultural importance of England was making Italian scholars increasingly more sensible of the impact of their activities in England, which had largely been ignored previously.[54] In the same year that Sprat's *History of the Royal Society of London* was published, there appeared in Florence the *Saggi di naturali esperienze* in which a decade of activity of the Academy of

49 Oldenburg to Finch, 7 December 1665, in *Oldenburg Correspondence*, iii, pp. 631–3.

50 Oldenburg to Finch, 10 April 1666, in *Oldenburg Correspondence*, iii, p. 86.

51 Oldenburg to Finch, 26 November 1667, and Oldenburg to Leopold, 26 November 1667, in *Oldenburg Correspondence*, iii, pp. 618–22. See also the 'Memoriall for Mr. Bosman going for Italy', *ibid.*, iv, pp. 119–20.

52 BNCF, MS. Gal. 278, number 49, fols 82ʳ–85ᵛ. See L. Giovannini, ed., *Lettere di Ottavio Falconieri a Leopoldo de' Medici*, series *Carteggio d'artisti dell'Archivio di Stato di Florence*, 10 (Florence, 1984), pp. 213–15.

53 Knowles Middleton, *The Experimenters*.

54 W.E. Knowles Middleton, 'Marchese F. Riccardi and A. Segni in England in 1668–9. Segni's diary', *Studi Secenteschi*, 21 (1981), 187–279.

Cimento was celebrated.[55] This book had the same celebrative intentions as Sprat's history and, on 11 December 1667, four copies of the *Saggi* were presented to Finch: one copy was for the King of England, one for Robert Boyle, one for Finch himself, and the last one for his inseparable friend, Baines.[56] In the following year, between February and April 1668, the secretary of the Cimento, Lorenzo Magalotti, visited England together with Paolo Falconieri with the specific aim of presenting volumes of the *Saggi* to the king and the Royal Society.[57]

Finch, from this point of view, did very little to create a connection between English and Italian scholars, and even the links that afterwards developed between the Royal Society and Italy grew up through essentially different channels.

Further research might explain what was the scientific value of the investigations by Finch and Baines who, during their lifetimes, did not publish anything. In the archive of the Finch family – now deposited in the Leicestershire Record Office – are kept nine miscellaneous volumes of medical and philosophical notes written by Finch and Baines over many years, that it would be worthwhile to study.[58] And possibly a study of their personal papers would show some difference of theoretical attitude between Finch and Baines, the latter apparently much more interested in more general philosophical problems than the first. It was not an accident that Baines was depicted by Carlo Dolci, in Italy, surrounded by books by Plato and Aristotle.[59] The opinions of their contemporaries were contradictory. The two men certainly had a very good reputation for being excellent anatomists from a technical point of view. Both of them were always held in the highest regard by

---

55   The *Saggi di naturali esperienze* was translated into English in 1684 by Richard Waller.

56   Finch to Leopold, 11 December 1667, in BNCF, MS. Gal. 278, number 72 , fols 112^r–113^v. Finch to Boyle, 28 January/6 February 1668, in Hunter, Clericuzio, and Principe, *Correspondence of Robert Boyle*, iv, p. 24.

57   On Magalotti's journey to England in 1688 see Knowles Middleton, *The Experimenters*, pp. 32, 291–5; Birch, *History*, ii, p. 286. See the letters from Oldenburg to Boyle of 11 February 1668, 10 March 1668, 17 March 1668, in *Oldenburg Correspondence*, iv, pp. 170, 234, 248.

58   Finch was described by Henry More in his *Divine Dialogues* (London, 1668), as 'a zealous but hairy-minded Platonist and Cartesian'. The nine notebooks are described in Historical Manuscripts Commission, *Report on the Finch Manuscripts*, II (London, 1922), pp. 500–4. The second one of them has been microfilmed (ref. MF 655) and a copy of the microfilm is in the Museo della Scienza di Florence. In this notebook there is also an ample catalogue of Finch's library. About his library, Finch once said: 'I am a pretender to some insight in books for all sort unless those of divinity of wch I have none in my library': The National Archives, MS. SP 98/11. An edition of the most important of Finch's manuscripts, an unpublished treatise of natural philosophy (Leicester Record Office, MS. Finch Papers, DG7 Box 4976 Lit. 9) is being prepared by Scott Mandelbrote, Sarah Hutton, and Robert Crocker.

59   C. McCorquodale, *Some Paintings and Drawings by Carlo Dolci in British Collections* (Florence, 1976), pp. 313–20.

their former tutor Henry More: he was certainly responsible for the belief of John Worthington and of Samuel Hartlib that the two friends could bring about great things in Italy.[60] Redi when he mentioned their presence 'in the Tuscan court' ('nella toscana corte') in his *Osservazioni sulle vipere* of 1664, spoke of them as 'illustrious and eminent subjects' ('soggetti ragguardevoli ed insigni') who had 'Pien di Filosofia la lingua e'l petto'.[61] Their activity was also discussed in a positive way by Claude Bérigard in his *Circoli Pisani*[62] and Robert Boyle spoke of Finch with great appreciation.

On the contrary side, we have already seen the judgement of the more original and passionate among the academicians of the Cimento. The discussion regarding the priority of discoveries regarding the optical nerve, in particular, had generated painful polemical ramifications. In that fiery year of 1664 in which Borelli composed a memoir in defence of Malpighi, he wrote that he was 'more than sure' of the two Englishmen's will to scrounge the credit for others' inventions ('loro volontà di scroccare l'invenzioni d'altri').[63] As late as 1680, Francesco Folli, who demanded for himself the merit of having thought of the idea of blood transfusion for the first time but who knew that it had been practised for the first time in England, expressed the suspicion that the news of his idea reached London from Tuscany ('di Toscana avesse navigato in Londra') and said explicitly that perhaps it was Finch – who without doubt had heard of Folli's work when he was in Florence – who had 'transport[ed]' it to his homeland.[64]

But apart from the polemical bitterness of Borelli, well-known for his frequent and violent outbursts, and of his friends, it is absolutely certain that in the battle between innovators and conservatives that was being fought in the Italian scientific environment, Finch sided many times and unambiguously with the latter. His role as a cultural mediator between the English scientific world and the Italian one was also disappointing. As we have seen, Finch, rather than becoming the celebrated promoter of exchanges between the Cimento and the Royal Society, was possibly

60 James Crossley, ed., *The Diary and Correspondence of Dr. Worthington*, 2 vols in 3 parts, The Chetham Society 13, 36, 114 (Manchester, 1847–6), i, pp. 339, 342.

61 See Redi, *Opere*, iv, p. 151. The lines in Italian are by Petrarch.

62 Claude Bérigard, *Circulus Pisanus...De veteri et peripatetica philosophia in Aristotelis libros octo physicorum, quatuor de coelo, duos de ortu et interitu, quatuor de meteoris et tres de anima* (Padua, 1661), p. 617; Targioni Tozzetti, *Notizie degli aggrandimenti*, i, p. 272; Fabroni, *Historiae*, iii, pp. 532–4.

63 Borelli to Malpighi, 16 May 1664, in *Malpighi Correspondence*, p. 212.

64 Francesco Folli, *Stadera Medica nella quale, oltre la medicina infusoria ed altre novità, si bilanciano le ragioni favorevoli e contrarie alla trasfusione del sangue* (Florence, 1680), pp. 37–8. See Antonella Sacchetti, 'Il cerchio della vita: filosofia e scienza nell'opera di Francesco Folli (1624–1685)', unpublished MA thesis in History of Science (Tesi di Laurea in Storia della Scienza), University of Siena, Curriculum of Philosophy, Arezzo (academic year 2000/2001), supervisor: Prof. Walter Bernardi.

even an obstacle to communication at a time when news of what was going on in the panoply of English science was anxiously sought in Italy.[65]

---

65   In general on the relationships between the Royal Society and Italy see Marie Boas Hall, 'The Royal Society and Italy 1667–1795', *Notes and Records of the Royal Society of London*, 37 (1982), 63–73; W.E. Knowles Middleton, 'What did Charles II call the Fellows of the Royal Society', *Notes and Records of the Royal Society of London*, 32 (1977), 13–16; Marta Cavazza, 'Bologna and the Royal Society in the seventeenth century', *Notes and Records of the Royal Society of London*, 35 (1980), 105–23.

Chapter 9

The Origins of the Royal Society Revisited

Mordechai Feingold

On 28 November 1660, a dozen men who regularly attended the Wednesday astronomy lectures read by Christopher Wren at Gresham College, London, retired (as was their custom) to continue discussing scientific matters informally. During that meeting:

> something was offered about a design of founding a college for the promoting of physico-mathematical experimental learning. And because they had these frequent occasions of meeting with one another, it was proposed, that some course might be thought to improve this meeting to a more regular way of debating things; and that, according to the manner in other countries, where there were voluntary associations of men into academies for the advancement of various parts of learning, they might do something answerable here for the promoting of experimental philosophy.[1]

The proximity of the event to the Puritan Revolution – the foundational meeting took place six months after Charles II's return to London – inevitably prompted historians to speculate on the possible effects exerted by the civil war and Interregnum on the institutionalization of English science. Were the founders of the Royal Society Puritans and/or Parliamentarians? Did 'puritan ideas on intellectual organization' inform the design of the architects of the Society? Was the Society a Baconian institution? These and related questions engendered heated debates but produced little light, primarily because the Society's origins were invariably assumed to be a particular case of a broader issue – the relation of English Protestantism to science. Such a preoccupation, I believe, resulted in misinterpretation of the evidentiary record and misunderstanding of the unique context out of which the Society emerged. The present essay intends to provide a more nuanced analysis of the relevant documents and the context within which they were written, and to

I wish to thank Michael Hunter and Scott Mandelbrote for their helpful comments.

1   Thomas Birch, *The History of the Royal Society of London* (4 vols, repr. Brussels, 1967), p. 3.

offer more solid ground to anchor the origins of the Royal Society in the Oxford meetings of the 1650s.

Wallis's account

Of the two near-contemporary accounts of the Society's origins – Thomas Sprat's rendition in the *History of the Royal Society* and John Wallis's *Defence of the Royal Society*, supplemented by his autobiography – Sprat's has generally been deemed the less reliable, primarily because of the underlying assumption that Sprat was concerned to conceal the collaboration of key members with the Cromwellian regime and thus sought to anchor the Society's pre-history in 'Royalist' Oxford rather than in 'Parliamentarian' London. As we shall see below, since it turns out that the same individuals figured in both accounts – and since the Oxford chancellor during most of the 1650s was Oliver Cromwell – such a conjecture is unwarranted. Wallis's account, in contrast, has never been subjected to anywhere near the same scrutiny as Sprat's and, consequently, the implications of Wallis's polemical purpose for his historical narrative have gone virtually unnoticed.[2]

The roots of Wallis's account can be traced back to 1659 when William Holder was asked to try to teach a boy who was born deaf – Alexander Popham – to speak. Holder appears to have made considerable progress with his charge and the youth was displayed before the King and the embryonic Royal Society in late spring 1660. Later that year Holder's work was interrupted following his elevation as prebendary of Ely, and Popham began losing his newly acquired skills. For his part, Wallis tutored in 1661 one Daniel Whaley, a man in his mid-twenties, who had lost his hearing at the age of five. Wallis, too, paraded his pupil before the Royal Society and the King,[3] and the ensuing publicity induced Popham's relations to send the deaf boy to Wallis for instruction. Holder did not pursue the matter further and gave his papers on the topic to John Wilkins, who intended to use the material in his *An Essay Towards a Real Character*. Wilkins's library burned down

---

2   Margery Purver was the only historian to recognize the significance of the polemical context, but her shaky command of the literature – as well as the exaggerated claims she made regarding Bacon and Sprat's version – obscured the point: *The Royal Society: Concept and Creation* (London, 1967). See, more generally, A. Rupert Hall and Marie Boas Hall, 'The intellectual origins of the Royal Society – London and Oxford', *Notes and Records of the Royal Society*, 23 (1968), 157–68; Christopher Hill, 'The intellectual origins of the Royal Society – London or Oxford', *Notes and Records of the Royal Society*, 23 (1968), 144–56; Charles Webster, 'The origins of the Royal Society', *History of Science*, 6 (1967), 106–28. The fullest account of the Interregnum period is to be found in Charles Webster, *The Great Instauration: Science, Medicine and Reform 1626–1660* (London, 1975) and Robert G. Frank, Jr., *Harvey and the Oxford Physiologists: A Study of Scientific Ideas and Social Interaction* (Berkeley and Los Angeles, 1980).

3   Birch, *History of the Royal Society*, i, pp. 83–4.

during the Great London Fire, and Holder was asked to rewrite his account. He consented and the narrative of his experience with Popham was published in the May 1668 issue of the *Philosophical Transactions*, and reprinted in Holder's *Elements of Speech*, published with the Society's imprimatur a year later.[4]

Wallis lost little time in staking his own claim for inventing the method of teaching speech to the deaf. A letter he had sent to Boyle in 1662, detailing his experience with Whaley, was now transmitted to Oldenburg, and the Secretary inserted it in the July 1670 issue of the *Philosophical Transactions* – along with an editorial comment that reminded readers of Whaley's limelight in London in spring 1662 as well as plugging a generous advertisement for Wallis's *Grammatica Linguae Anglicanae*.[5] No mention was made of Holder. A couple of years later a translation of Wallis's account appeared in the appendix to the first volume of the Leipzig periodical *Miscellanea curiosa*, with an addendum by Wallis. Then, in 1674, Wallis produced a new edition of his *Grammar*, where he inserted for the first time a report of his success in speech therapy.[6] Holder took offence, not only because Wallis had abrogated credit for inventing such a method, but because of the insinuation in the same editorial comment that Wallis alone had taught Popham to speak. Immediately Holder sought redress. According to John Aubrey, who was present when Holder confronted Oldenburg, the Secretary admitted that it was Wallis who had in fact written the editorial comment. The matter was raised at a Council meeting of the Society, probably in late spring 1675, and it was 'ordered that acknowledgement must be made in the transactions, for this abuse'.[7] Holder promptly composed his version of the events, and Oldenburg prepared a brief preface in which he justified publication out of a desire 'to avoid partiality on his part'. However, President Brouncker, Wallis's intimate friend, refused to license publication unless Holder softened his language.

While events in London unfolded, there appeared in Oxford in early 1677 Robert Plot's *The Natural History of Oxford-Shire*, which relied on Wallis for information regarding his own work and the work of others. The Savilian professor availed himself of the opportunity to further bolster his case, and Plot dutifully pronounced that it had been none other than Wallis who 'first observed and discovered the *Physical* or *Mechanical* Formation of all *Sounds* in *Speech*, as plainly appears from his Treatise *de Loquela*, prefix'd to his *Grammar* for the *English* Tongue, first publish'd in the year 1653'. By following this method, Plot

---

4   Birch, *History of the Royal Society*, ii, p. 272; *Philosophical Transactions* (number 35) iii, 665–8. Oldenburg immediately reviewed the book: *Philosophical Transactions* (number 47) iii, 958–9.

5   *Philosophical Transactions* (number 61) iv, 1087–97 (Wallis's letter); 1098–9 (editorial comment). No manuscript copy of Wallis's letter to Boyle survives.

6   John Wallis, *Grammar of the English Language*, ed. J.A. Kemp (London, 1972), p. 117.

7   *The Correspondence of Thomas Hobbes*, ed. Noel Malcolm (2 vols, Oxford, 1994), ii, pp. 753–4. No record of this affair is recorded in the Journal Book – in line with most other contentious matters.

added, Wallis 'also found out a way whereby he hath taught *dumb Persons*…to *speak* and *read* intelligibly'. True, the account continued, Wilkins also addressed 'the distinct manner of forming all *sounds* in *speech*' in his *Essay*, as did Holder. 'Yet whether either of these, with advantage of what Dr. Wallis did before, have with more accuracy of judgment performed the same, I dare not by any means take upon me to determine'.[8] Such an escalation of the controversy obviously did not contribute to Holder's willingness to temper his charges against Wallis. Nor was the rapidly accelerating schism within the Society between Brouncker and Oldenburg, on the one hand, and a growing sector of the membership, on the other, conducive to the resolution of the affair.

An account of the rift goes beyond the scope of this paper; suffice it to say that the ringleaders of the opposition were Robert Hooke and Sir Christopher Wren. And as Holder was Wren's brother-in-law and Hooke's friend – while Wallis was Brouncker's friend and protégé – the priority dispute became inextricably entangled in the Society's politics. Many opposition members were deeply antipathetic toward Wallis. As Aubrey informed Hobbes in 1675, Hooke 'has been as much abused by Dr Wallis as any one', for Wallis made 'it his Trade to be a common-spye. steales from every ingeniose persons discourse, and prints it: viz from Sr Chr: Wren God knows how often, from Mr Hooke etc. he is a most ill-natured man, an egregious lyer and back-biter, a flatterer, and fawner on my Ld Brouncker & his Miss: that my L^d may keepe up his reputation'.[9] Ultimately, the rupture resulted in the ousting of Brouncker from the presidency in November 1677 and in the election of a Council that included, in addition to Hooke, Wren, and Holder, such close allies and friends of theirs as Thomas Henshaw, Thomas Hill, Sir John Hoskyns, Sir Jonas Moore, Nehemiah Grew, and Seth Ward.

Since the fate of the *Philosophical Transactions* was thrown into limbo following Oldenburg's death in September 1677 and the ensuing coup, Holder decided to publish an expanded version of his attack on Wallis elsewhere, entrusting the task to Hooke's friend, Henry Brome. *A Supplement to the Philosophical Transactions* appeared in early 1678, in a format designed purposely to imitate the original *Transactions*. In narrating the events described above, however, Holder was not at all concerned with the issue of the Society's origins; he invoked the Oxford Club only because he wished to name several members as

8   Robert Plot, *The Natural History of Oxford-Shire* (Oxford, 1677), pp. 281–2. The book was licensed by Ralph Bathurst on 13 April 1676.

9   As an illustration of the sort of treachery of which Wallis was capable, Aubrey charged that when Wallis was entrusted with the printing of William Oughtred's *Clavis Mathematicae*, he became dissatisfied with the generous encomium bestowed on him by the author – 'a sharp-witted, pious, and hard-working man, very well versed in all literature of the more recondite sort, and perceptive in mathematical matters' – so he added a sentence of his own composition: 'and with astonishing ability to unravel and explain writings which have been hidded and concealed in the most elaborate of cyphers': *The Correspondence of Thomas Hobbes*, ed. Noel Malcolm (2 vols, Oxford, 1994), ii, pp. 753–4.

witnesses to the events that occurred in 1659. Thus, he prefaced his narrative with a brief comment on the group:

> Some years immediately before His Majesties happy Restauration, divers ingenious persons in *Oxford* used to meet at the Lodgings of that excellent Person, and zealous promoter of Learning, the late Bishop of *Chester*, Dr. *Wilkins*, then Warden of *Wadham* College, where they diligently conferred about Researches and Experiments in Nature, and indeed laid the first Ground and Foundation of the Royal Society.

After this factual preamble, Holder shifted gears, as the period that directly concerned him: 'In that time, *viz.* in the Year 1659', Popham was recommended to his care by Wilkins, Seth Ward, and Ralph Bathurst, partly because these three were 'desirous to serve the Ends, and contribute something to the design of that Worthy Company before-mentioned, *viz.* Improvement of natural knowledge and publick benefit'.[10]

Wallis retaliated immediately via an open letter addressed to Brouncker dated 6 March 1677/8, which shrewdly tied his own apologia to a defence of the Society's old guard. In Holder's pamphlet, Wallis thundered, he found 'great complaints of the *Royal Society*; of the *Philosophical Transactions*;...Of the Publisher thereof, Mr. *Oldenburg*...but, most of all, of *my self*. Clearly, Wallis contrived to characterize Holder's charges against him as an integral part – albeit by other means – of the cabal against Brouncker and Oldenburg. Consequently, in addition to fending off charges of improper conduct in the matter of speech therapy, Wallis sought to depict Holder and his allies as betrayers of the 'genuine' Royal Society; and since the opposition party was intimately involved with the Oxford Club, the casual remark made by Holder was turned by Wallis into a central issue in his pamphlet. Hence its title: *A Defence of the Royal Society*.

Anthony Wood once noted that Wallis, 'at any time, can make black white, and white black, for his own ends, and hath a ready knack of sophistical evasion, as the writer of these matters [Wood] doth know full well'.[11] Such tactics are in evidence everywhere in his critique of Holder. To confine myself to the matter at hand, note how Wallis deliberately reversed the sequence of Holder's narrative cited above, and strung together sentences in order to produce a claim regarding the Society's origins that Holder never made: 'In that time, *viz.* in the Year 1659', Wallis cited Holder as saying, 'divers ingenious persons in *Oxford* used to meet at the Lodgings of Dr. *Wilkins* ['that excellent Person, and zealous promoter of Learning, the late Bishop of *Chester*' is silently omitted], then Warden of *Wadham* College, where they diligently conferred about Researches and Experiments in

---

10   William Holder, *A Supplement to the Philosophical Transactions* (London, 1678), p. 4. Holder also mentioned that Sir Charles Scarborough incorporated an account of his method in the anatomical lectures he delivered at the College of Physicians.

11   Anthony Wood, *Fasti Oxonienses*, ed. Philip Bliss (2 parts, London, 1815–20), ii, p. 245.

Nature, and indeed laid the first Ground and Foundation of the Royal Society'. Such textual reconstruction enabled Wallis to charge Holder with committing gross errors of fact, if not with the intention to deceive. After all, he triumphantly pointed out, by 1659 Wilkins had already left Oxford and the meetings at Wadham College had been suspended. He had to acknowledge, of course, that meetings had been held *earlier* at Wadham College, 'and that those Meetings might be somewhat conducing to that of the *Royal Society* which now is'. But, Wallis added, 'without disparagement to Bishop *Wilkins*', these meetings were 'not, that *first Ground and Foundation of the Royal Society*...Which I take to be much earlier than those Meetings there'. It was at this juncture that the famous account of the Society's origins is introduced:

I take its *first Ground and Foundation* to have been in *London*, about the year 1645. (if not sooner) when the same Dr. *Wilkins*...Dr. *Jonathan Goddard*, Dr. *Ent*... Dr. *Glisson*, Dr. *Scarbrough*... Dr. *Merrit*, with my self and some others, met weekly, (sometimes at Dr. *Goddards* Lodgings, sometimes at the *Mitre in Wood-street* hard by) at a certain day and hour, under a certain Penalty, and a weekly Contribution for the Charge of Experiments, with certain Rules agreed upon amongst us. Where (to avoid diversion to other discourses, and for some other reasons) we barred all Discourses of Divinity, of State-Affairs, and of News, (other than what concern'd our business of Philosophy) confining our selves to Philosophical Inquiries, and such as related thereunto; as Physick, Anatomy, Geometry, Astronomy, Navigation, Staticks, Mechanicks, and Natural Experiments. We there discoursed the Circulation of the Blood, the Valves in the Veins, the Copernican Hypothesis, the Nature of Comets and new Stars, the Attendants on Jupiter, the Oval shape of *Saturn*, the Inequalities and Selenography of the *Moon*, the several Phases of *Venus* and *Mercury*, the Improvement of Telescopes, and grinding of Glasses for that purpose, (wherein Dr. *Goddard* was particularly ingaged, and did maintain an Operator in his house for that purpose) the weight of the Air, the Possibility or Impossibility of Vacuities, and Natures abhorrence thereof, the Torricellian Experiment in Quicksilver, the Descent of Heavy Bodies, and the Degrees of Acceleration therein; with others of like nature. Some of which were then but new Discoveries, and others not so generally known and embraced as now they are.

These Meetings we removed, soon after, to the *Bull-head* in *Cheap-side*; and (in Term-time) to *Gresham*-Colledge, where we met weekly at Mr. *Foster's* Lecture, (then Astronomy-Professor there) and, after the Lecture ended: repaired, sometime to Mr. *Foster's* Lodgings, sometimes to some other place not far distant, where we continued such Inquiries; and our numbers encreased.

About the years 1648, 1649, some of our Company were removed to *Oxford*; (first, Dr. *Wilkins*, then I, and soon after, Dr. *Goddard*;) whereupon our Company divided. Those at *London* (and we, when we had occasion to be there) met as before. Those of us at *Oxford*, with Dr. *Ward*...Dr. *Petty*...Dr. *Bathurst*, Dr. *Willis*, and many others of the most inquisitive Persons in *Oxford*, met weekly (for some years) at Dr. *Petty's* lodgings on the like account; (to wit, so long as Dr. *Petty* continued in *Oxford*, and for some while after;) because of the conveniencies we had there, (being the House of an Apothecary) to view, and make use, of Drugs and other like matters, as there was occasion.

Our Meetings there, were very numerous, and very considerable. For, beside the diligence of Persons, studiously Inquisitive, the Novelty of the Design made many to resort thither; who, when it ceased to be new, began to grow remiss, or did pursue such Inquiries at Home.

We did afterwards (Dr. *Petty* being gone for *Ireland*, and our numbers growing less,) remove thence. And (some years before His Majesty's Return) did meet, (as Dr. *Holder* observes) at Dr. *Wilkin's* Lodgings, in *Wadham*-Colledge.

But, before the time he mentions, those *set Meetings* ceased in *Oxford*, and were held at *London*. Where (after the death of Mr. *Foster*) we continued to meet at *Gresham*-Colledge (as before,) at Mr. *Rook's* Lecture, (who succeeded Mr. *Foster*,) and from thence repaired to some convenient place, in or near that Colledge.[12]

Wallis's account is remarkable for several reasons. Not only does it aggrandize the London meetings at the expense of the Oxford meetings, but it ascribes to the former an elaborate organizational structure that developed only in Oxford. Indeed, Wallis goes so far as to relegate the Oxford meetings to the level of a provincial club, the members of which focused primarily on a narrow range of the medical sciences – in contrast to the very impressive cosmopolitan range of studies that engaged the attention of Londoners. Wallis also insinuates that the Oxford Club flourished only during William Petty's brief sojourn at the University (1649 to 1652), with but intermittent meetings at Wadham thereafter. Conversely, the London meetings are depicted as vibrant and continuous throughout the period 1645–1660 and, therefore, alone worthy of being considered as the true precursor of the Royal Society. Furthermore, Wallis is careful to exclude from his account those members of the Oxford Club who lent a hand to the dethroning of Brouncker. Thus, for example, no mention is made of either Hooke or Wren among those 'most inquisitive Persons' at Oxford. Even more conspicuous in his absence is Hooke's patron and friend Robert Boyle – except when mentioned as the recipient of the letter in which Wallis detailed the progress he had made with Whaley.

Most striking, however, is the wilful belittling of Wilkins's centrality to both the London and Oxford meetings. Wallis's ploy can be inferred from his protesting too loudly that correcting Holder's account is made 'without disparagement to Bishop *Wilkins*', as well as from his deletion of the praise Holder showered on Wilkins. Equally telling is the minor role accorded to the Wadham College meetings – certainly when compared to those taking place at Petty's lodgings. Even more pernicious, however, is the subtle affront to Wilkins's originality in devising a theory of artificial language. Wallis had already helped Plot to a lengthy account of Dalgarno's ideas on the subject and to the information that the latter 'met with no *Man* that took so much Pains to understand the *Novelty*, or so Zealous to have it

12   John Wallis, *A Defence of the Royal Society* (London, 1678), pp. 7–8.

finished and come abroad', as Wilkins. In the *Defence*, Wallis repeats the claim that it was Dalgarno's 'enterprise' that 'gave occasion to Dr. *Wilkins*...to pursue the same Design (as [he] himself intimates in his Epistle)'. Wallis then proceeds to take credit for assisting Dalgarno to formulate his ideas, and concludes that it was his ideas on the matter of sounds that informed both Wilkins's and Holder's writings on the subject.[13]

The reasons for denigrating Wilkins are many and diverse. Within the immediate polemical context, Wallis obviously felt it necessary to contradict Holder's statements regarding Wilkins's centrality for Oxford, as he did on any other issue raised by his opponent. Even more important, however, was the fact that Wilkins was the patron saint of the Hooke-Wren party both in Oxford and London. For that reason, undermining the significance of the Oxford meetings, and of Wilkins's role more generally, was a calculated rebuttal to the narrative offered by Thomas Sprat – yet another protégé of the late bishop. On a more personal level, Wallis may well have been peeved at the greater encomium Holder received in Wilkins's *Essay*. While Wallis's *Grammar* had simply been credited as having 'with greatest Accurateness and subtlety...considered the Philosophy of Articulate sounds', Wilkins lavished a warm personal tribute on Holder and Lodwick: 'I must not forget to acknowledge the favour and good hap I have had, to peruse from their *private* papers, the distinct Theories of some other Learned and Ingenious persons, who have with great judgment applyed their thoughts to this enquiry; in each of whose Papers, there are several suggestions that are new, out of the common rode, and very considerable'.[14]

The minor corrections Wallis made in his 1697 narrative of the events further substantiate the polemical context that informed his 1678 account. Two decades later he could afford to be more conciliatory toward Holder, albeit still claiming priority in the matter of speech therapy. As for the origins of the Society, Wallis now omits the allegation that the London meetings introduced the organizational structure he claimed for them in his former account, as well as acknowledging that club meetings took place at Robert Boyle's lodgings after Wilkins left Oxford. He remains adamant, though, about minimizing the latter's contribution, still portraying the Wadham meetings as subsidiary to, and less frequent than, those taking place at Petty's lodgings. More significant still is the claim made by Wallis for the first time, namely that it was Theodore Haak who 'gave the first occasion, and first suggested those meetings'.[15] Likewise, he refrains even now from mentioning

---

13   Plot, *Oxford-Shire*, pp. 282–5; Wallis, *Defence*, pp. 16–19. Wilkins did not make such an open admission in the preface to his *Essay*; this was the first time Wallis claimed he had had discussions with Dalgarno.

14   Wilkins, *Essay*, p. 357. Though Wilkins appears to have been instrumental in securing for Wallis the Savilian professorship of geometry, their relations at Oxford and subsequently appear to have been cordial at best. Wallis's Presbyterianism and personality were among the issues that separated them.

15   Christoph J. Scriba, 'The autobiography of John Wallis, F.R.S.', *Notes and Records of the Royal Society*, 25 (1970), 17–46, at pp. 39–40.

Wren and Hooke – the latter of whom he had locked horns with for the previous two decades.

The Oxford meetings

Contextualizing Wallis's account is not intended to serve as a prelude to any rejection of the reality – or the relevance – of the London meetings, rather to argue that, for reasons to be detailed below, the Oxford meetings were the more relevant for the foundation of the Royal Society. Contemporaries certainly viewed matters in such a light. On 9 January 1660/1, for example, the day he was admitted Fellow of the Royal Society, John Evelyn noted in his diary that the group had 'begun some years before at *Oxford*, & interruptedly here in *Lond[on]* during the Rebellion'. Eight years later Oldenburg, too, emphasized the centrality of the Oxford meetings when dedicating the fourth volume of the *Philosophical Transactions* to Seth Ward: 'We ought to remember, that 'tis now about 15 or 16 years, since your Lordship Geometrized Astronomy...And that you added Life to the *Oxonian* Sparkles, I mean that Meetings, which may be called the *Embryo* or First Conception of the *Royal Society*'. For his part, Aubrey was convinced that Wilkins 'was the principall reviver of experimentall philosophy (secundum mentem domini Baconi) at Oxford, where he had weekly an experimentall philosophicall clubbe, which began 1649, and was the incunabula of the Royall Society. When he came to London, they mett at the Bull-head taverne in Cheapside, (e.g. 1658, 1659, and after), till it grew to[o] big for a clubb, and so they came to Gresham colledge parlour'.[16]

Sprat, then, was not alone in privileging the Oxford meetings as most relevant to the foundation of the Royal Society; indeed, in all likelihood, it was this very consensus that made it unnecessary for him to dwell on the London meetings in the brief historical narrative he intended to provide. Certainly, his list of key participants is almost identical to the one drawn up by Wallis, including those who allegedly 'collaborated' with Parliament – Wilkins, Petty, and Goddard. Besides, notwithstanding the perception today, there was little that was novel in the 1645 meetings. Like other European countries, England had witnessed the proliferation of learned associations at least since Elizabethan times. One of the more celebrated groups was the Society of Antiquaries, founded in the mid-1580s, which held weekly Friday meetings in London during term, in addition to a yearly feast day on All Souls Day. Topics were set in advance, with specific members charged with the presentation of papers; discussion and debate was expected to follow. The Society was dissolved in around 1607, and an attempt to revive it in 1614 failed owing to

16   *The Diary of John Evelyn*, ed. E.S. de Beer (6 vols, Oxford, 1955), iii, p. 266; John Aubrey, *Brief Lives*, ed. Andrew Clark (2 vols, Oxford, 1898), ii, p. 301. Significantly, Aubrey locates the meetings at the 'Bull-head taverne in Cheapside' in the late 1650s whereas Wallis claimed those took place in 1645.

unspecified opposition by James I.[17] The failure of such a semi-formal association did not put an end to the desire of antiquarians to congregate. During the late 1610s and 1620s Edmund Bolton sought tirelessly to interest the Stuart monarchs and their courtiers in his ambitious schemes to establish a Royal Academy.[18] Other individuals settled for more modest arrangements. In 1638, for example, Sir Edward Dering, Sir Christopher Hatton, Sir Thomas Shirley, and William Dugdale bound themselves into a formal association, aimed at facilitating their respective antiquarian studies. They agreed to share resources, to collaborate, and to communicate with each other, while at the same time agreeing upon a method that would ensure recognition of individual discoveries. The group appears to have evolved into a London club that held regular meetings, and it was probably to papers delivered at those meetings that Hartlib referred in 1641 when he noted in his diary that Hatton 'hase a whole volume of Conferences held some years agoe here in England'.[19] This club, or a descendant of it, continued well into the 1650s, and Elias Ashmole recorded attending 'the Antiquaries Feast' on Friday, 2 July 1658.[20]

Clubs and associations

Literary men and general scholars were avid socialites indeed. Of the many groups whose identity has come down to us mention may be made of the early 1610s meetings at the Mitre Club at Fleet Street, which overlapped with (or transformed into) the meetings of the 'Sireniacal Gentlemen' at the Mermaid Tavern on the first Friday of each month.[21] These were administered by a 'seneschal', and a fine was imposed on those who failed to attend the club's 'feast'. Even more famous is the Great Tew circle, the club that met during the 1630s at the Oxfordshire seat of Lucius Cary, 2nd Viscount Falkland.[22] Numerous other gatherings mushroomed in London and beyond, like the soirées at Archbishop John Williams's palace, to which Theodore Haak and John Pell were invited in 1638 'for the freer discourse of all sorts of literature and experiments', or the 'Order of the Fancy' – a literary circle organized by Sir John Mennes and James Smith – or the literary club

17   Joan Evans, *A History of the Society of Antiquaries* (Oxford, 1956), pp. 10–13.
18   Joseph Hunter, 'An Account of the Scheme for the Erecting a Royal Academy in England, in the Reign of King James the First', *Archaeologia*, 32 (1847), 132–49.
19   L.B.L., 'On the Surrenden Charters', *Archaeologia Cantiana*, 1 (1858), 50–65, at pp. 55–8; Evans, *A History of the Society of Antiquaries*, pp. 22–3; Sheffield, Sheffield University Library MS. Hartlib Papers, 30/4/73A, Ephemerides (1641).
20   C.H. Josten, ed., *Elias Ashmole (1617–1692)* (5 vols, Oxford, 1966),ii, p. 737.
21   I.A. Shapiro, 'The 'Mermaid' Club', *Modern Language Review*, 45 (1950), 6–17; Pascal Brioist, 'Que de choses avons nous vues et vécues à la Sirène', *Annuaire du Département d'Histoire et Civilisation*, 1 (1992), 89–132.
22   Hugh Trevor-Roper, 'The Great Tew Circle', in *Catholics, Anglicans and Puritans* (London, 1988), pp. 166–230.

organized by John Cleveland and Samuel Butler in the 1650s, in or around Gray's Inn.[23]

Mathematicians and natural philosophers were perhaps even more eager to form associations, given the recondite nature of their studies and the general predilection for humanistic studies. During the early years of Elizabeth's reign, John Dee proved pivotal to such efforts; soon additional groups were formed, most notably those revolving around William Gilbert and Thomas Harriot. By the 1630s we find such active groups as the Cavendish circle – which included Sir Charles Cavendish, Thomas Hobbes, John Pell, Robert Payne, and William Oughtred – and Christopher Towneley's circle of northern astronomers. However, from the early years of the seventeenth century onward, Gresham College in London became increasingly the focal point of scientific gatherings, by virtue of the central (and permanent) meeting place it offered, and the calibre and enthusiasm of its professors of mathematics – so much so, that Archbishop Laud mistook Gellibrand's meetings in the 1630s for 'Conventicles'.[24] But the College was not only a rendezvous for mathematicians. Sir Kenelm Digby resided at the College intermittently during the 1630s, where he not only diverted himself 'with his chymistry, and the professors' good conversation', but proceeded to erect a laboratory. Johannes Bánfi Hunyades was in charge of the project and remained at Gresham for several years, describing himself in 1642 as a master of chemistry.[25]

It was thus that venerable and vibrant setting of Gresham College that facilitated the formation of the so-called 1645 group. The catalyst behind the galvanization was John Wilkins, who gathered around him a core group of former Oxford students and friends – such as Jonathan Goddard, Walter Charleton, Christopher Merrett, Theodore Haak, and Daniel Whistler, and a few Cambridge men like Charles Scarborough, who arrived to London after a sojourn in Oxford and formed a broad-ranging scientific club. Wilkins's centrality was due partly to his close personal ties with most members, and partly to his being arguably the most influential scholar in London in the mid-1640s, not least because he served as chaplain to Charles Louis, Elector of the Palatinate. The significance of the group, however, was not in inaugurating a new form of meetings but in its attempt to

---

23 Aubrey, *Brief Lives*, ii, p. 129; i, p. 175; Timothy Raylor, *Cavaliers, Clubs, and Literary Culture: Sir John Mennes, James Smith, and the Order of Fancy* (Newark, NJ, 1994).

24 William Prynne, *Canterburie's Doome* (London, 1646), p. 182; Francis R. Johnson, 'Gresham College: precursor of the Royal Society', *Journal of the History of Ideas*, 1 (1940), 413–38; Mordechai Feingold, 'Gresham College and London practitioners: the nature of the English mathematical community', in Francis Ames-Lewis, ed., *Sir Thomas Gresham and Gresham College: Studies in the Intellectual History of London in the Sixteenth and Seventeenth Centuries* (Aldershot, 1999), pp. 174–88.

25 Mordechai Feingold, *The Mathematicians' Apprenticeship: Science, Universities and Societies in England, 1560–1640* (Cambridge, 1984), pp. 166–89; Sheffield University Library, MS. Hartlib Papers, 30/4/51B, Hartlib, Ephemerides (1640).

synchronize the meetings of a variety of specialized clubs that operated in the capital during those years.

Chief among these was the College of Physicians which was represented by Charleton in 1657 as a research institute closely resembling Bacon's Solomon's House, owing to the way the private and collaborative researches of the members interlocked: 'when they meet together in Consultations, they are so candid and liberal in the communication of their single observations and discoveries, that no one of them can long be ignorant of the notions of all the rest: and the noble Emulation that hath equally enflamed their ingenious breasts, makes them unanimous in cooperating toward the Common design, the erecting an intire and durable Fabrick of solid Science'. The College became even more important following the departure of Wilkins and friends to Oxford. In 1648 'some of the Club resolve to moove the Colledge for erecting of a Laboratory in which all Chymical Medecins may the better bee prepared every Dr taking his turne to attend it', and two years later Hartlib was told that Whistler and Merrett 'have promised to make a Club for the perfecting of Mechanical Arts and to meete and correspond with Mr Worsley about it'.[26]

A related group was a club of mathematical practitioners, the members of which in the late 1640s included Scarborough, Jonas Moore, Samuel Foster and Thomas Wharton. In the following decade it broadened to include newcomers to London, comprising by the late 1650s many of the key members of the future Royal Society, as is made clear from a chance survival of a letter that Anthony Thompson sent John Pell on 22 November 1658 (the eve of Cromwell's funeral) inviting him to attend: 'There is this day a meeting to bee in the Moore Fields of some mathematical friends (as you know the custome hath beene) there will bee Mr. Rook and Mr. Wrenn, my Lord Brunkerd. Sir Paul Neale, Dr. Goddard, Dr. Scarburow, etc. I had notice the last night of your being in towne from some of the gentellmen now named, and of there desire to injoy your company; there will bee no such numbers as you usually have seene at such meetinges; 12 is the number invited. Sir, I hope you will excuse the short warning, for it was shorte to mee'.[27] The date indicates that the mathematicians met on Mondays, while the Gresham meetings continued to be held on Wednesdays or Thursdays, and the antiquarians stuck to Fridays, thus avoiding conflict as much as possible.

The late 1640s and 1650s saw an exponential rise in the number of such clubs. They ranged from the semi-secretive private 'Invisible College' group of Robert

---

26   Walter Charleton, *The Immortality of the Human Soul, Demonstrated by the Light of Nature* (London 1657), pp. 34–43; Sheffield University Library, MS. Hartlib Papers, 31/22/21B–22A, Hartlib, Ephemerides (1648); 28/1/77A, Hartlib, Ephemerides (1650).

27   James Orchard Halliwell, ed., *A Collection of Letters Illustrative of the Progress of Science in England from the Reign of Queen Elizabeth to that of Charles the Second* (repr. London, 1965), pp. 95–6.

Boyle, Benjamin Worsley, and friends,[28] to the chemical society (with utopian overtones), which Thomas Henshaw and Thomas Vaughan established in the former's house in Kensington. The latter comprised Henshaw's Oxford teachers Abraham Woodhead and Obadiah Walker, as well as Sir Robert Paston (a future member of the Royal Society), Robert Child, George Starkey, and two obscure practitioners Webbe and Goodwin.[29] To these active groups we may add numerous failed attempts to establish formal organizations, such as Thomas Bushell's scheme for a new 'Solomon's House' and Samuel Morland's 1655 project of a 'College of Arts'. John Evelyn's well-known 1659 scheme 'to Errect a [Philosophic] *Mathematical College*' also belongs to this tradition.[30]

The umbrella-like structure that was briefly experimented with in London was carried by Wilkins and friends to Oxford and immediately implemented, as is made clear from a 1649 letter of Petty informing Hartlib that he had been admitted 'into several clubs of the virtuous'. Similarly, Seth Ward told Sir Justinian Isham in February 1652 that in addition to their 'Greate Clubb' they had 'a combination of a lesser number' of groups as well.[31] The Oxonians were allowed a full decade to perfect such a structure and the experience they harvested proved invaluable to the foundation of the Royal Society. They experimented with other procedural matters as well. A set of rules governing their meetings was drafted in October 1651 and it detailed such procedures as balloting members, the necessary quorum for decisions, admission fees, and penalties for non-attendance and non-performance of tasks.[32] It was also at Oxford that the focus on scientific matters, to the exclusion of theological and political topics, was quite strictly enforced.

Again, these procedural matters were not invented in the 1650s. We learn from Spelman's account, for example, that as early as 1614, when the antiquaries sought to regroup, they 'conceiv'd some rules of Government and limitation to be observ'd amongst us; whereof this one was one, That for avoiding offence, we

---

28   Charles Webster, 'New light on the Invisible College: the social relations of English science in the mid-seventeenth century', *Transactions of the Royal Historical Society*, 5th ser., 24 (1974), 19–42.

29   Donald R. Dickson, *The Tessera of Antilia: Utopian Brotherhoods & Secret Societies in the Early Seventeenth Century* (Leiden, 1998), pp. 186–207.

30   Sheffield University Library, MS. Hartlib Papers, 28/2/75B–76A, Hartlib, Ephemerides (1653); 29/5/18B Hartlib, Ephemerides (1655); *The Diary of John Evelyn*, ed. de Beer, iii, p. 232. For the recreation of the Towneley group, see Charles Webster, 'Richard Towneley (1629–1707), the Towneley group and seventeenth century science', *Transactions of the Historic Society of Lancashire and Cheshire*, 118 (1966), 51–76.

31   G.H. Turnbull, 'Samuel Hartlib's influence on the early history of the Royal Society', *Notes and Records of the Royal Society*, 10 (1953), 101–30, at p. 113; H.W. Robinson, 'An unpublished letter of Dr. Seth Ward relating to the early meetings of the Oxford Philosophical Society', *Notes and Records of the Royal Society*, 7 (1950), 68–70, at p. 69.

32   Douglas McKie, 'The origins and foundation of the Royal Society of London', *Notes and Records of the Royal Society*, 15 (1960), 1–37, at pp. 25–6.

should neither meddle with matters of State, nor of Religion'. They also appointed one of their members to serve as a 'Register'. Other pre-revolutionary schemers, notably Bolton and Sir Francis Kynaston, introduced recommendations that were only picked up by the Oxford Club and the Royal Society.[33] Hence, we should not be misled into assuming that the mere setting up of a scientific club was sufficient to assure the success of the sort of organization that the architects of the Royal Society sought to implement in 1660. Only the decade of routine club life at Oxford made it possible to experience first-hand what was involved in managing such an enterprise and what pitfalls stood in the way of success.

Foremost among these pitfalls was that which contributed to the failure of all previous attempts to establish professional societies: invariably, the novelty wore off. Spelman noted in 1628 that the Society of Antiquaries languished after 1607 'as all good uses commonly decline; so many of the chief Supporters hereof either dying or withdrawing themselves from *London* into the Country; this among the rest grew for twenty years to be discontinu'd'. Wallis concurred. In reference to the London meetings of the 1640s he wrote: 'Our Meetings there, were very numerous, and very considerable. For, beside the diligence of Persons, studiously Inquisitive, the Novelty of the Design made many to resort thither; who, when it ceased to be new, began to grow remiss, or did pursue such Inquiries at Home'.[34] Hence, Wilkins and his colleagues quickly foresaw that reliance on weekly contributions and the good will of members was insufficient to ensure lasting success, and thus attempted more radical means to ensure permanence. In late 1653, the instrument-maker Ralph Greatorex informed Hartlib that members of the Club 'are now erecting a Colledge for Experiments et Mechanicks at Oxford towards which Dr Wilkins hath given 200lb. It is over the Schooles or in the long Gallery. where all the Models of Inventions Arts etc are to bee reserved with a Treatise added to each of them shewing the structure and vse of it'. Greatorex was in a position to know as it was he who had been picked to serve as 'keeper of that College'. In the following year, Seth Ward hurled at John Webster the information that there was 'a reall designe amongst us, wanting only some assistance for execution, to erect a Magneticall, Mechanicall, and Optick Schoole, furnished with the best instruments, and Adapted for the most usefull experiments in all those faculties'.[35] The efforts to institutionalize science at Oxford ultimately failed, too, partly because of the growing hostility toward Wilkins among certain of the godly party at the University. The experience fortified further the resolve of Wilkins and his colleagues to establish the institution in perpetuity. This they would seek to accomplish not just by

---

33   *Reliquiae Spelmannianae. The Posthumous Works of Sir Henry Spelman* (Oxford, 1698), pp. 69–70; Hunter, 'An account of the scheme for the erecting a Royal Academy'; Ewald Flügel, 'Die älteste englische Akademie', *Anglia*, 32 (1909), 261–8; Francis Kynaston, *The Constitution of the Musaeum Minervae* (London, 1636).
34   *Reliquiae Spelmannianae*, p. 69; Wallis, *Defence of the Royal Society*, p. 8.
35   Sheffield University Library, MS. Hartlib Papers, 28/2/78B, Hartlib, *Ephemerides* (1653); [John Wilkins and Seth Ward], *Vindiciae academiarum* (Oxford 1654), p. 36.

enlisting the support of the returned monarch, but by codifying their elaborate procedures and rituals into a chartered corporation.

The Oxford experience was crucial for other reasons as well. To a large extent, those who attended the London gatherings of the 1640s were busy divines and physicians who managed once or twice a week to devote spare hours to scientific activity. But their other occupations, and the constraints on their time, turned the meetings into a discussion club, similar to other scholarly groups in London.[36] For that reason Anthony Wood concluded quite rightly that the London meetings were not 'a foundation for a Society but merely for diversion sake'. Wallis himself admitted that it was only after he had arrived to Oxford that '*Mathematicks* which had before been a pleasing Diversion, was now to be my serious Study'.[37] That proved to be true for other members of the Oxford Club as well, for the University environment offered them a unique opportunity for prolonged and uninterrupted periods of research and collaboration with individuals who lived within a few hundred yards of each other. Additionally, since many of them served as professors and heads of house, it became possible to raise a new generation of talented researchers and committed patrons who would prove instrumental to the initial success of the Royal Society. Furthermore, not only was science pursued on a more professional basis at Oxford; the nature of the enterprise was radically transformed there. Whereas the participants of the 1640s London group were primarily recipients of continental ideas and experimental results, the process of assimilation came to a close at Oxford, and it was here that Englishmen produced their original contributions to mathematics, astronomy, physics, and the life sciences.

John Aubrey, then, perceptively discerned the dawn of a new era when he pinpointed the advent of experimental philosophy to the period after 1649, not because England was hitherto devoid of science and practitioners, but because the pursuit of science assumed new meaning and dignity. 'The searching into Naturall knowledge began but since or about the death of King Charles the first', Aubrey wrote. Previously, "twas held a strange presumption for [any] man to attempt improvement of any knowledge whatsoever...they thought it not fitt to be wiser then their fathers & not good manners to be wiser then their neighbours; and a sin to search into the wayes of nature'. Earlier, learning was 'Paedantry, i.e. criticall learning...Their stile pedantique, stuff't with Latin, & Greeke sentences'. True, during Elizabethan and Jacobean times there 'were very learned men in their kinds', who merited respect as forerunners for 'they made the rough waies smooth

---

36   It went unnoticed that in his autobiography Wallis prefaced his description of the London group with an encomium of the theological/scholarly discussion group he frequented as well: 'I do own myself to have received much advantage by the Conversation and the learned Debates of so many Grave, Reverend and Learned Divines, on all points of Divinity.' Obviously he regarded them as part of the same milieu. Scriba, 'The Autobiography of John Wallis', p. 31.

37   Anthony Wood, *The History and Antiquities of the University of Oxford*, ed. John Gutch (2 vols in 3, Oxford, 1792–6), ii, pp. 632–3; Scriba, 'The autobiography of John Wallis', p. 40.

and removed the rubbish; but yet that was but a sad, & slavish labour', while 'Mathematics & experimentall Philosophy [were] understood not as by men, but boyes'. In other words, he added elsewhere, before 1640 'the studies in fashion were poetry, and controversies with the church of Rome'.[38] It was necessary for that fashion to dissipate, Aubrey and other contemporaries were convinced, if the new science was to come into vogue.

Aubrey, Wallis, Sprat, and other observers understood that it was a coincidence that the new astronomy, mathematics, and physics – developed by mostly Catholic savants – came into being during the era of the English Revolution. If they contemplated a more causal relation between the new political order and the reception of the new science in England, the correlation was negative, for in retrospect they realized that the pursuit of science became a form of escapism to numerous individuals – and not only Anglicans – who under different circumstances would have pursued other careers or studies. Sprat made the point explicit when describing how Oxonians 'who had begun a *free way* of reasoning', were joined by 'some *Gentlemen*, of Philosophical Minds, whom the misfortunes of the Kingdom, and the security and ease of a retirement amongst Gown-men, had drawn thither. Their first purpose was no more, then onely the satisfaction of breathing a freer air, and of conversing in quiet one with another, without being ingag'd in the passions, and madness of that dismal Age'.[39] Sprat did no more than articulate the private and public opinions of numerous colleagues. Walter Charleton had commented on the trend in print a decade earlier: 'our late Warrs and Schisms, having almost wholly discouraged men from the study of theologie; and brought the Civil Law into contempt: the major part of young Schollers in our Universities addict themselves to Physick'. For his part, Ralph Bathurst reminded Seth Ward in 1664 that he had turned to medicine twenty years earlier to 'serve for a livelihood, (as indeed I never desired to have it, being only my refuge in bad times, and not my primitive designe)', while Isaac Barrow pursued a similar route since 'he found the times not too favourable to one of his opinion in the affairs of Church and State'. Samuel Rolle, Barrow's contemporary at Trinity, also acknowledged years later that he had been driven to study medicine 'by the great Suspition which [he] had of the Approaching ruine of Schollars in the late time'.[40] The same held true for members of the upper class. 'I shall therefore bring over with me no ambitions at all to be a states-man, or meddle with the unlucky Interests of Kingdomes', John Evelyn wrote on the eve of his return to England, 'but shall very contentedly submit to the losse of my education, by which I might have one day

38   Michael Hunter, *John Aubrey and the Realm of Learning* (London, 1975), pp. 41–2; Aubrey, *Brief Lives*, i, p. 150.

39   Thomas Sprat, *History of the Royal Society*, ed. Jackson I. Cope and Harold W. Jones (St. Louis and London, 1959), p. 53.

40   Charleton, *The Immortality of the Human Soul*, p. 49; Thomas Warton, *The Life and Literary Remains of Ralph Bathurst* (London, 1761), p. 54; *The Theological Works of Isaac Barrow*, ed. Alexander Napier (9 vols, Cambridge, 1859), i, p. xi; A.G. Matthews, ed., *Calamy Revised* (Oxford, 1934), p. 416.

hoped to have bin considerable in my Country. A Friend, a Booke, and a Garden shall for the future perfectly circumscribe my utmost designes'.[41]

Other individuals who turned to science or medicine rather than to church or state included Seth Ward, Thomas Willis, and John Wallis, to name only those who left direct testimony of the fact. But what began as a diversion soon gained momentum and turned into a consuming passion in its own right. It was the determination to preserve and further promote that passion that was foremost in the minds of former members of the Oxford Club when they conspired in the months following the Restoration to establish a new Society in London. As has been observed, their creation 'represented a new type of institution, a public body devoted to the corporate pursuit of scientific research, something unprecedented either in this country or elsewhere: though parallels may be found for facets of both its activity and its organization, the combination was unique'.[42]

41   Cited in Michael Hunter, 'John Evelyn in the 1650s: a virtuoso in quest of a role', in Hunter, *Science and the Shape of Orthodoxy: Studies in Intellectual Change in Late Seventeenth-Century Britain* (Woodbridge, 1995), p. 70.
42   Michael Hunter, *Establishing the New Science: The Experience of the Early Royal Society* (Woodbridge, 1989), p. 1.

Chapter 10

The 'Great Projector': John Cary and the Legacy of Puritan Reform in Bristol, 1647–1720

Jonathan Barry

In *The Great Instauration*, Charles Webster established the origins of the Puritan reform proposals of the 1640s and 1650s in the utopian religious ideals of the Hartlib circle. One set of interlocking proposals were for workhouses, combining education for the young with the provision of work for the poor, and health and welfare support for the sick and infirm, in the context of ambitious proposals to stimulate trade and manufactures.[1] These ideals informed practical measures such as the London Corporation of the Poor and the first Navigation Acts. However, Webster eschewed the task of tracing the impact of this legacy. Although he noted the revival of the 'reformers' programme for a well-educated, articulate class of craftsmen and labourers' with 'the emergence of workhouse schemes in the later seventeenth century', he judged that 'increasingly these proposals were motivated by purely economic considerations, rather than by a genuine humanitarian belief in the value of education'. Though the Quaker John Bellers 'was indeed actuated by a desire to relieve the poor', 'Locke and his friends moved in a world of Leviathan political economy...Training was conceived merely in terms of economic exploitation'.[2] This essay seeks to question this specific judgment by applying Webster's general approach to the workhouse proposals of John Cary, the leading figure in establishing Bristol's pioneering Corporation of the Poor in 1696. Though Cary corresponded with Locke and could be considered a 'political economist', writing extensively on trade and manufactures from a mercantile perspective, his proposals were driven by more than 'purely economic considerations', reflecting similar Protestant and civic ideals as animated Samuel Hartlib's circle.

The Corporation of the Poor was one of several initiatives in Bristol responding to the wars against France and the threat of Jacobitism within a politically and religiously pluralist city. These shared the aim of a 'reformation of manners',

---

1   Charles Webster, *The Great Instauration: Science, Medicine and Reform 1626–1660* (London, 1975), pp. 207–17, 244–5, 360–9, 454–65.
2   *Ibid.*, pp. 244–5.

required because only an industrious and virtuous nation could hope to defeat its enemies, economically and militarily, not least because such victory was dependent on the blessings of God, who would desert the British cause if provoked beyond endurance by national vice and irreligion. The threats posed to 'manners' – that is to say, to the fabric of urban society, which was assumed to depend on a common culture based on household, religion and public order – by the tensions caused by revolution, war and religious difference, were the common currency of urban politics. They found their focus in recurrent debates about how to rid the town of 'beggars' – those whose dependence and idleness challenged the model of independent and industrious householders – and of the vices of swearing and cursing. Yet, at the same time, begging, swearing and cursing all appeared the inevitable counterparts of ideological division and party politics. Political and religious leaders became dependent on the people for support, while seeking to buy or coerce their votes. The recurrent use of oaths to consolidate political support and exclude opponents made oath-taking a central issue; the bitterness of partisan politics made opponents seem damnable. To many contemporaries the closest parallel to this state of affairs was the turbulence of civil war and republic when, indeed, many of the same issues had been fought out. The reform schemes of that earlier period clearly provided a reference point for many of the post-1689 plans, yet the association of these reforms with radical republicanism made them deeply suspect to many. Publicly, it was hardly possible to justify the borrowing of ideas from that source, although privately Cary and others may have cherished the connection, or even hoped such schemes would hasten the return of the republic.[3]

The Cary family and reform

Cary has attracted considerable scholarly attention, both as a writer on 'economics' and for his poor relief activity. Mary Fissell and Paul Slack have sketched out the 'radical Whig' context of his proposals on the poor, but his career within Bristol radical politics has not been properly elucidated.[4] He was born about 1647 into a

---

3   London, British Library (BL), Additional MSS 5540 (Cary's papers), fol. 26r, includes a 'Calves Head' song (but fol. 26v copies verses on the death of Queen Mary by a Jacobite). Cary was a close friend of the Customs Collector John Dutton Colt, who was charged (*ibid.*, fol. 52) with proposing oaths 'to our sovereign lord the people, for we can make a king or queen when we please': see D.W. Hayton et al., eds, *History of Parliament: The House of Commons 1690–1715* (5 vols, Cambridge, 2002), iii, pp. 660–6; Daniel Ballard, *To the Honourable the Commons of England in Parliament Assembled* (London, 1700).

4   Mary Fissell, 'Charity universal? Institutions and moral reform in eighteenth-century Bristol', in Lee Davison et al., eds, *Stilling the Grumbling Hive: The Response to Social and Economic Problems in England, 1689–1750* (Stroud, 1992), pp. 121–44; Paul Slack, *From Reformation to Improvement: Public Welfare in Early Modern England* (Oxford, 1999), pp. 102–27. E.E. Butcher, ed., *Bristol Corporation of the*

long-established family of Bristol drapers; his mother, from the regicide Scrope family, died when he was very young. He had two brothers, Richard, who became a London merchant, and Thomas (1650–1711) who was one of the city's leading clergymen (rector of St Philip and St Jacob from 1675 to his death, and of All Saints as well from 1701). His father, Shershaw (d.1681), was a merchant with strong West Indian connections, which led him into sugar refining in Bristol; he was active in the Society of Merchant Venturers, serving as Master in 1671–2. John was freed in 1672 as the apprentice of a linen-draper, Walter Stephens. He was a member of the Mercers and Linen-drapers' Company for about a decade from the late 1660s, acting as Warden in 1675–6 (when Stephens was Master), but after his father moved to Lisbon in 1673–4, John operated increasingly as a merchant. He was Warden of the Society of Merchant Venturers in 1683–4 and became their chief lobbyist in Parliament and elsewhere by the 1690s, probably also representing other interest groups; in 1697 the Mercers and Linen-drapers paid him £5 for 'activity against the woollen bill in Parliament'.[5] In the 1690s he was an active political agent for the Whigs, as well as a militia captain and deputy lieutenant, and twice stood as a parliamentary candidate for Bristol, though he withdrew before the poll in 1695 and only polled 279 votes in 1698.[6] From 1700 onwards he shifted his interests increasingly to Ireland, acting initially as a commissioner under the Resumption Act, and, although he did not die until around 1720, he played little further part in Bristol politics.

John's most important writings date from the period 1695 to 1700. A whole series of pamphlets covering different trades, based on his *Essay on the State of England in Relation to its Trade, its Poor and its Taxes, For carrying on the present War against France* (printed in small numbers in Bristol in 1695), were published by London publishers and these led him into a series of controversies with defenders of foreign imports from the East Indies.[7] These writings were

Poor, 1696–1834, Bristol Record Society III (1932); Monica M. Tompkins, 'The two workhouses of Bristol 1696–1735', University of Nottingham MA thesis (1962).

5 The old *Dictionary of National Biography* entry on Cary contains several errors, which have been corrected in the new entry, by Kenneth Morgan, in the *Oxford Dictionary of National Biography*. See H.T. Lane, 'The life and writings of John Cary', Bristol MA thesis (1932); Bristol, Bristol Archives Office (BAO), 10531 (Shershaw's letters); Bristol, Bristol Central Library, Bristol Collection, 4939 (Mercers and Linen-drapers Company Papers); BL, Add. MSS 5540, fols 78 onwards; I.V. Hall, 'Bristol's second sugar house', *Transactions of the Bristol and Gloucestershire Archaeological Society*, 68 (1949), 110–64 (Cary family tree between pp. 110 and 111).

6 W.J. Hardy, ed., *Calendar of State Papers Domestic, 1694–5* (London, 1906), p. 235; Hayton, *History of Parliament*, ii, pp. 212–13.

7 John Cary, *A Discourse concerning the Trade of Ireland and Scotland* (London, 1696); idem, *A Discourse concerning the East-India Trade* (London, 1696 and 1699); idem, *A Discourse of the Advantage of the African Trade to this Nation* (London, 1712); Anon., *The Linnen Drapers Answer to that Part of Mr Cary his Essay on Trade, that concerns the East India Trade* (London, 1696); John Cary, *A Reply to a*

regularly reprinted thereafter, largely through their inclusion in the revised and expanded *Essay towards Regulating the Trade and Employing the Poor of this Kingdom* (1717, second edition 1719), which was reissued in 1745 as *A Discourse on Trade*; his writings were still regarded as sufficiently significant to merit both French (Paris, 1755) and Italian (Naples, 1757) translations. He published two books on issues of coinage, credit and the national debt in 1696 and he followed these with proposals on banking and public debt.[8] In 1698 he attacked William Molyneux's arguments for Irish parliamentary autonomy in *A Vindication of the Parliament of England* (London; second edition, London, 1700); he is also generally assumed to have written the anonymous, *An Answer to Mr Molyneux His Case of Ireland* (London, 1698). Both reflect his long-running insistence that Irish trade interests must not damage England's, especially its cloth trade: his broadsheet on this, *To the Freeholders and Burgesses of the City of Bristol* (1698), suggests that this may have been central to his 1698 electoral campaign. Once in Ireland he began encouraging alternative Irish manufactures, having been 'desired by the ministry to give my thoughts of such an undertaking'. His final publications arose from his personal troubles in an Irish Chancery case and his subsequent arrest by the House of Lords for contempt of its warrant.[9]

His scheme for the Bristol Corporation of the Poor, which became a blueprint for provincial workhouse schemes, was widely known. Cary continued to press the case for poor law reform, not only in his *Account of the Proceedings of the Corporation of Bristol* (London, 1700, reprinted at Dublin in 1704) but in a pamphlet and broadsheet arguing for a national reform on the same model in 1699–1700; in about 1710 he published a further *Proposal To Raise 150000L per annum and to give Employment to the Poor.*[10]

Advocates of such proposals were often labelled 'projectors', as contemporaries were quick to detect self- or trade-interest, especially if such advocates were not from the landed elite. In 1711 an opponent described Cary as 'the great

Paper Delivered to the Right Honourable the Lords Spiritual and Temporal entituled, The Linnen-drapers Answer (London, 1696); Anon., An Answer to Mr Cary's Reply (London, 1696).

8   *An Essay on the Coyn and Credit of England: as they stand with respect to its Trade* (Bristol, 1696); *An Essay towards the Settlement of a National Credit* (London, 1696); *A Proposal for the Paying off the Publick Debts by Erecting a National Credit* (London, 1719).

9   *Some Considerations relating to the Carrying on the Linnen Manufacture in the Kingdom of Ireland by a Joint Stock* (Dublin, 1704); *John Cary Esq. Appellant* (London, 1710); *The Rights of the Commons in Parliament Assembled Asserted and the Liberties of the People Vindicated* (London, 1718); *The Case of John Cary Esq.* (London, 1719).

10 *A Proposal offered to the Committee of the Honourable House of Commons, appointed to consider of ways for the better providing for the Poor and setting them on work* (London, n.d. [c.1699]); J.C., *Reasons for Passing the Bill for Relieving and Employing the Poor of this Kingdom humbly offered* (London, n.d. [c.1699]).

projector', although, as we shall see, he saw Cary's motives as more political than financial. Cary's policy preferences clearly fitted the interests of a provincial out-port involved in the Atlantic trade and in manufactures based both on the traditional cloth industry and new industries involving the processing of colonial products (tobacco, sugar) or imported techniques (glass, metalware). They reflect-ed his lobbying work and his family's own careers in linen-drapery, sugar-refining and trade. Cary himself disliked 'the name of a projector, which I carefully endea-vour to avoyd', insisting of his work that 'there is noe Room left in it for Self Interest, which is the overthrow of all publique affairs'. None of his schemes in-volved his direct personal gain, and all were aimed at winning parliamentary support and statutory authority to create public bodies or alter national policy on trade, taxation, or poor law provision. He invited John Locke 'to judge whether I have not done as became an English Gentleman; I love my Country, and will spend my time and spirits to serve it; but to help to carry on a private design, where I cannot see any prospect of answering the end I aim at, I doe not think myself obliged, or to set forth Projects only to be made the discourses of Coffeehouses, which are intended for soe great an Assembly [i.e. Parliament], and neglected by them'.[11] Both the Tory Edmund Bohun ('your book of trade is by far the best I have ever read and written with so disinterested an air that no man can possibly tell where your trade loses by it') and Locke ('I see noe party or interest you contend for but that of truth and your country. Such a man carrys authority and evidence in what he says') delighted Cary by endorsing his self-image as a gentleman patriot, not a mercantile lobbyist.[12]

Nor was Cary's agenda simply economic. Although apparently an Anglican (serving as churchwarden for St John Baptist parish in 1678 and 1680, and for his brother's parish of St Philip and St Jacob in 1685, and baptizing six children in the latter during the 1680s), Cary came from a family of radical Whigs, and his connections were with low-church Anglicans, and dissenting Protestants – Presbyterian, Independent and even Quaker. In his *Essay* Cary assumes that 'liberty of conscience' is both a good thing and a stimulus to trade. In February 1688, when James II turned from the Tories to Whigs and dissenters, John was made a Bristol common councillor (while Walter Stephens became an alderman), before the restoration that autumn of the former Tory corporation.[13] Cary was

11 Anon., *Some Considerations offered to the Citizens of Bristol relating to the Corporation for the Poor in the said City* (London, 1711), p. 12; Edmund de Beer, ed., *Correspondence of John Locke* (8 vols, Oxford, 1979), v, pp. 626, 746, 726.

12 Beer, *Correspondence of John Locke*, v, p. 626; BL, Add. MSS 5540, fols 56–65. Modern commentators agree: see J.A.W. Gunn, *Politics and the Public Interest in the Seventeenth Century* (London, 1969), pp. 261–2; Perry Gauci, *The Politics of Trade: the Overseas Merchant in State and Society* (Oxford, 2001), p. 217.

13 J.J. Simpson, 'St Peter's Hospital', *Transactions of the Bristol and Gloucestershire Archaeological Society*, 48 (1926), 221–2; Cary, *Essay on the State of England in Relation to its Trade, its Poor and its Taxes, For carrying on the present War against*

bitterly critical of this restored corporation and of Tory parish élites who used their power over the poor. His Corporation of the Poor struck at both, by removing all poor relief from parish to civic level and providing for government of the Corporation of the Poor by Guardians, who would take over the magistrates' responsibilities as justices overseeing parish decisions. Not only were these Guardians elected by all those ratepayers who paid at least 1d per week towards the poor rates (so offering a 'democratic' alternative to the corporate and vestry procedures whereby existing members decided who should fill any vacancies), but the Guardians, like the ratepayers, included dissenters excluded from public office under the Test Acts. Cary's 1699 proposal for a national scheme urged 'that no officer in these Corporations, by reason of such office, shall be liable to the penalties mentioned in an act made 25 Car 2 for the preventing of the dangers which may happen from popish recusants; because this may keep out many people who may be very instrumental in carrying on this work'. It thus mirrored the blueprint for revived civic democracy which Cary had drawn up 'for my private satisfaction' in 1691 which proposed the election of aldermen for life by scot-and-lot voters in the wards, as well as of the common council by the people. As the Tory attack on the Corporation of the Poor, published in 1711, noted:

> I cannot but wonder that they [the Mayor and Aldermen] so tamely suffered themselves to be divested of all their power formerly. Indeed the intrigue was managed with privacy and not above one of them (if I am rightly informed) joined heartily; the rest that knew of it, was either averse to it or stood neuter...I fancy when the great projector [i.e. Cary] had brought all this to pass, it was very pleasing to him to see that he had raised a considerable government in the city, independent in a great measure of the common magistrate.[14]

The Corporation of the Poor also reflected Cary's eagerness to reform the manners of the poor. His discussion of the poor in his *Essay* focused on beggary and idleness. 'When the nation comes to see that the labour of its people is its wealth, 'twill put us on finding out methods to make every one work that is able, which must be done either by hindring such swarms from going off to idle or useless imployments, or by preventing such multitudes of lazy people from being maintained by begging'. The original Act saw the problem as not only a growth in the number of poor but also 'idleness and debauchery amongst the meaner sort' for 'want of workhouses to put them to work' and 'sufficient authority' to compel them.[15]

France (Bristol, 1695), p. 42; John Latimer, *The Annals of Bristol in the Seventeenth Century* (Bristol, 1900), p. 447.

14   BL, Add. MSS 5540, fols 37–42; Cary, *Proposal offered to the Committee*, p. 8; Anon., *Some Considerations offered to the Citizens*, p. 12.

15   Cary, *Essay on the State of England*, p. 136; Butcher, *Bristol Corporation of the Poor*, p. 179.

However, Cary did not just blame the poor, but also attacked aristocratic and metropolitan luxury, both in itself and in its effects. 'Much proceeds from imitation', by those without land, of the 'useless way of living' of gentry with estates who had left the country for London; the former were then 'forced to betake themselves to play [i.e. gambling] or begging'. Too many sought an income in parasitic occupations such as the revenue, the law, medicine, or even buying and selling, which 'cannot be said to augment the riches of the nation, only live by getting from one another'. Cary opposed driving down the cost of labour, arguing that 'it hath been a constant observation grounded on reason that this nation never thrives more than when the labour of the poor is at such prices as they may live comfortably by it'. Wages must relate to cost of provisions so 'you cannot fall wages unless you fall product [i.e. reduce cost of agricultural products] and if you fall product you must necessarily fall land'. Manufacturers could cut prices without cutting wages as 'new projections are every day set on foot to render the making of our manufactures easie, which are made cheap by the heads of the manufacturers, not by falling the price of poor peoples labour; cheapness creates expense [i.e. expenditure] and expense gives fresh imployments, so the poor need not stand idle if they could be perswaded to work'.[16] In 1700 he criticized 'two objections raised against the poor, viz, That they will not work and that they spend what they get in fine feeding. But we soon found that the great cause of begging did proceed from the low wages for labour; for after about eight month's time our children could not get half so much as we expended in their provisions'. He recommended a compulsory pension scheme 'to be collected by a society of honest men in each port', funded from freight charges and seamen's wages, for the relief of old and disabled sailors, and similar provision for military and naval pensioners and their families; and praised almshouses when 'they are designed to relieve impotent old age or educate youth; not to maintain idle beggars or ease rich parishes, but to provide for those who have been bred up in careful imployments, though not able to stem the current of a cross fortune', claiming that 'almshouses raised for [old sailors, their wives and young children] are as great acts of piety as building of churches'. He opposed taxes that fell on the poor, 'their province being more properly to labour and fight than to pay', criticizing the hearth tax, poll taxes, and general excise 'besides the great charge and oppression of officers'.[17]

Cary wished to see the poor given an opportunity to live independently. English freedom was a key value, and he praised the status of freeholders and the 'great spirit' this created of raising oneself by industry. Encouraging youth:

> in an early delight of labour would keep up a true English spirit in them and create
> a desire to secure a property in what they have, whereas a slothful dependence on
> another's bounty makes men slavishly give up all at the will of their benefactors,
> and having no properties of their own to secure, are easily perswaded to part with

16 Cary, *Essay on the State of England*, pp. 153–6, 6–7, 55, 145, 147.
17 Cary, *Account of the Proceedings of the Corporation of Bristol* (London, 1700), p. 13; Cary, *Essay on the State of England*, pp. 167–9, 173–4.

their liberties; this a former reign knew well, when the ministers of that court found an inclination in the people to sell their priviledges for luxury and ease.

He recognized the importance of education in making this possible. The alternative, leaving the young poor on the streets, was that 'beggary is now become an art or mystery, to which children are educated from their cradles', whereas if better employed they 'might be more useful to the Common-wealth'.[18] His *Account of the Proceedings of the Corporation of Bristol* portrayed 'our undertaking being nothing less, than to put to work a great number of people, many of which had been habited to laziness and beggary; to civilize such as had been bred up in all the vices that want of education could expose them to; and to clothe, lodge and feed them well, with the same sum of money which was distributed among them when they begg'd, lay in the streets and went almost naked' and he summarized the achievements as follows:

> We are freed from beggars; our old people are comfortably provided for; our boys and girls are educated to sobriety and brought up to delight in labour; our young children are well lookt after and not spoilt by ill nurses; and the face of our city is so changed already that we have reason to hope these young plants will produce a virtuous and laborious generation, with whom immorality and prophaneness may find little incouragement; nor does our hopes [sic] appear to be groundless, for among three hundred persons now under our charge within doors, there is neither cursing nor swearing, nor prophane language to be heard, though many of them were bred up in all manner of vices, which neither Bridewell nor whippings could fright them from, because, returning to their bad company for want of employments, they were rather made worse than bettered by those corrections, whereas the change we have wrought in them is by fair means.[19]

Cary's account was not entirely accurate (whipping *was* used, for example), but the surviving records do suggest that the aim to reform manners was an institutional, not just a personal, priority.

John Cary's own writings focus on the secular implications of this reformation, although his militant Protestantism is clear. Cary's papers include a set of 'propheticall verses I had in my custody before any part of it came to pass' predicting the downfall of James II in 1688, and he lambasted the 'tyrannical oppressions of the late King James'.[20] His writings share with other political arithmeticians an underlying aim of creating the conditions for a successful war against France: 'When I consider the necessity of the war we are now engaged in, and the consequences of its event (the liberty of Christendom and the security of the Protestant religion depending on the success thereof) I think it the duty of every

18 Cary, *Essay on the State of England*, pp. 166, 153, 15.
19 Cary, *Account of the Proceedings*, pp. 4, 19–20.
20 BL, Add. MSS 5540, fols 21v (reproduced in P. McGrath, ed., *Merchants and Merchandise in Seventeenth-Century Bristol*, Bristol Record Society XIX (1955), p. 169), 39v.

good subject to offer his advice' since 'we cannot preserve at too high a rate those inestimable jewels of liberty and property'. Hence the subtitle of his *Essay, For carrying on the present War against France*, and the justification of each proposal as contributing to the war effort; if poor law reform ensured that 'every person did by his labour get one half penny per diem to the publick' then it 'would pay the charge of the war'. His writings on Ireland, while critical of the short-sighted Protestant gentry there, took it for granted that they should be supported by England against the 'papists', noting 'the vast charges we have been at for its reduction and delivery out of the hands of foreign powers and popish cut-throats'. Throughout his work he praised the Dutch and attacked France:

> France being like a Tavern, with whom we spend what we get by other nations; tis strange we should be so bewitch'd to that people, as to take off their growth which consists chiefly of things for luxury.

The Dutch suffered no beggars while 'our inhabitants seem to encourage them in an idle way of living, contrary both to their own and the nation's interest' since:

> Idleness though it cannot be called the image of the Devil, who is a busie active spirit, yet sits for any impression, for whilst people neglect by some honest labour to serve the publick good, they too often fall on such courses as render them publick evils.

The principal cause of beggary was 'sloath and a desire of ease leading to such ways of living as our fathers would have been ashamed of', whereby:

> religion is despised and vice promoted...Nor is God more honoured among any than he is among those industrious people, who abhor vice on equal principles of religion and good husbandry, labour being usually a barrier against sin, which does generally come in at the doors of idleness.[21]

Thus Cary would not have accepted a distinction between the principles of 'religion and good husbandry' and his writings regularly invoke God's blessing and wisdom, but equally they are conspicuously lacking in religious quotations or arguments from religious duty or advantage. For a fuller statement of their possible religious meaning one has to look to his brother's sermon at the monthly fast for national success against the Jacobites and the French, published in 1691. This contains an extended call for 'an impartial reformation from all orders and degrees', which God required to ensure the successful defence of the revolution, that providential rescue from 'two intolerable evils, Popery in the church and slavery in the state'. This had only come after sin had brought them 'so near unto destruction', for it was for 'contempt of God's word and worship, for profaning the Lord's day, dishonouring his sacred name, by customary swearing and cursing, for

21   Cary, *Essay on the State of England*, pp. 170, 163, 98, 125, 131, 151, 153, 166.

drunkenness, adultery, pride and dissolute living that we were likely to lose our religion, our liberties and our properties'. Like the ancient Jews of his text (from Ezra) 'we are a rebellious and an unthankful people', and though 'he hath miraculously preserved us to demonstrate to the AntiChristian world that we profess his true religion, although we do not live up to it', 'it was more for the sins of the papists than for the righteousness of the Protestants, that God so providentially appeared for us'. Thomas insisted that we should not 'impute it to chance or fortune, or to our own wisdom and endeavours, or to the policy and craft of statesmen, or to the renowned instrument of it, that illustrious Prince (whom God hath in mercy to us exalted to the throne) but wholly to the providence of the Almighty'. The required response was not merely moral reform but also 'peace and unity', the character of the 'primitive and purest' Christian church. In fact, the two were identical, for 'internal holiness is absolutely necessary to salvation; let us thus live in peace, love one another and honour the Gospel with holy lives, and then we shall answer God's end in our Great Deliverance'. Such unity clearly excluded the 'mystical Babylon' of the 'Roman yoke' which he proceeded to attack for every crime, but particularly for encouraging sin, slavery and 'ignorance'. He urged Protestants 'not to be more zealous for the rites and ceremonies of religion than for the substantial and indispensable duties of it'. They should not 'contend about the shell and part with the kernel of Christianity, the love of God and our neighbours; let us all endeavour to exceed one another in practicing the substantial duties of piety, justice, sobriety and charity and then we shall not differ much about indifferent things'.[22]

This emphasis on Protestant unity fits well with Thomas's career. He had become vicar of Sts Philip and Jacob in 1675 by corporation appointment only after the incumbent, arch-Tory Thomas Godwyn, had been subjected (according to his own account) to a campaign of denigration and harassment led by Thomas Day, involving both legal disputes and heated struggles within the church building when both clerics claimed to be the lawful clergyman. Godwyn identified Thomas as the protégé of the leading Whig clergyman Thomas Palmer (whose son was apprenticed to John Cary), and in 1680 Thomas married the daughter of James Harris, a Whig merchant, signatory of a 1696 letter to the city MPs supporting the passing of the Act for the Corporation of the Poor (another daughter married Sir William Daines, Whig MP for Bristol from 1702). One example of Thomas Cary's close ties to dissenters is the gift to him (as well as the Presbyterian minister) of £20 in 1703 in the will of Michael Pope, grocer and member of a leading Presbyterian

22 Thomas Cary, *A Sermon preached at St Philip and St Jacob 15 July 1691, being the Monthly Fast* (London, 1691), pp. 19, 10, 6, 7, 8, 10, 14, 15–18, 13. Cary's other surviving sermon, *A Sermon Preached August 27ʰ 1691 being the Anniversary Festival of the Natives of that City* (London, 1691), invited Bristolians to seek happiness only in God, as 'there is no true happiness without union with God by faith and love', since the riches of this world 'shall shortly be found nowhere, but in the ashes of an universal dissolution' (pp. 31–2).

family, the executor of the will being Nathaniel Wade, another radical Whig involved in both the Rye House plot and Monmouth's rebellion.[23]

Thomas's sermon was delivered during a visit by the Earl of Macclesfield, to whom he dedicated it as his chaplain. After the Revolution of 1688 the Whig Earl had replaced the former Lord Lieutenant, the Duke of Beaufort, who had used the city militia to disarm and harass dissenters and Whigs. In October 1689 the Tory-led common council complained that the militia was in 'the hands of dissenters and those obnoxious to the Church and government of England'. Sir Thomas Earle retaliated by writing to Secretary Shrewsbury denouncing Mayor Arthur Hart, Sir John Knight and others as 'most zealous Jacobites'. Subsequently (according to an attack on Earle) he and other common councillors, acting in 'their military capacity' as deputy lieutenants, entered the Council House and demanded the common council records 'in purpose to bring in accusations against the mayor, to pry into the secrets of this city and to reflect upon the government thereof'. John Cary was a militia captain (and himself a deputy lieutenant by 1695) and in 1691 he accused the corporation of snubbing the Earl (as well as the judges on circuit), 'not so much as by taking any notice of him at his coming to town, or by paying him a visit whilst here, but have in the House [i.e. common council] made votes reflecting on his Honour in purpose to set the people against the Government', a vote according to Cary opposed by a great part of the common council 'but yet the faction prevailed against them'. After the 1690 election Bristol's deputy lieutenants, together with some Whig aldermen and common councillors, wrote to the Earl on behalf of Cary, who had been falsely accused of trading with the French by Knight and his supporters because, they claimed, Cary was 'making a great interest for the other candidates' against the successful Tory candidates Knight and Hart. On 14 May 1690, Knight used a parliamentary debate to denounce the Earl and his personal force of 'auxiliaries'.[24]

Down to 1696 the militia was active in rounding up suspected Jacobites, including the town's leading Tories. It was under these conditions, and exploiting the tensions created by the assassination plots against William, that the Whigs assured their ascendancy both in the corporation and in parliamentary elections. In 1693 the Whigs managed to win over the neutrals on the council and ensure the mayoralty of Robert Yate (1693–4), followed by Thomas Day (1694–5) and Samuel Wallis (1695–6). Following their election as Bristol's MPs in 1695, Day

23 Thomas Godwyn, *Phanatical Tenderness* (London, 1684), pp. 6, 13–21; Lane, 'Life and writings', p. 24; Jonathan Barry, 'The politics of religion in Restoration Bristol', in Tim Harris, Paul Seaward and Mark Goldie, eds, *The Politics of Religion in Restoration England* (Oxford, 1990), pp. 163–89 at p. 171; Hayton, *History of Parliament*, iii, p. 822; London, Dr Williams Library, MS. 89.13, G. Lyon Turner, typescript history of Bristol Independency in the seventeenth century, appendix on Weekes's congregation, pp. 20–1.

24 See Hayton, *History of Parliament*, ii, pp. 203, 209–15 (Bristol); iv, pp. 289–90 (Hart), 331–2 (Henley) and 574–8 (Knight: quotation on p. 575); v, pp. 949–53 (Yate); McGrath, *Merchants and Merchandise*, pp. 162–3.

and Yate were to push through the legislation that created the Corporation of the Poor, while Wallis, as mayor, supported its foundation and in 1699 gave £100 to fund a sermon at its annual meeting. Furthermore, by using the Association Oath to exclude up to eleven Tories from voting in crucial common council elections in September 1696, the Whigs established control over the corporation and the future rota of magistrates. In addition, Robert Henley and Thomas Edwards had been sent to Whitehall to prevent the release of Knight (imprisoned for treason after the attempted assassination of the King), as this would be fatal to efforts to establish a 'good succession of magistrates'.[25] The grand jury presentment of midsummer 1696, which congratulated Mayor Wallis and the aldermen for their execution of the laws against profanity, also congratulated the deputy lieutenants and militia officers for their zeal after 'the late horrid and detestable plot', rejoicing that all the officers had taken the oaths and subscribed to the Association, as there was 'no higher assurance amongst men' than such oaths and associations. After praising the efforts to create the new Corporation of the Poor, it ended by claiming that 'nothing can conduce more to the glory of God, preservation of the Protestant religion, as now established by law, safety of his Majesty's government or this city than choosing such religious and loyal men as Mr Mayor'. Although the next mayor elected, John Hine, a former radical, proved an 'unexpected Remora', in Cary's words, blocking the Corporation of the Poor completely during his year of office, his sheriffs, Saunders and Whitchurch, supported it.[26]

The relief of the poor

Cary's manuscripts show him considering a reform of the poor relief system in around 1691, noting that it was important to see representative pressure brought on the aldermen to see justice done in the poor rates, especially between the poorer and richer parishes. This may reflect his own experience as a resident of Temple and Sts Philip and Jacob and churchwarden for the latter, which was the largest suburban parish and faced the additional jurisdictional hurdle of being partly within the city (the in-parish) and partly in Gloucestershire (the out-parish). The Bristol Act covered only the in-parish, and the growing problems of the out-parish, due to 'a great resort of weavers and other manufacturers', led to an unsuccessful attempt to obtain a workhouse in 1729. Cary was to be particularly responsible for St Philip and St Jacob's poor under the Corporation of the Poor. Cary's old master Walter Stephens left £3 13s 4d per annum in 1695 to be distributed to the poor of the in-parish of St Philip and St Jacob weekly for ever. Cary was the executor of the 1686 will of Samuel Hale, another Whig (suspected of involvement in the Rye House plot) who had left money for apprenticing the poor in seven poorer parishes. It is

25   Hayton, *History of Parliament*, iv, p. 577.
26   BAO, 04452(1), Grand Jury Presentment Midsummer 1696, printed copy in British Library, 816 m.16(28); Cary, *Account of the Proceedings*, p. 3.

tempting to associate Hale with the Gloucestershire family of Sir Matthew Hale, whose 1659 proposal for poor relief, which presaged much in Cary's writings, was first published posthumously in 1683 and then reprinted in 1695.[27] In his *Essay* Cary argued for:

> taking care that the poor's rates be made with more equality in cities and trading towns than now they are, especially in the former, where the greatest number of poor usually residing in the suburbs or out-parishes are very serviceable by their labours to the rich in carrying on their trades, yet when age, sickness or a numerous family makes them desire relief, their chief dependence must be on people but one step above their own condition, by which means those out-parishes are more burthened in their payments than the in-parishes are, though much richer, and is one reason why they are so ill-inhabited, no one careing to come to a certain charge; and this is attended with another ill consequence, the want of better inhabitants makes way for those disorders which easily grow among the poor; whereas if cities and towns were made but one poor's rate, or equally divided into more, these inconveniences might be removed and the poor maintained by a more impartial contribution.

By January 1696 he had prepared proposals 'for employing and maintaining the poor, grounded on that part of my essay'.[28]

Cary's method of argument, itself a radical one, was to ignore authority and precedent and to justify his recommendations purely in terms of current secular requirements. He does not offer, therefore, any indication of models which may have influenced him. It is tempting to relate his work to London's first Corporation of the Poor, supported by Hartlib, which was abolished in 1660. Two features of the scheme seem also to have Hartlib as their most recent progenitor. One was the collection of data about the poor. Before commencing, the Guardians noted 'the names of all the poor' and 'the qualifications of all, either as to age, health, civility etc, what each person did or could get by the week, and in what employment'. The second was the considerable emphasis on health: 'To such as were sick, we gave warrant to our physician to visit them; such as wanted the assistance of our surgeons were directed to them and all were relieved till they were able to work', and on diet:

> we took the advice of our physician and bought the best of every sort ... the effect on their change of living, nature being well supported, threw out a great deal of

27　*Journal of the House of Commons*, 21 (1727–32), pp. 656, 684; Simpson, 'St Peter's Hospital', p. 222; Sir Ralph Bigland, *Historical, Monumental and Genealogical Collections relative to the County of Goucester*, Pt 4, Uley-Yate, intro. and indexes, ed. Brian Frith (Gloucester, Alan Sutton, 1995), p. 1554; Latimer, *Annals of Bristol in the Seventeenth*, p. 419; Lane, 'Life and writings', pp. 21, 26; Slack, *From Reformation to Improvement*, pp. 89, 100.
28　Cary, *Essay on the State of England*, pp. 167–8; Beer, *Correspondence of John Locke*, v, pp. 634–5.

foulness, so that we had generally twenty down at a time in the measles, smallpox and other distempers; but by the care of our physician and the blessing of God on his endeavours, we never buried but two, though we had seldom less than one hundred in the house at any time.

The physician in question was Dr Thomas Dover, inventor of Dover's Fever Powder. The medical facilities of the Corporation thus predated by almost forty years the establishment of the first voluntary hospital in Bristol, and continued to operate on a large scale throughout the eighteenth century.[29]

Cary spent considerable time in London lobbying Parliament and moving in Whig circles, regularly meeting Locke's friends, so he was doubtless aware of the London precedents for a Corporation of the Poor. However, he must also have known about previous Bristol schemes, particularly an earlier effort to establish a city workhouse in the Bridewell, where a linen manufacture was financed by the corporation in 1679, since this was established by the Company of Linen-drapers and Mercers and by 1684 was being run by 'Walter Stephens and Company'. Cary's master, Stephens, had, together with his father of the same name, been a founder member of the Company and was a leading figure until his death. Furthermore, the 1679 scheme was put forward by James Holloway, who was executed for treason in 1684 for his part in the Rye House plot (Holloway was married to 'Martha Stevens' of Bristol, possibly related to Walter). The parallels between Holloway and Cary are striking: the former had become involved in London politics through going to London to lobby for a national scheme to promote linen manufacture, building on this local proposal. In addition to employing 'five hundred spinners of the inhabitants of the city', the undertakers were also to bring in 'twelve women to teach to spinne and twelve men to teach to weave'.[30]

The 1679 scheme was itself a revival of an idea mooted in March 1654 'to set the poore on worke within this Citty in spinning of Yarne, knitting of stockin's and other manufactures', which also involved a salary for 'women to teach such children as shalbe sent to work there'. The parishes were to be entitled, with the agreement of the mayor and aldermen, to send their poor, so that the parishes would be 'very much eased of their charges', but the initial capital was to be raised by a levy on the parishes. Parish poor who 'cannot without inconvenience to their familyes or for other reasons come to Worke at the Workehouses' were to be allowed to work on the materials at home, provided security was given. There is no direct reference in the city records to the role of the Company of Linen-drapers and Mercers, but this had been incorporated only in 1647 and was well-represented in the corporation (Walter Stephens senior having been sheriff 1645–6 with John

29   Slack, *From Reformation to Improvement*, pp. 84–9; Cary, *Account of the Proceedings*, pp. 7, 8, 12; J. Johnson, *Transactions of the Corporation of the Poor in the City of Bristol* (Bristol, 1826), pp. 108–9.
30   Latimer, *Annals of Bristol in the Seventeenth*, pp. 394, 423–4; *The Free and Voluntary Confession of James Holloway* (London, 1684); J.F. Nicholls and J. Taylor, *Bristol Past and Present* (3 vols, Bristol, 1881–2), iii, pp. 75–6.

Young, its first Master), so it may well have sponsored this scheme. It is notable that of the six non-merchants among the first assistants of the Corporation of the Poor in 1696, four were mercers or linen-drapers (Callowhill, Batchelor, Millerd and Codrington). This company had a deep interest in the success of woollen manufacture in Bristol, which Cary continued to see as key to employment, as well as to trade.[31]

Another possible influence on Cary's scheme was a Quaker one. The Bristol Quaker Benjamin Coole had corresponded with Cary in September 1695 about Cary's *Essay*, enclosing a book which must have been John Bellers's *Proposals for Raising a Colledge of Industry*, just published. Cary replied saying that he liked the design but that it would be difficult to find so many well-disposed persons to form such a society 'which is to be upheld only by virtue and good government'. He also doubted 'whether seminaries for trade may not at last turn into seminaries for religion, so instead of being hives for industrious bees become nests for idle drones', since, whether the religion was good or bad, once people were maintained on a foundation this led only to idleness and laziness, his example being deans and chapters. The beehive became the official seal of the Bristol Corporation of the Poor, with the motto 'Hiemis memores aestate laborant' (mindful of winter, they work in summer). Two leading Quakers (Charles Jones and Thomas Goldney) were among eight signatories of the letter urging the MPs to obtain the Act in March 1696. The Quaker Guardians on the Corporation of the Poor, who were later active in the Society for Reformation of Manners, were also leading figures in the establishment of a Quaker workhouse in 1697 (which included a school) and their workhouse was eventually erected in 1700 on land purchased from Nathaniel Wade, who, though an Independent in religion, was married to a Quaker, Anne Vickris, the granddaughter of Cary's aunt Alice.[32]

A final parallel, if not exactly a model, which may be noted is the Society for the Reformation of Manners, started in 1699, many of whose members were also active in the Corporation of the Poor. The Society was another interdenominational body which acted as a pressure group outside the civic and parochial structure, while using its influence within those bodies to enforce reform. Working in conjunction with grand jury presentments for reform, and using sympathetic magistrates and chief constables, the Society exerted a pressure downwards on ward constables and other 'inferior officers' to force them to do their duty, and to support, both financially and by 'countenancing' and encouragement, those who did so willingly. The Society's other role was to exercise pressure upwards on the mayor and aldermen to play their part as the city's magistrates. In other words, like

---

31 BCL, Bristol Collection, 4939; Latimer, *Annals of Bristol in the Seventeenth*, p. 218.
32 BL, Add. MSS 5540, fols 74–5; R.S. Mortimer, 'Quakerism in seventeenth-century Bristol', University of Bristol MA thesis (1946), pp. 239–49; W.M.D. Wigfield, ed., *Monmouth's Rebellion* (Bradford-upon-Avon, 1980), pp. 151–71 (Wade's confession).

the Corporation of the Poor, it used city-wide institutions and the ward structure to offer an alternative (if a highly elite one) to the parochial and civic establishment.[33]

The Corporation of the Poor and the politics of religion

The way the Corporation of the Poor was established reflected an effort to bypass, and also to pressurize, the city corporation, as well as the parishes. The scheme was first discussed in a series of meetings in leading taverns and coffeehouses in January 1696, which led to a 'meeting of the citizens' to establish a set of proposals, and only then were these put to the common council, on 3 February 1696. Despite 'many oppositions' the proposal, with accompanying petitions from 'a great number of the substantial inhabitants', was passed on to the MPs in a letter signed by eight Bristolians, of whom only Nathaniel Wade, now steward of the sheriff's court (effectively deputy town clerk), held a formal position of power in the city. By March the bill was before Parliament; the first meeting of the new body was held on 19 May 1696.[34] From early on the Corporation of the Poor was to face hostility from some parochial officers and from Tories. Refusal by both Mayor Hine and some churchwardens to collect funds was overcome by new statutory provisions which allowed the Guardians to proceed even if parish or city officers refused to co-operate. By 1699, the Corporation of the Poor was fully established, but even then it remained controversial. On 3 August 1703 the Guardians debated abandoning the scheme in favour of the old system, but decided unanimously against. The Tories made a fresh attempt to abolish the Corporation of the Poor in 1711, though on 16 February the common council decided, after long debate but unanimously, to back a new Act to increase the funding that could be raised. Tory MPs in Parliament then brought in amendments, which both added churchwardens for each parish as ex-officio Guardians, and imposed a religious test for office-holders, against the opposition of the MP Joseph Earle; this may be one reason for his break with the Tory party in Bristol, so that in 1715 he stood as a Whig candidate. This test was subsequently repealed by a Whig Parliament in 1718 (when the junior churchwardens were also removed as Guardians) on the grounds that a large number of the most active Guardians had been excluded from service by its requirements.[35]

33 J. Barry, ed., 'The Society for the Reformation of Manners 1700–5', in J. Barry and K. Morgan, eds, *Reformation and Revival in Eighteenth-Century Bristol*, Bristol Record Society XLV (1994), pp. 3–5.

34 Lane, 'Life and writings', pp. 168–74; *Proposals for the Better Maintaining and Employing the Poor in Bristol* (Bristol, 1696); John Cary, *A Discourse on Trade* (London, 1745), pp. 117–21; Johnson, *Transactions of the Corporation of the Poor*, pp. 4–6; Hayton, *History of Parliament*, iii, pp. 864–5 and v, pp. 950–1; BL, Add. MSS 5540, fol. 100.

35 John Latimer, *The Annals of Bristol in the Eighteenth Century* ([Frome], 1893), pp. 54–5, 103; Hayton, *History of Parliament*, iii, pp. 953–4; *Journal of the House of*

Religious qualifications and oath-taking were central to the politics of the period. Cary's father had refused a place on the common council in 1664–5, unwilling to take the oaths then required, and John himself was a member only during the period in 1688 when all such requirements were suspended. However, as we have seen, it was not only Whigs who had scruples about oath-taking: in 1695 Sir John Knight had opposed a bill for the enforcement of oaths to King William, and Tory unwillingness to take the Association Oath of 1696 had helped the Whigs. Intriguingly, in October 1696, the common council was asked by Bristol's Quakers if, in line with the Affirmation Act, they might take an amended version of Bristol's burgess oath, thus entitling them to trade in the city and to vote in parliamentary elections as Bristol freemen. This was put to a committee which finally reported in favour only on 18 November 1697, the delay suggesting a considerable struggle. In his *Essay* Cary noted that:

> it were to be wisht some way might be found out to make methods of trade more easie to the Quakers than now they are; I am apt to think that he who appears in the face of a court to give evidence on his word if he be a man of conscience looks on himself equally obliged to speak the truth as if he was sworn, and nothing will deter a dishonest man like the fear of punishment.[36]

Like oaths, other religious forms caused major problems to any inter-denominational body. The Corporation of the Poor struggled with the format of religious services or how to provide religious education to the children in its care. Cary's account of their activities stressed that the children went to church on Sundays and had prayers twice a day but noted that the girls 'were taught their catechisms at home'. The Tory attack in 1711 alleged (with heavy sarcasm) that:

> At last they agreed on a more infallible way, it seems, by requesting a divine of the town to compose a form [of prayer] for them, which he accordingly did. If the piece does not speak the author, please to know, 'twas the Reverend Mr T.C. [i.e. Thomas Cary]. But it was put to the judgement of a person learned in the law [presumably the lawyer Nathaniel Wade] before it went to the press, who it seems lopped off several branches, and being an enemy to forms in general, thought, I suppose, if there must be an evil, the less the better.

Hugh Waterman, Tory rector of St Peter's (where the Mint workhouse was located), argued in the first annual sermon in 1699 for 'contriving that such poor as shall be placed in these Houses, be instructed in matters of religion', insisting that it was not enough 'just to learn them to read and to repeat a catechism, though this

Commons, 17 (1711–14), pp. 529–30, 609, 625, 644, 672 and 18 (1714–18), p. 670; Butcher, *Bristol Corporation of the Poor*, pp. 92–3.

36   Latimer, *Annals of Bristol in the Seventeenth*, p. 330; Nicholls and Taylor, *Bristol Past and Present*, iii, p. 117; Hayton, *History of Parliament*, iv, p. 577; Mortimer, 'Quakerism', pp. 79, 345–7; Cary, *Essay on the State of England*, pp. 42–3.

may be of advantage; but they should be made to understand the Fundamentals of the Christian Religion'. In June 1718 the house committee invited him to provide a form of prayer out of the Book of Common Prayer to be used daily among the people, but until 1767 laymen, including inmates, conducted the prayers and services.[37]

Controversy over religion and the role of the established church within reform movements not only affected the Corporation of the Poor, but also prompted an alternative, clergy-led model of Anglican civic reformation which, from 1705 to 1715 in particular, provided a militant alternative to John and Thomas Cary's lay-led and non-denominational vision. This also sought to provide a city-wide solution to pressing problems, but did so through revitalizing the existing parochial system. I have explored this elsewhere, but it is worth noting the attitudes taken to the Anglican reform schemes by the Carys. Arthur Bedford, Whig vicar of Temple, pursued a series of reform schemes from 1700 as chief correspondent and agent in Bristol for the Society for Promoting Christian Knowledge (SPCK). He sought to establish a Clergy Society, and when this failed, through Thomas Cary's opposition, joined the Society for the Reformation of Manners and persuaded it to promote Sunday evening sermons for reformation at St Nicholas church, and, after some reluctance, to fund schooling (provided no church catechism was used) in most parishes from 1702 to 1705. Bedford and the SPCK saw Thomas Cary as a key figure to influence and although he refused to become a SPCK correspondent and rejected their efforts to involve him in establishing parochial charity schools in 1705 (after Bedford's scheme had failed), they continued to send him their circulars. Bedford then looked to Edward Colston, the Bristol-born London merchant who poured his money into a range of projects to strengthen the Anglican church. From 1709 Colston supported parochial church schools in five parishes, including Temple, which Bedford and his SPCK friends organized. Bedford told the SPCK in 1709 that only 3 of 232 eligible children in his parish were helped by the Corporation of the Poor, 'though the pretences of their teaching the children had hitherto hindered all endeavours of that nature at Bristol'. The Tory pamphleteer of 1711 saw the education of the poor as potentially the most attractive of the corporation's activities, but claimed that it was totally failing in the task, which would be best performed by parish charity schools.[38]

Colston also sought to strengthen Anglican educational provision at city level. In 1702 he gave £500 to rebuild the city school for boy orphans, Queen Elizabeth's

37   Cary, *Account of the Proceedings*, pp. 11, 17; Anon., *Some Considerations offered to the Citizens*, p. 6; Hugh Waterman, *A Sermon preached before the Court of Guardians of the Poor in the City of Bristol at St Peter's Church April 13th 1699* (Bristol, 1699), pp. 12–14; Butcher, *Bristol Corporation of the Poor*, pp. 20, 94; Johnson, *Transactions of the Corporation of the Poor*, p. 50.

38   Barry, 'The Society for the Reformation of Manners', pp. 6–13; Barry, 'Hell upon earth or the language of the playhouse', in Stuart Clark, ed., *Languages of Witchcraft: Narrative, Ideology and Meaning in Early Modern Culture* (Basingstoke, 2001), pp. 139–58; Anon., *Some Considerations offered to the Citizens*, pp. 5–6.

Hospital, and in 1705 he proposed to extend the school from 44 to 90 endowed places, if the corporation paid for suitable accommodation, but this was refused, ostensibly on grounds of civic poverty. The Society of Merchant Venturers (already managers of his almshouse) then agreed to manage a new school, Colston's Hospital, for 100 poor boys. The strictly Anglican nature of this school may explain why the city corporation declined to support it, and when Colston's nephew stood as Tory candidate in 1705, the Whig slogan was apparently 'No alms houses, No Churchmen, No Jacobites'. Colston referred to 'being hardly censured...even by some of the magistrates', since such establishments are 'only a nursery for beggars and sloths, and rather a burthen than a benefit to the place', which suggests a tension between supporters of the Corporation of the Poor as a place to train poor children in work as well as teaching them, and those who favoured a purely educational establishment.[39]

Colston also made numerous gifts not only to the city's churches to improve the edifices or install organs or altarpieces, but also to provide sermons and prayers at Bristol's Newgate prison and (from March 1708) an annual series of Lent sermons, to be preached in turn by the city's clergy each Wednesday and Friday, which combined a catechetical purpose with a call to penitence. He gave £2,000 to the Queen Anne's Bounty commissioners through his agent Thomas Edwards, and later bequeathed £6,000 to increase the salaries of poor clergymen nationally; locally he gave money to All Saints church (one of Cary's livings) to fund prayers. Meanwhile Bristol's Anglican clergy sought to address the problem of small parishes and poor livings by petitioning in 1710–11 for an Act of Parliament to establish a rating system for the city. In its attempt to equalize the value of parochial livings according to the work involved, on the basis of a city-wide property rating, the scheme was repeating the formula of the Corporation of the Poor, though with the aim of strengthening, rather than weakening, the city's parochial structure. The scheme also appealed to the need to provide the clergy with a security that raised them above dependence on their parishioners, so that the bill's supporters could provide the proper moral leadership in a reformed city: 'can you reconcile the most precarious condition of life, mere begging, to honour?' Although Thomas Cary signed the initial agreement to apply for an Act, he did not contribute with the other clergy to the costs, was accused by Waterman of arguing for a deferral as an excuse for inaction, and did not sign the petition to Parliament. Although the proposal won some support from across the political and religious spectrum, it was opposed by most of the corporation and aroused a storm of controversy. Its opponents accused the clergy of seeking dominion over the city, foreshadowing other actions against dissenters.[40]

39   Hayton, *History of Parliament*, ii, p. 213; Barry, 'The Society for the Reformation of Manners', pp. 11–12.
40   BAO, P/Tem E4 (1–19), especially 3–5, and 19 for Cary; *An Apology for the Clergy of the City of Bristol* (quotation on p. 33); Philo-Bristolii, *Letter from a Freeman of Bristol to Joseph Earl* (London, 1712); *Reasons Offer'd to the Inhabitants of Bristol Against a Tax Solicited for by the Clergy Thereof* (London, 1712; John Cary's

However, it would be too simple to present a contrast between Whig and Tory, lay and Anglican, radical and conservative plans for reform. The clerical mainten-ance scheme revived a republican project, sponsored by Parliamentarians who, after 1660, became leading dissenters and Whigs. A series of ordinances and acts were passed between 1648 and 1657 establishing a levy on the city's inhabitants to support a preaching clergy, together with the use of dean and chapter revenues and (in 1657) a merging of parishes to form 12 larger parishes. Each attempt met with vociferous opposition and parochial non-co-operation and the proposal lapsed in 1660, but the idea remained, to be revived (unsuccessfully) both in 1664 and in 1677. In 1711–12, opponents of the proposal played on its republican precedents, by reprinting the petition of over 400 freemen of Bristol (most, they claimed, 'true sons of the church of England in her persecuted state') against the measure in 1651. Perhaps aware of the ecclesiastical contradiction (as noted by the supporters, who argued that it could not be dismissed as the work of a 'high-flying spirit' since it only repeated the proposals made in the 1650s), they argued that it threatened the rights of Bristol's freemen to freedom from tithes. To support the scheme was to betray the rights which all Bristol freemen had sworn to uphold and thus a violation of a sacred oath.[41]

It is dangerous to read the rage of party between 1705 and 1715 back into the politics of the previous decade. Bedford's first report to the SPCK on Bristol's educational provision in 1700 praised the schooling provided for about 250 boys and girls in the two workhouses. The Tory attack in 1711 was forced to counter the Corporation of the Poor's claims to bipartisan support, namely that 'some of the Church-party, nay even pinnacle-men, as they are pleased to call them, appear as zealous in this matter as any dissenter'. Granting there were 'a few such', the Tory pamphleteer urged them to recognize that they had been made:

> the tools of ill-designing men while they stand behind the curtain, and sneer at the tragi-comedy. However it is certain they make use of this handle to divide us, and 'twas a late saying of a pious a Whig, disputing on this matter, 'D-n the Mint, if we can but divide them, it will in a great measure answer the end'.[42]

By the 'few such', he may have been referring to Colston and his lawyer and business agent in Bristol, Thomas Edwards (whose son, married to Colston's niece, was Tory MP 1713–15). Although Colston was to become an active Tory, branded a Nonjuror and crypto-Jacobite by a Whigs in the heated party strife of 1710–15, until about 1705 he was part of a broad anti-Jacobite alliance in London and

annotated copy is Oxford, Bodleian Library, Gough Somerset 50 (6)); Latimer, *Annals of Bristol in the Eighteenth*, pp. 77, 92–4.

41   Dr Williams Library, MS. 89.13, chap. 3, pp. 444, 52, 73; chap. 5, pp. 22–46; chap. 6, p. 60, and chap. 10 on Jeremy Holwey; Latimer, *Annals of Bristol in the Seventeenth*, pp. 208, 221, 227, 273–4; Nicholls and Taylor, *Bristol Past and Present*, iii, pp. 28–30, 39, 68; BAO, EP/A/28/1.

42   Anon., *Some Considerations offered to the Citizens*, pp. 8–9.

Bristol, which overrode the distinctions of churchmanship. Until the 1690s Edwards's chief connections were with dissenters and Whigs, and he was a key anti-Jacobite figure, closely linked to Yate and to Yate's brother-in-law Robert Henley, who had stood as a Whig candidate in 1679. Edwards had been active in the Corporation of the Poor from the start, giving substantial donations, and also acted for the low-church Bishop Hall (the 'last Puritan bishop'), passing to the Corporation of the Poor a £50 gift from the Bishop for Bibles. Colston also gave generously in the Corporation of the Poor's early years, having been a partner, with Day and Wade, in the sugarhouse which was converted first to the Mint and then into the Corporation of the Poor's main workhouse.[43] Cary's *Essay* praised almshouses for the old (not for 'idle beggars'), especially one 'magnificently built and suitably endowed by a certain gentleman near a great city [identified in a printed marginal note as 'Mr Edward Colston near Bristol'], for which he deserves to be honoured though perhaps he may scarce be imitated'. Admittedly Cary's patrons, the Society of Merchant Venturers, administered this almshouse and he also praises their other almshouse as 'a worthy pattern', but the reference to Colston seems enthusiastic. Moreover, in the 1717 edition the reference was amended to include Colston's Hospital for 100 boys 'to be educated in principles of virtue and afterwards put out to trades', adding that it was 'so free from ostentation' that he was fully satisfied with its management.[44]

Finally, we should note that there could also be tensions within the Whig reformist tradition, as well as alliances with other anti-Jacobites. In July 1695, Henley described Cary to Robert Harley as an 'inconsiderable and inconsiderate prating man'.[45] This probably reflected frustration at Cary's attempts to create a separate political base. As noted, Cary initially stood in the 1695 election against Day and Yate and then used his position in the Society of Merchant Venturers to try to control the actions of Day and Yate as Bristol's MPs over issues such as the Council of Trade.[46] Lacking their wealth, gentry status (although at this time the Carys were establishing their claim to be a cadet branch of the Devonshire Carys) and position in the corporation, and perhaps with a more radical version of the Whig agenda, Cary had to exploit his city connections to establish his claim to authority in Bristol reform, and one could reasonably read his ventures into print as a further strategy by which he established his own independent voice. In his correspondence with Locke, Cary clearly anticipated a time when he could speak directly in Parliament.[47]

43 Barry, 'The Society for the Reformation of Manners', p. 11; K. Morgan, *Edward Colston and Bristol* (Bristol, 1999); Hayton, *History of Parliament*, iii, pp. 652–3.

44 Cary, *Essay on the State of England*, pp. 167, 169; Cary, *Discourse on Trade*, pp. 113–14.

45 Hayton, *History of Parliament*, ii, p. 212.

46 McGrath, *Merchants and Merchandise*, pp. 163–8.

47 I.V. Hall, 'The grant of arms to the Cary family', *Transactions of the Bristol and Gloucestershire Archaeological Society*, 70 (1951), 155–6; Beer, *Correspondence of John Locke*, v, p. 634: 'when I have the honour to sit there' (9 May 1696).

Having failed yet again to become a MP in 1698, Cary transferred his efforts
to Ireland, although with even less success, and he clearly died an embittered man.
Meanwhile his Corporation of the Poor, once so controversial in itself, became,
after 1710, a part of the civic establishment over which the rival parties fought for
control. In a final irony, over subsequent decades the Corporation of the Poor
became a focus of Tory and parochial opposition to the largely Whig and strongly
Presbyterian corporation, and by the 1750s it was being invoked, during the Bristol
Watch-Bill debate, as the bastion of civic ratepayer views against the self-selecting
Whig oligarchy.[48] To be successful, reform measures must tap into deep concerns
and structural issues. This means that they will inevitably bear family resemb-
lances, both to earlier reform proposals and to alternative schemes for reform circulating at the same period; and that, once established, they will be subject to
development in very different directions from their original conception. But, as
Webster has shown, it is always worth attempting to understand the initial vision of
those proposing reform.

---

48   Jonathan Barry, 'The parish in civic life: Bristol and its churches 1640–1750', in
     Susan Wright, ed., *Parish, Church and People* (London, 1988), pp. 168–9.

Chapter 11

Medicine, Race, and Radicalism in the Later Scottish Enlightenment

Colin Kidd

In place of the long-unquestioned assumption among Scottish historians that nationhood enjoyed an enduring and dominant salience throughout their country's past, students of late eighteenth- and nineteenth-century Scotland have begun to rediscover an obsessive preoccupation with race, which – to the exclusion even of national identity – entranced several generations of Scottish intellectuals. Indeed, during the nineteenth century a Lowland-based intelligentsia deconstructed the Scottish nation into two distinct racial groups, a super-race of Teutonic Lowlanders and an inferior population of Celtic Highlanders. This vein of racial theorizing had real – and sometimes pernicious – social consequences. An anti-Celtic Teutonism manifested itself most obviously in Lowland insensitivity towards Gaelic victims of the Highland famine of the 1840s and in opposition to mass Irish immigration into Glasgow and its industrial hinterland.[1] In addition, racial stereotyping compounded the problem of Protestant sectarianism, a potent combination which persisted as a vital force in Scottish society into the interwar period.[2] During the nineteenth century racialism worked against the grain of nationalism, whose potential was sublimated into an anti-Celtic nativism, while for many North British intellectuals the Union of 1707 represented the welcome integration of kindred Teutonic peoples.[3] Nationalist historiography was virtually non-existent; instead several historians and archaeologists embraced an overtly racialist interpretation of

I should like to thank Jacqueline Jenkinson and the staffs of the Royal Medical Society in Edinburgh and the Royal College of Physicians and Surgeons of Glasgow (RCPSG) for help with this topic.

1   Krisztina Fenyo, *Contempt, Sympathy and Romance: Lowland Perceptions of the Highlands and the Clearances during the Famine Years, 1845–1855* (East Linton, 2000); J.E. Handley, *The Irish in Modern Scotland* (Cork, 1947), esp. pp. 104–8; L.P. Curtis Jr., *Apes and Angels: the Irishman in Victorian Caricature* (revd edn, Washington D.C., 1997), pp. 96–8.
2   See e.g. S.J. Brown, '"Outside the covenant": the Scottish Presbyterian churches and Irish immigration, 1922–1938', *Innes Review*, 42 (1991), 19–45.
3   Colin Kidd, 'Teutonist ethnology and Scottish nationalist inhibition, 1780–1880', *Scottish Historical Review*, 74 (1995), 45–68.

the Scottish past.[4] The sense of a racial cleavage between Celts and Teutons has even been detected within the politics of the Free Church, and assigned a prominent role in creating the conditions for the Free Presbyterian schism in 1893.[5] Nineteenth-century racial prejudice, underpinned by a self-confident science of race, it is now recognized, clearly played a significant role in shaping the response of Lowland Scotland to political, social and religious trends. However, little attention has been paid to the roots of this phenomenon.

Indeed, the Scottish Enlightenment seems a most improbable seedbed for racial science. The various interconnected achievements of the moral philosophers, jurists and philosophical historians of the Scottish Enlightenment, in the emergent spheres of what came to be known as sociology, anthropology and political economy, rested upon the assumed uniformity of human nature.[6] In particular, the stadialist theory of mankind's progress through four broad stages of socio-economic development from primitive rudeness to commercial refinement was incompatible with notions of racialist differentiation; indeed it was bound up with a comparative sociology predicated upon the presumed similarity of manners in modern 'savage' and prehistoric European societies. The aspiration towards a historical sociology which was universal in scope was rooted in the assumption that the basic motivations of mankind were the same in all ages and places. This did not preclude, as some scholars have noted, a little dabbling with alternative approaches. In a footnote to an essay on national character David Hume revealed his belief in a racial hierarchy, a prejudice echoed in William Smellie's racist articulation of the Great Chain of Being; while there were also excursions into physical anthropology, with Lord Kames opening one of his treatises with an argument for polygenesis (the theory of man's plural origins in a variety of races) and Lord Monboddo famously exploring the relationship of orang-utans to the human family.[7] Nevertheless, there was no systematic investigation of racial issues; this begs the question of why so many intellectuals in the later Scottish Enlightenment came to incorporate a racial dimension into the study of human nature.

The stock answer locates the source of Scottish racialism in the sphere of philology. John Pinkerton, a major figure in the late eighteenth-century Scots literary revival, has won considerable notoriety as the founding father of Scottish

4   See e.g. D.V. Clarke, 'Scottish archaeology in the second half of the nineteenth century', in A.S. Bell, ed., *The Scottish Antiquarian Tradition* (Edinburgh, 1981), pp. 130–1; Kidd, 'Teutonist ethnology'.

5   J.L. MacLeod, *The Second Disruption* (East Linton, 2000).

6   Paul Wood, 'The natural history of man in the Scottish Enlightenment', *History of Science*, 28 (1990), 89–123.

7   See e.g. John Immerwahr, 'Hume's revised racism', *Journal of the History of Ideas*, 53 (1992), 481–6; W.F. Bynum, 'The great chain of being after forty years: an appraisal', *History of Science*, 13 (1975), 1–28: pp. 5, 7; Robert Wokler, 'Apes and races in the Scottish Enlightenment: Monboddo and Kames on the nature of man', in Peter Jones, ed., *Philosophy and Science in the Scottish Enlightenment* (Edinburgh, 1988), pp. 145–68.

racialism. A strident critic of the cult of Ossian, and indeed of all things Gaelic, Pinkerton instead promoted the Scots dialect of the Lowlands, which he mistakenly identified as the tongue of the ancient Picts and claimed as the aboriginal language of Scotland. Indeed, Pinkerton also contended that ancient Europe had been peopled by two distinct races, an inferior Celtic stock, the provenance of the Gaelic Highlanders, and the industrious Goths, or Scythians, from whom – in defiance of the facts – he asserted the Picts were descended. For Pinkerton linguistic methods offered a route into the problems of human biological variation. Textual hermeneutics underpinned his racialism: Pinkerton openly challenged the orthodox scripture doctrine that all mankind was descended from a single human pair, arguing instead that polygenesis best explained human racial diversity.[8] Pinkerton's racialist ideas – if not the religious heterodoxy which accompanied them – enjoyed a wide circulation within the Scots literary and lexicographical revival, receiving the imprimatur of the Reverend Dr John Jamieson in his *Etymological Dictionary of the Scots Language* (1808). Although it seems plausible that anti-Celtic racism rose in tandem with the campaign to boost the Lowland Scots dialect and its rich tradition of medieval Scots literature, it is much less certain whether the origins of Scottish racialism can be ascribed exclusively – or even primarily – to the field of philology.

For Pinkerton's ideas appeared to reach their culmination in the work of another infamous Scots racial theorist and Celtophobe, the anatomist Robert Knox, known to posterity both for his involvement in the Burke and Hare scandal and as the author of a virulently racist treatise, *The Races of Men* (London, 1850; 2nd edn, 1862). Historians of anthropology are also familiar with the fact that the leading champion of monogenist racial science during the first half of the nineteenth century, the Bristolian physician James Cowles Prichard, began his study of race during his medical education at Edinburgh where his MD dissertation of 1808 explicitly addressed the origin of human varieties.[9] Scottish phrenologists – led by the brothers George and Andrew Combe – were also associated with racial classification on the basis of cranial measurement.[10] Clearly, medicine, in the broadest sense, was implicated, in some as yet undefined way, with the establishment of racial science in nineteenth-century Scotland. Nevertheless, how far, and in what ways, did medicine contribute to the initial rise, and then consolidation, of racial science in Scotland? Did anatomists merely follow where Pinkerton led, or did the medical profession generate its own distinctive set of interests in racial questions, whether

---

8   John Pinkerton, *Ancient Scotish Poems* (2 vols, London, 1786), i, pp. xxiv–xxvi; Pinkerton, *A Dissertation on the Origin and Progress of the Scythians or Goths* (London, 1787).

9   H.F. Augstein, *James Cowles Prichard's Anthropology* (Amsterdam, 1999).

10 Nancy Stepan, *The Idea of Race in Science: Great Britain 1800–1960* (London, 1982), pp. 20–8. The fullest discussion is in Bruce Armstrong, 'Wha's like us? Racism and racialization in the imagination of nineteenth-century Scotland', unpublished Glasgow University Ph.D. thesis (1994), chap. 7.

inspired by conventional medicine or by phrenology? Indeed, did the ideological significance of race differ between medical and philological circles?

Rejection of polygenesis

The Scottish obsession with race, within the medical field at least, appears to have emerged out of an orthodox concern to rebut the polygenist theories aired by Kames in his *Sketches of the History of Man* (1774). The Biblical account of the origins of mankind from a single pair of humans struck Kames as incompatible with the facts of biology and geography. The 'very frame of the human body', including colour, hair type, and physiognomy, seemed to point to aboriginal racial differences. Nor did Kames believe that climatic variation accounted for racial differences: 'Let a European for years expose himself to the sun in a hot climate, till he be quite brown, his children will nevertheless have the same complexion with those in Europe'. In addition, native Americans and Australasians presented particularly acute problems of racial provenance, as their respective continents seemed never to have been connected by any land passage to Europe, Africa or Asia. Not only did this geographical remoteness make it unlikely that America had been peopled 'from any part of the old world', but the 'external appearance of the inhabitants' made 'this conjecture approach to a certainty'. The bodies of the Americans were hairless, their faces were beardless, and their 'copper colour' differed 'from the colour of all other nations'. To Kames the heterodox idea of a series of 'local creations' seemed much less implausible than the orthodox theory of monogenesis, which depended both on the global dispersion of Adam's and Eve's descendants and on the remarkable variations they experienced in racial traits in response to environmental differences. Having exploded the orthodox account of the peopling of the earth, Kames nevertheless backtracked from his heterodoxy, proposing an alternative anthropology based on the 'terrible convulsion' at the Tower of Babel, which not only confounded the languages of mankind, but also brought about an immediate change of bodily constitution, without which the dispersed 'builders of Babel could not possibly have subsisted in the burning region of Guinea, nor in the frozen region of Lapland'.[11] However, this last-minute evasion of the heterodox logic of his own argument did not hoodwink Kames's readers, and his name became a by-word for polygenist heterodoxy.

Kames's polygenism drew an immediate response from the prominent Scottish scientist John Anderson, who delivered a paper to the Glasgow Literary Society in 1774 which addressed the issue of racial variation. In particular, Anderson rejected the argument that, because whites and blacks seemed to retain their colouring in different climates, this led inexorably to polygenist conclusions, 'for this plain reason, that a cause may produce an effect which will continue to produce similar

11   Henry Home, Lord Kames, *Sketches of the History of Man* (2 vols, Edinburgh, 1774),
       i, pp. 10–15, 32–43; ii, pp. 70–6.

effects while the first cause is removed'. In this way environmental changes could have 'lasting effects upon the body which are transmitted to posterity'. For example, the ancient inhabitants of 'Negroland' might have become black by way of some local disease or environmental cause, as a result of which perhaps a 'mucus' might have 'lodged in their skin', this 'effect' remaining and being 'so wrought into the constitution as to make a variety in the human kind'.[12] Another prompt rebuttal of Kames's speculations on race came in the 1775 Edinburgh MD thesis of John Hunter (d. 1809), *De Hominum Varietatibus*, a work which empha-sized not only the role of climate but also the thickness of the skin in determining colour.[13] From the outset of the Scottish debate over polygenesis medical speculation was pressed into the service of theological orthodoxy.

The most influential response to Kames issued from Samuel Stanhope Smith, a prominent academic at Princeton, the transatlantic outpost of the Scots Presbyterian Enlightenment. Published in Philadelphia in 1787, Smith's *Essay on the Causes of Complexion and Figure in the Human Species* immediately attracted attention back in the mother country, and was published the following year in an Edinburgh edi-tion which carried a preface by Benjamin Smith Barton, an American medical student. Smith not only propounded an environmentalist account of racial varia-tion, but he also displayed an understanding – heavily indebted to the sociology of the Scottish Enlightenment – of the ways in which the 'state of society' further affected the impact of climatic factors on the human form.[14]

Over the following decades the challenge of polygenesis – and the popularity of Smith's response – pushed the study of racial differences towards the top of the Scottish medical agenda. The origins of race became a staple topic of discussion at the leading forum for medical students in the Scottish Enlightenment, Edinburgh's Royal Medical Society. The most celebrated of these papers – a version of his dissertation – was given by Prichard in session 1807–8, but it is interesting to note that this early formulation of the Prichardian monogenesis which was to dominate nineteenth-century British anthropology followed a series of staunchly anti-polygenist papers within the Royal Medical Society by Richard Millar, Stanhope Smith's champion Smith Barton, James Buchan, John Bradley, E. Holme, William Webb, R.D. Mackintosh, and Joseph Reade, and that the same session also witnessed a powerful attack on Kames, 'the daring advocate of the doctrine of diversity of species', by Richard Dyett. This line was continued in session 1811–12 by Nicholas Pitta who denounced the vulgar scientist error of assuming that polygenism was more intellectually rigorous 'simply because it opposes a tenet of

12   John Anderson, 'Discourses of natural and artificial systems in natural history; and of the varieties in the human kind', Glasgow, Strathclyde University Library Special Collections MS 9, fols 30–1, 33.
13   John Hunter, 'Inaugural dissertation', in T. Bendyshe, ed., *The Anthropological Treatises of Johann Friedrich Blumenbach* (London, 1875).
14   Samuel Stanhope Smith, *An Essay on the Causes of Complexion and Figure in the Human Species* (1787; Bristol, 1995), see esp. pp. 71–2.

religion'.[15] Indeed, Millar argued that medical science rested upon an assumption of monogenetic unity.[16]

These papers retail the standard scientific arguments against polygenesis. Albinism and white negroes were favourite monogenist subjects,[17] as was the racial makeup of the Jewish population. Why, they asked, drawing on an argument of Buffon's which was also employed by Smith,[18] did the Jews – who were clearly of one stock, given their prohibition on intermarriage with other groups – have different complexions in different climates?[19] Inevitably, attention was also focused on medical explanations, such as Pitta's 'carbonaceous pigment', which might account for changes in skin colour – from a primitive white to black, obviously. Borrowing heavily from Stanhope Smith, Pitta noted that fair-skinned people contracted freckles when exposed to the sun. As these were only gradually removed and became indelible in time, Pitta claimed that 'the dark colour of many nations, may be justly considered an universal freckle'.[20] Reade had similarly concluded that colour was 'only an accidental variety in warm climates'.[21] However these papers also throw into relief the anxieties and weak points in the monogenist case, such as the possibility that the women of the Cape of Good Hope had a racially

---

15   Archives of the Royal Medical Society, Bristo Square, Edinburgh: Richard Millar, 'How far can the varieties of the human species that are observable in the different countries of the world, be accounted for from physical causes?', MS Records vol. 19 (1785–6), 144–77; Benjamin Smith Barton, 'An essay towards a natural history of the North American Indians. Being an attempt to describe, and to investigate the causes of some of the varieties in figure, in complexion etc among mankind', 23 (1788–90), 1–17; James Buchan, 'Whether are moral and physical causes sufficient to account for the varieties which occur in the human species?', 26 (1790–1), 302–22; John Bradley, 'Whence the varieties of the human species?', 27 (1791–2), 95–105; E. Holme, 'To the operation of what causes are we to ascribe the variety of complexion in the human species?', 29 (1792–3), 366–82; William Webb, 'Are the diversities among mankind the effect of physical and moral causes?', 32 (1794–5), 134–67; R.D. Mackintosh, 'Upon what do the physical varieties of the human body in different characters depend?', 42 (1798–9), 31–69; Joseph Reade, 'What are principally the causes of variety in the human species?', 44 (1800–1), 99–114; James Cowles Prichard, 'Of the varieties of the human race', 58 (1807–8), 87–133; Richard Dyett, 'Is there any original difference of intellectual ability amongst mankind?', 58 (1807–8), 215–36; Nicholas Pitta, 'What is the influence of climate on the human species? And what are the varieties of men which result from it?', 66 (1811–12), 283–307.
16   Millar, 'Varieties', p. 149.
17   Mackintosh, 'Varieties', p. 57; Reade, 'Variety', pp. 107–9; Prichard, 'Varieties', pp. 92–3.
18   Smith, *Essay*, p. 36.
19   Bradley, 'Varieties', pp. 97–8; Mackintosh, 'Varieties', pp. 39–40; Prichard, 'Varieties', p. 112; Pitta, 'Climate', p. 289.
20   Pitta, 'Climate', pp. 289, 302.
21   Reade, 'Variety', p. 110.

distinctive conformation of the pudenda, the notorious 'Hottentot apron'.[22] Furthermore, a number of papers tackled the puzzle of why there was no regular gradation of colour by latitude. Buchan, Bradley and Holme invoked geographical factors, including the influence of prevailing winds, the nature of the soil, and its elevation, to explain why West Africans were darker than other peoples at the same latitude, and why even adjacent peoples were markedly lighter.[23]

Uniquely among the various speakers on racial origins at the Royal Medical Society, Alexander Robertson, who delivered a paper during the session of 1798–9, stands out as a self-declared 'proselyte to the opinion of Lord Kames',[24] the only other talk to eschew advocacy of the monogenist position being R.E. Taylor's in 1793–4, which concluded on a note of scepticism that 'in the present state of our knowledge, I think, we are by no means authorized to conclude that mankind are originally descended from one pair'.[25] Robertson wondered why 'we seek in vain for negroes in the burning climates of Asia or America'. The answer lay in the racial distinctiveness of blacks: 'No other race of men seems capable of ever receiving the deep black colour, though exposed to the same degree of heat'.[26] Despite the force of Robertson's objections to monogenesis and Taylor's agnosticism, it seems clear that for contemporaries the theological claims for the unitary origins of mankind generally trumped the scientific case for polygenesis.

The dominant motive behind the initial rise of a racially-focused science during the Scottish Enlightenment – in the province of theology, Hume excepted, a very tepid affair – was the conservation of scriptural authority. At one extreme Webb's paper endorsed the 'tradition of Moses' as a reliable 'historical record',[27] yet even where the substance of argument was medical and scientific the issue was nevertheless framed by the parameters of religious orthodoxy. These parameters were shifting in other spheres. For instance, Dr James Hutton's account of deep geological time, delivered at the Royal Society of Edinburgh during the 1780s, overthrew the traditional chronology of the earth, which conservative Biblical exegesis put at around six thousand years;[28] but this strain of revisionism was more easily assimilated to mainstream opinion than was polygenesis, which posed an immediate threat to central elements in the Christian faith, including the Fall, the

---

22   Millar, 'Varieties', pp. 170–2; Mackintosh, 'Varieties', p. 54.
23   Buchan, 'Varieties', p. 311; Bradley, 'Varieties', pp. 99–100; Holme, 'Complexion', pp. 369–78.
24   Alexander Robertson, 'Do the varieties which we observe among mankind arise from the action of moral and physical causes, or are there different races of men?', Royal Medical Society MS Records, 40 (1798–9), pp. 201–17, at p. 202.
25   R.E. Taylor, 'What are the causes of the variety of complexion in the human species?' Royal Medical Society MS Records, 31 (1793–4), pp. 274–88, at p. 288.
26   Robertson, 'Varieties', p. 209.
27   Webb, 'Diversities', p. 167.
28   James Hutton, 'Theory of the earth', *Transactions of the Royal Society of Edinburgh*, 1 (1788), 209–304.

transmission of original sin, and Christ's redemption of all mankind. Polygenist racialism struck at the fundamental beliefs of a Christian society.

In spite of the radical implications of polygenesis, rendered more vivid during the 1790s by contemporary fears about the infiltration of Jacobin infidelity, the ideological profile of racial issues remained uncertain, ambiguous and cross-grained. Presbyterian orthodoxy did not necessarily serve to inhibit the exploitation of other races. Scotland's remarkable economic development in the eighteenth century had been catalysed by Glasgow's tobacco trade with the Chesapeake, while Scots based south of the border had been active in the slave trade.[29] Of course, the contemporary evangelical campaign against the slave trade meshed conveniently with the defence of scriptural anthropology; but, more awkwardly, conventional racist slurs were sometimes to be found in works ostensibly devoted to attacking polygenesis. Anderson, for example, found the natives of 'Negroland', in respect of 'scent' and bodily 'effluvia', to be no more 'offensive' than the 'inhabitants of St. Kilda'.[30] As neither racialism nor anti-racism was as yet programmatic, an instinctive sense of white racial superiority was far from incompatible with a clear rejection of polygenist heresy (a theological position logically unconnected in itself to any particular racial attitude).

Moreover, the controversy generated by the work of Pinkerton, whose racialist history of Scotland was published in 1789,[31] linked the wider issue of mankind's origins with the more particular concern of Scotland's own racial identity. Indeed, the borders between philology and physiology were porous, and the dispute over Scotland's ethnic composition spilled over into the mainstream of medical science. In his MD thesis Prichard divided the nations of Europe into three racial groups, the Celts, Goths and Slavonic Sarmatians. Significantly, despite his monogenist opposition to Pinkerton's polygenist racialism, Prichard divided the peoples of Scotland along Pinkertonian lines into two sections. The Gaels – 'Scoti proprii' – Prichard placed among the dark Celtic peoples, while he contended that the lighter, blue-eyed Germanic race also included the Picts from whom, following Pinkerton, he believed the Lowlanders had descended: 'In media Europa magna Germanica natio, quae oculis coeruleis, crinibus flavis vel rutilatis, cute pulchra et rubicundiore ubique insignis est, Suedos, Norvegios, Icelandicos, Danos, Germanos et antiquos et hujus aevi, Saxones et Anglos, Caledonios vel Pictas, et ab iis oriundos Scotos planitiei, Belgas, Vandalos, Gothos, aliosque continet'.[32] Indeed, throughout his distinguished career Prichard would deploy philological as well as

29   T.M. Devine, *The Tobacco Lords* (Edinburgh, 1975); David Hancock, 'Scots in the slave trade', in Ned Landsman, ed., *Nation and Province in the First British Empire: Scotland and the Americas, 1600–1800* (Lewisburg, PA, 2001), pp. 60–93.

30   Anderson, 'Discourses', MS 9, fol. 40.

31   John Pinkerton, *An Enquiry into the History of Scotland* (2 vols, London, 1789).

32   James Cowles Prichard, *Disputatio inauguralis de generis humani varietate* (Edinburgh MD thesis, 1808), pp. 103–4.

physiological arguments in defence of monogenetic truth.[33] Although racial theorists seemed oblivious of disciplinary demarcations, the argument was raised on the medical side that biological science could resolve the question of Scotland's racial composition with a greater degree of authority than other branches of knowledge. Had more racial philologists, wondered John Macculloch, MD, FRS, 'been equally physiologists', the field might have been spared a great deal of 'fiction and nonsense'. In that spirit, Macculloch set out to provide a 'physiological' corrective to Pinkerton, though accepting some of the broad outlines of the original thesis: 'As well might we hope to see a Negro race become white', claimed Macculloch, 'as to find a Goth converted into a Celt, through any descent'. Macculloch claimed that Pinkerton's philological errors had led to mistaken conclusions about the respective places of Germano-Pictish and Celtic peoples in Scotland's chequered ethnogenesis.[34]

Monogenist medical science

However, the pressures of theological orthodoxy did more to shape the contours of Scottish racial science than the Pinkertonian controversy. Even as the immediate challenge posed by Kames receded, the defence of monogenesis retained a significant purchase on Scottish medical discourse and – given the attraction beyond Scotland of Edinburgh and Glasgow as centres of medical education – its wider British hinterland.[35] The English physician Thomas Jarrold used his Glasgow MD thesis on variations in the forearm to tackle the extreme views of the Manchester-based surgeon Charles White, set out in *An Account of the Regular Gradation in Man* (1799), that the negro was closer in bodily form to the ape than to the white European, and returned to this attack on White's racialism in his *Anthropologia* (1808).[36] Though conceding White's argument that the blackness of the negro did not arise from climatic factors, Charles Bell (1774–1842) – educated at Edinburgh and later professor of surgery there – argued that White misunderstood the colouring process in the *rete mucosum*.[37] Elsewhere Bell's influential work on human physiognomy eschewed polygenism, and he acknowledged the role of

33 Augstein, *Prichard's Anthropology*, chap. 6.
34 John Macculloch, *The Highlands and Islands of Scotland* (4 vols, London, 1824), iv, pp. 255, 257, 263–5, 279, 281, 291–2, 294–5.
35 Steven Shapin, '"Nibbling at the teats of science": Edinburgh and the diffusion of science in the 1830s', in Ian Inkster and Jack Morrell, eds, *Metropolis and Province: Science in British Culture, 1780–1850* (London, 1983), pp. 151–78.
36 Thomas Jarrold, *Disputatio medica inauguralis, de longitudine brachii* (Glasgow, 1802); Jarrold, *Anthropologia: or dissertations on the form and colour of man* (London, 1808).
37 Charles Bell, 'Rete mucosum', in John and Charles Bell, *The Anatomy of the Human Body* (3rd edn, 3 vols, London, 1811), iii, p. 207.

supernatural design in anatomy.[38] William Cooper's paper on albinos at the Glasgow Medical Society in 1818 included the assertion that most of the differences which distinguished the varieties of mankind could largely be accounted for by climate, and 'after being once produced become hereditary', requiring 'an indefinite number of generations for their obliteration'; which disposed of the standard polygenist objection that when members of each race were transplanted from their native environments their offspring retained the original colour of the parents.[39] Albinism, moreover, was evidence of a type of colour change which was independent of environmental conditions. William Charles Wells (1757–1817), South Carolina-born of a Scots loyalist family and educated at Dumfries and the Edinburgh medical school before settling in London, concluded from his study of a white Sussex woman whose left arm was covered in black skin, that 'great heat' was 'not indispensably necessary to render the human colour black'. Suggestively, Wells also postulated how minor variations in susceptibility to disease might operate in different climates in the primitive ages of mankind to shape distinctive – but 'accidental' – racial populations.[40] The conservative physician and leading Scots health reformer, W.P. Alison, included an attack on polygenesis in his textbook, *Outlines of Human Physiology*. One noted weak point in pluralist theories of human origins lay in determining just how many separate races had been created. Contemplating the view that there were three distinct races of mankind, the Caucasian, Ethiopian and Mongolian, Alison reflected that 'when we compare all the actual varieties of the species with these standards, we find great difficulty in fixing the proper place of many, and may be led ultimately to think it as probable that they are all derived from one as from those original stocks'.[41]

Racialist assumptions nevertheless became more pronounced within the dominant culture, even when unaccompanied by explicit polygenism. Jarrold's *Anthropologia* earned a scathing review in the *Edinburgh Medical Journal*, not least on the grounds of his alleged assessment 'that the perfection of the human colour is the negro blackness'.[42] In his student textbook, *Outlines of Comparative Anatomy* (1813), Andrew Fyfe endorsed what he perceived to be the thesis of the Dutch anatomist Petrus Camper (1722–89), that a hierarchy of intelligence could be determined from the facial angle. In the 'human adult *European*', noted Fyfe, the

---

38   Charles Bell, *Essays on the Anatomy of Expression in Painting* (London, 1806); Bell, *The Hand, its Mechanism and Vital Endowments as Evincing Design* (Bridgewater Treatise IV, London, 1833).

39   William Cooper, 'Of albinoes', Glasgow Medical Society, Essays, vol. 3 (1818), RCPSG MS 2/1/6, fol. 1.

40   William Charles Wells, *Two Essays...and An Account of a Female of the White Race of Mankind, Part of whose Skin Resembles that of a Negro; With Some Observations on the Causes of the Differences in Colour and Form between the White and Negro Races of Men* (London, 1818).

41   W.P. Alison, *Outlines of Human Physiology* (3rd edn, Edinburgh and London, 1839), p. 453.

42   *Edinburgh Medical Journal*, 5 (1809), 98–102.

facial angle was 85 degrees, in the orang-utan it was 67 degrees and among the quadrupeds it sank as low as twenty degrees.[43] Similarly, Dr Perry, addressing the Glasgow Medical Society in 1825, noted that the facial angle was widest 'where the intellect was highest, as in the best heads of the Europeans'.[44]

This common racialist misreading of Camper, who, as Miriam Meijer has shown,[45] was himself a monogenist with no intention of establishing the facial line as a measure of intelligence, serves as a reminder that Scotland's cosmopolitan medical community absorbed – and sometimes misconstrued – a growing body of work on race by continental scientists. Scottish medical writings of the period demonstrate a familiarity with the works of Camper, Johann Friedrich Blumenbach (1752–1840) of Göttingen, who classified humanity into five racial groupings, four of which were degenerations from the original Caucasian stock, Samuel Thomas Soemmerring (1755–1830), also of Göttingen, who explored the role of the nervous connection between the brain and the rest of the body in determining perceived differences in intelligence between Europeans and Africans, and Georges Cuvier (1769–1832), who classified the human race into three distinct varieties.[46] At the very least this corpus of work lent a growing legitimacy to the notion that studies of racial differences were now an integral component of medical science, but a science moreover which – in spite of its customary monogenist bias – did nothing to dent complacent assumptions of white European superiority.

Indeed, in an attack on the explicitly anti-racialist theories of the Heidelberg anatomist Friedrich Tiedemann (1781–1861), the Scots phrenologist Andrew Combe cited an apparent consensus on negro inferiority constituted by Camper, Soemmerring and Cuvier.[47] Tiedemann had found no significant differences in cranial capacity between negroes and Europeans, much to the dismay of Combe, who lambasted Tiedemann's methodological failings, primarily 'taking absolute size of the brain as a measure of intellectual power only', without any discrimination between the sizes of the different regions of the brain and their respective mental functions, moral, emotional and affective, as well as intellectual. According to Combe, if Tiedemann were to establish the negro as the intellectual equal of the European, he would need to demonstrate 'not only that the two brains are equal in

43 Andrew Fyfe, *Outlines of Comparative Anatomy* (Edinburgh, 1813), p. 5.
44 Dr Perry, 'Remarks on phrenology as connected with the structure of the brain', 19 April 1825, Glasgow Medical Society, Essays, vol. 12, RCPSG MS 2/1/14, fol. 4.
45 Miriam C. Meijer, *Race and Aesthetics in the Anthropology of Petrus Camper (1722–1789)* (Amsterdam, 1999).
46 See e.g. Prichard, *Disputatio inauguralis*; Fyfe, *Outlines*, 'Advertisement'; Cooper, 'Albinoes', fol. 6. Later, the Scottish medical profession would also become acquainted with the racial theories of the Swedish craniologist Anders Retzius: see A. Retzius, 'On the bony frame of the head in different nations', *Edinburgh Medical and Surgical Journal*, 74 (1850), 99–114.
47 Andrew Combe, 'Remarks on the fallacy of Professor Tiedemann's comparison of the Negro brain and intellect with those of the European', in George and Andrew Combe, eds, *On the functions of the cerebellum* (Edinburgh, 1838), p. 292.

absolute size, but that the anterior lobe, or seat of the intellect, is equally developed in both'.[48]

Combean phrenology

Combean phrenology itself, which flourished in Scotland from 1815 onwards, with phrenological societies springing up in many towns, their members' enthusiasm carried along by a wave of indigenous publications devoted to this new branch of knowledge, played a far from marginal role in consolidating racial attitudes, even within the milieu of conventional medicine. Although the leaders of Scotland's intellectual establishment, from the *Edinburgh Review* to the Royal Society of Edinburgh, had, from its first appearance in Scotland, little truck with this charlatan pseudo-science, the insights of phrenology were not at first unwelcome in respectable professional and intellectual circles, and supporters included doctors (Andrew Combe himself held an Edinburgh MD), surgeons, prominent clergymen (for a time), and even the editor of *The Scotsman*, Edinburgh's new radical newspaper.[49] Phrenology was, for example, a regular topic of discussion during the mid-1820s at the Glasgow Medico-Chirurgical Society and the Glasgow Medical Society, and won a sympathetic hearing in the *Glasgow Medical Journal*.[50]

Race, it should be remembered, was not itself at the heart of the initial Combean project, at bottom an unconventional science of the mind which also embraced a popular health movement and wider reformist goals in society;[51] nevertheless various factors drew phrenologists into the battlefield of racial science. Craniology provided a crucial link between phrenological interests and a major topic in racial science. Moreover, Scottish phrenology defined itself as a corrective to the dominant native philosophy of mind represented by the Common Sense school, whose exponents, such as Thomas Brown, Sir William Hamilton, and Dugald Stewart, were among the most vociferous critics of the new science. George Combe pointedly differed from Stewart's maintenance of the Enlightenment doctrine that the capacities of the human mind were universally the same, claiming that 'if we glance over the history of Europe, Asia, Africa, and America, we shall find distinct

---

48   *Ibid.*, pp. 293–5.
49   G.N. Cantor, 'The Edinburgh phrenology debate, 1803–1828', *Annals of Science*, 32 (1975), 195–218; Steven Shapin, 'Phrenological knowledge and the social structure of early nineteenth-century Edinburgh', *Annals of Science*, 32 (1975), 219–43; Cantor, 'A critique of Shapin's social interpretation of the Edinburgh phrenology debate', *Annals of Science*, 32 (1975), 245–56.
50   Minute Book of the Glasgow Medico-Chirurgical Society, 10 June, 7 July, 27 October, 11 November, 25 November, all 1824, RCPSG MS 5/1/1, fols 41, 43, 49, 51–2; Perry, 'Remarks'; Mr Hood, 'Essay on Phrenology', 7 February 1826, Glasgow Medical Society Essays, vol. xiii, RCPSG MS 2/1/15; *Glasgow Medical Journal*, 1st ser. 4 (1831), 270–9.
51   Roger Cooter, *The Cultural Meaning of Popular Science: Phrenology and the Organization of Consent in Nineteenth-Century Britain* (Cambridge, 1984).

and permanent features of character which strongly indicate natural differences in their mental constitutions'.[52] In a similar vein of combativeness, the work of Prichard, the leading British figure in the field of racial science and a prominent critic of phrenology, was subjected to robust criticism from the phrenological camp.[53] In his *Introduction to Phrenology in the Form of Question and Answer* Robert Macnish, a member of the Faculty of Physicians and Surgeons of Glasgow, spelled out the racialist implications of the new science: 'Which nations possess the most intellectual form of head? Those undoubtedly which are denominated the white or Caucasian variety'. Other races were 'so deficient in intellect' that it was 'found impracticable to educate them'. Prejudice was given a specious veneer of phrenological explanation: 'When the frontal and coronal regions of the brain are generally well developed in a nation, its tendency will be towards intellectual and moral pursuits; and unless some strong external counteracting agency is at work the people will speedily become civilized'. On the other hand, populations 'where the posterior and basilar regions predominate' were destined to be 'governed by the lower propensities', calling into question the civilizing process.[54]

However, phrenologists did not consider themselves to be crude defenders of existing racial prejudices. Rather they considered the novel insights of phrenology to be capable, if properly deployed, of effecting a revolution in racial science. According to James Straton, secretary of the Phrenological Society of Aberdeen, 'the doings of ethnologists' were 'sad specimens of scientific bungling. The tendencies are in the right direction, however; a little farther on they will discover that ethnology, apart from Gall's discoveries, is the shadow apart from the substance'. Phrenology, Straton contended, might shed its own light on 'the question of Celt and Saxon, about which so much has of late years been spoken and written, and of which so little of the clear and definite organic distinctions, if any such exist, is yet known'. Deviating from the Pinkertonian school, Straton divided Scotland into three distinct 'ethnological districts'. The peoples of the eastern coastal region between the Forth and Shetland, Straton argued, were of mixed Norman, Danish and Celtic blood; those south of the Forth-Clyde line were predominantly of Saxon blood; while those of the north-west Highlands and islands were largely of Celtic origin.[55]

Such distinctions – however trivial they now seem – carried a heavy ideological freight; for Scots phrenologists explicitly linked racial character with the capacity for democracy and self-improvement. The potential for radicalism

52   George Combe, *A System of Phrenology* (3rd edn, Edinburgh, 1830), p. 600.
53   Andrew Combe, 'Dr Prichard and phrenology', in Combe and Combe, eds, *On the Functions of the Cerebellum*, pp. 248–90.
54   Robert Macnish, *An Introduction to Phrenology in the Form of Question and Answer* (Glasgow, 1836), pp. 157–8.
55   James Straton, *Researches in Cerebral Development* (London, 1851), pp. 17, 20, 26. Cf. Straton, *Contributions to the Mathematics of Phrenology* (Aberdeen, 1845), pp. 14–18, 20–1, 31.

rested in part upon the phrenological capacities of the Saxon race, Combeans claiming that polities were shaped by the mental characteristics of their peoples.[56] George Combe contended that 'independence, civilization, and political freedom, are the results of large aggregate sizes of brain', features common to such Teutonic peoples as the 'British, Anglo-Americans and Swiss'.[57] On the other hand, the Celts of western Europe seemed to Combe to lag behind their Teutonic counterparts in the progress of civilization.[58] Not that the Celts were alone in such failings. Andrew Combe argued that 'independence must, in the nature of things, precede liberty'. For liberty presupposed 'moral energies' and 'enlightened views of [man's] social and public relations', qualities conspicuously lacking in many peoples, and, most unfortunately it seemed to Combe, in the newly independent states of Latin America.[59]

However, this racially-based liberalism constituted only one dimension of the radical worldview propagated by phrenologists. Its theological heterodoxy also loomed large. Critics found Combean natural law to be incompatible with the Fall of Man. William Scott, for example, denounced phrenological accounts of human development as a reversal of the Christian truth of man's original perfection and subsequent degeneracy,[60] while William Gillespie claimed that, read theologically, Combean phrenology was implicitly Pelagian and Socinian.[61] Nor did man's future state seem to be reconcilable with the materialist reckoning of the Combeans that death involved the mere dissolution of the body. Contrary to the gospel message, Combeans seemed to hold out the promise of self-perfectibility to those who complied with the requisite physiological and phrenological conditions. Moreover, Combean awareness of racial limits to the capacity for progression, brought race once again into unhappy conjunction with religious norms. 'Will any one now be surprised to learn from Mr. Combe', pondered Gillespie, 'that we cannot, by any means, make Christians of native American savages, or native New Hollanders? – or, by parity of reasoning, of any other tribes of savages as they?'[62] Whereas the

56   See e.g. G. Lyon, 'Essay on the phrenological causes of the different degrees of liberty enjoyed by different nations', *Phrenological Journal and Miscellany*, 2 (1824–5), 598–619.

57   George Combe, 'Phrenological remarks on the relation between the natural talents and dispositions of nations, and the development of their brains', in S.G. Morton, *Crania Americana* (Philadelphia and London, 1839), p. 283.

58   *Ibid.*, p. 271.

59   Andrew Combe to Mrs Henry Siddons, 3 December 1830, in George Combe, *The Life and Correspondence of Andrew Combe MD* (Edinburgh, 1850), p. 198.

60   William Scott, *The Harmony of Phrenology with Scripture: Shewn in a Refutation of a Philosophical Error contained in Mr. Combe's Constitution of Man* (Edinburgh, 1836).

61   William Gillespie, *An Exposure of the Unchristian and Unphilosophical Principles set forth in George Combe's work, entitled The Constitution of Man* (2nd edn, Edinburgh, 1836), pp. ix, 66.

62   *Ibid.*, pp. ix–x.

justification of overseas missions rested upon the psychic unity of mankind and a universal capacity for civilization, the phrenologists considered the mind to be a mere aggregate of mental powers, physically limited in its potential for progress by the natural endowment of faculties. Like polygenesis, a doctrine with which its proponents flirted,[63] phrenology appeared to present an unpalatable view of human nature sharply at odds with Christian teaching.

Religious issues (in tandem, as noted, with a receptivity to the concerns of continental racial anatomists) had inspired the Scottish medical profession's fascination with racial difference, and religious controversy continued into the second third of the nineteenth century to dog phrenological engagement with the topic. Nevertheless, on the topic of race, the phrenologists shared several attitudes with conventional medical science. Robert Knox, the anatomy lecturer whose career in Edinburgh was cut short by the Burke and Hare scandal,[64] espoused a Saxonist racial liberalism similar to that of the Combes, as well as their contempt for the Celtic peoples.[65] Nor in the first decades of the nineteenth century was there any major gulf between medical theorists of race and the philological school championed by Pinkerton. Anatomy and language seemed to correspond, and in the context of Scottish ethnology both groups recognized – and valued – the same ethnic categories. The differences in methodology between the philologists and physiologists to which Macculloch drew attention were marginal. Medical and pseudo-medical knowledge largely reinforced the original analysis put forward by the philologists, and adopted by archaeologists and historians, that Scotland was a racially-divided nation. In this way, medical science worked in tandem with other disciplines to thwart the emergence of a coherent ethnic nationalism within the nineteenth-century Scottish intelligentsia. Similarly, the cult of Saxonist liberalism clouded any potential linkage between radicalism and nationalism.

However, as should now be clear, the ideological salience of the race issue did not pertain primarily to the differences between unionism and nationalism (important as these were in the particular case of Scotland), but to the radical implications for Christian orthodoxy – and for the conservative social order which it upheld – of innate racial differences. Racialism's radical significance also extended to a keen awareness of inherent *racial* capacities for freedom and democracy, and, through phrenology, to schemes for popular self-improvement. The experience of the later Scottish Enlightenment pricks the modern assumption that race is automatically a tool of the political Right, or of nationalists.

Yet the dominant motivation behind racial science in late Enlightenment Scotland was conservative: to conserve the monogenetic paradigm upon which Christian truths depended. Scottish culture witnessed a rather lopsided division between a monogenist majority and a polygenist fringe, with the split between monogenists and polygenists appearing *within* rather than between academic

63   Armstrong, 'Wha's like us?', pp. 233–4.
64   Owen Dudley Edwards, *Burke and Hare* (1980; Edinburgh, 1993).
65   Robert Knox, *Races of Men* (London, 1850), esp. pp. 18–19, 27, 59.

disciplines. Orthodox philologists were just as keen to establish an aboriginal universal language as were their medical counterparts to demolish polygenist explanations of racial variation.[66] Nevertheless, as the scale and depth of anti-Celtic prejudice fomented in nineteenth-century Scotland indicate, the dominant strain of monogenist science, no less than the polygenist heterodoxy it opposed, fostered a racialist mindset.

---

66   See e.g. John Callander, *Two Ancient Scottish Poems* (Edinburgh, 1782), pp. 4–5, 24–6, 95, 98; John Jamieson, *Hermes Scythicus* (Edinburgh, 1814), pp. 5–7.

Chapter 12

After the Revolution: Scientific Language and French Politics, 1795–1802

Pietro Corsi

As Charles Webster has shown, important intellectual factions within the constellation of the pro-Parliamentary and Cromwellian intelligentsia saw the question of language – its foundation, nature, the possibility of establishing universal languages, and the key importance of a pedagogical effort to teach modern European languages to tradesmen and citizens – as an integral part of the cultural and moral reform they wished to promote. He has also reconstructed the short-lived, albeit intense debate on the proposals to reform weights and measures, and to introduce a decimal system.[1] A century and a half later, in revolutionary France, the two issues were again at the forefront of heated epistemological, linguistic and political debates. Many of the solutions proposed, such as the adoption of the metric system on a decimal base, or the criteria to be followed in order to reform the language of science, are still with us today. Yet, if the difficulties faced by the adoption of the metric system are well known and easy to understand – local resistance to worrying novelties, and the unpalatable connection with the revolutionary fervour that had launched the Project – the reform of scientific language has almost been taken for granted.

In particular, the close connection between the debate on the language of science and the rapidly changing political situation during the decade 1795–1805 still awaits clarification. In other words, although from the beginning of the nineteenth century it has been a commonly accepted practice to forge new names in science by using mostly Greek or Latin words (a choice that would have horrified Webster's heroes), French scientists at the turn of the century had to work hard to make contemporaries overlook the attitudes and arguments used to establish this principle. The need for a new language for science, as well as for philosophy, and politics, was vociferously advocated and theorized by several actors of the revolutionary decades. These included Antoine-Laurent Lavoisier (1743–1794) and his followers, the young Georges Cuvier (1769–1832) and, surprisingly, Jean-Baptiste

---

1 Charles Webster, *The Great Instauration: Science, Medicine and Reform 1626–1660* (London, 1975), pp. 411–20 and *passim*.

Lamarck (1744–1829). Though a stern opponent of the neologisms introduced into the vocabulary of chemistry by Lavoisier and his followers, and of contemporary proposals for reforming the language of science in general, between 1800 and 1802 Lamarck did not hesitate to propose new 'Greek' terms such as hydrogeology or biology. In the realms of philosophy and politics, the innovative linguistic fervour of the 'Idéologues' has been closely studied, and a recent study of Emmanuel-Joseph Sieyès (1748–1836) has pointed out the terminological preoccupations underlying his meditations on the reform of politics, which, in his eyes, required a reform of political language.[2]

As is well known, in France the debate on the language most appropriate to science long preceded the revolutionary storm. This point was explicitly acknowledged by key protagonists of this debate during the 1790s, who referred to works by John Locke (1632–1704), Etienne Bonnot de Condillac (1715–1780), and Carl Linnaeus (1707–1778), or to the *Méthode de nomenclature chimique* published by Lavoisier and his followers in 1787, as the authoritative foundation for their proposals.[3] What was new was the intense and openly political dimension that the debate took on during the last decade of the eighteenth century, as well as the normative proposals that many participants hoped would be endorsed by educational and administrative authorities.[4] Moreover, it has rarely been mentioned that

2   Harry B. Acton, 'The philosophy of language in revolutionary France', *Proceedings of the British Academy*, 14 (1959), 199–221; Maurice Crosland, *Historical Aspects of the Language of Chemistry* (London, 1962); Sergio Moravia, *Il pensiero degli Idéologues: scienza e filosofia in Francia (1780–1815)* (Florence, 1974); Geroge Gusdorf, *La conscience révolutionnaire, les Idéologues* (Paris, 1978); Olivia Smith, *The Politics of Language, 1791–1819* (Oxford, 1984); François Azouvi, ed., *L'institution de la raison. La révolution culturelle de Thermidor* (Paris, 1992); Jacques Guilhaumou, *Sieyès et l'ordre de la langue: l'invention de la politique moderne* (Paris, 2002). For the revival, and criticism, of the French debate on language and science in early nineteenth-century England, see Pietro Corsi, 'The heritage of Dugald Stewart: Oxford philosophy and the method of political economy, 1809–1832', *Nuncius*, 2 (1987), 89–144.

3   Lia Formigari, *Signs, Science and Politics: Philosophies of Language in Europe 1700–1830* (Amsterdam, 1993); Wilda Anderson, *Between the Library and the Laboratory: The Language of Chemistry in Eighteenth-Century France* (Baltimore, 1984) and her 'Scientific nomenclature and revolutionary rhetoric', *Rhetorica*, 7 (1989), 45–53; Umberto Eco, *Kant and the Platypus: Essays on Language and Cognition* (London, 1999); Marco Beretta, *The Enlightenment of Matter. The Definition of Chemistry from Agricola to Lavoisier* (Canton, MA, 1993). For a recent, penetrating survey of the literature, see Jessica Riskin, 'Rival idioms for a revolutionized science and a republican citizenry', *Isis*, 89 (1998), 203–32.

4   See for instance W. Randall Albury, 'The order of ideas: Condillac's method of analysis as a political instrument in the French Revolution', in *The Politics and Rhetoric of Scientific Method. Historical Studies*, ed. John A. Schuster and Richard R. Yeo (Dordrecht and Boston, 1986), pp. 203–25 and Jessica Riskin, *Science in the Age of Sensibility. The Sentimental Empiricists of the French Enlightenment* (Chicago,

after 1795, in the space of five to seven years, public discussion on the most appropriate language to be adopted in science quickly reached a peak and rapidly faded away. By 1802–1804, the fashion for neologisms had become an object of acrimonious derision from conservative writers on science.

It is appropriate to emphasize at this point that the purpose of this paper is not to reconstruct in detail the debate on science and language during the last decades of the eighteenth century, an issue historians of several disciplines and intellectual practices have dwelt upon; nor to cover again the ground of the political debate on science, its utility and indeed essential ideological role for the political authorities emerging after the fall of Robespierre in July 1794. The seminal work by Roger Hahn on the Académie des sciences, an institution suppressed in 1793, the equally important work on Cuvier's early career by Dorinda Outram, and, most recently, Jean-Luc Chappey's masterly reconstruction of the political tight-rope on which the founders and supporters of the 'Société des Observateurs de l'Homme' had to balance themselves during the short life of their association (1800–1804), have done much to highlight the political and institutional background to this essay.[5] It will be our task to show how political considerations were also responsible for the embarrassed silence on the issue of the relationship between linguistic and scientific innovation that followed the consolidation of Napoleon's power after 1800.

After the storm: scientific expectations

A passage in an unpublished letter from Antoine-François Fourcroy (1755–1809) to the pharmacist and entrepreneur Henri-Albert Gosse (1753–1816) in Geneva will at once plunge us into the charged atmosphere of the months following the fall of Robespierre. As a member of the 'Comité d'instruction publique' (he had taken the seat left vacant by Jean-Paul Marat), Fourcroy had been an eminent representative of the revolutionary Republic. He was now in charge of the complex institutional engineering meant to provide a meritocratic justification for the regime in power after 1794, intent on steering a difficult route between the dangers of an

2002), chap. 7. See Beretta, *The Enlightenment of Matter*, and Riskin for the issue of the language of science and its political dimension before the period here examined.

5   Roger Hahn, *The Anatomy of a Scientific Institution: The Paris Academy of Sciences, 1666–1803* (Berkeley, 1971); Dorinda Outram, 'Politics and vocation: French science 1793–1830', *British Journal for the History of Science*, 13 (1980), 27–43; Outram, 'The ordeal of vocation: the Paris Academy of Sciences and the Terror, 1793–95', *History of Science*, 21 (1983), 251–73; Outram, *Georges Cuvier: Vocation, Science and Authority in Post-Revolutionary France* (Manchester, 1984); Jean-Luc Chappey, *La Société des Observateurs de l'Homme (1799–1804). Des anthropologues au temps de Bonaparte* (Paris, 2002). See also Janis Langins, *La République avait besoin des savants* (Paris, 1987) and Nicole and Jean Dhombres, *Naissance d'un pouvoir: sciences et savants en France, 1793–1824* (Paris, 1989).

ultra-democratic resurgence and menacing attempts at pro-monarchical armed insurrection. Scientific achievements and proficiency were to guarantee the public and the private good. The republican hierarchies, solidly empowered by their intellectual merit, were going to ensure the prosperity of the state through a systematic exploitation of scientific practices and a massive effort at scientific and technological education:

> You will learn with pleasure that we are giving a great impulsion to the sciences, the arts, to public education, to industry and agriculture, with a force and urgency equal to the ones vandalism has deployed to destroy them. Schools of health, of public works, a special school to train teachers are being established this very moment. We take care of arts and sciences everywhere, we help, call upon, encourage all educated men; the Convention honours and repays them, with money, for the losses and the shameful neglect they were subjected to for too long. Long live the republics where Knowledge and virtue are valued. Within a few years, France will no longer be recognizable.[6]

In spite of Fourcroy's optimism, times remained hard. Career, and indeed, life prospects were dramatically uncertain, and good intentions were severely hampered by economic difficulties. As late as December 1796, the witty Déodat de Gratet de Dolomieu (1750–1801) still complained to Marc-Auguste Pictet (1752–1825) that 'nothing new happens in science; those who cultivate it are slowing down this winter. *Knowledge freezes without money*, one could say. This lack of money introduces a pronounced lethargy in any undertaking that requires some activity'.[7]

6   Henri-Albert Gosse, 'Lettres adressées à Henri-Albert Gosse', Geneva, Bibliothèque publique et universitaire, MS. 2628, fol. 138v, Fourcroy to Gosse, 26 January 1795: 'Tu apprendras avec plaisir que nous donnons avec autant de force et d'empressement que le vandalisme n'avait mis à la détruire, une grande impulsion aux sciences, aux arts, à l'instruction publique, aux manufactures et à l'agriculture. Des Écoles de santé, des travaux publics, une école normale pour former des Professeurs sont établis en ce moment. On s'occupe partout des arts et des sciences, on soigne, on appelle, on encourage les hommes instruits; la Convention les honore et les indemnise par des sommes des pertes et de l'oubli honteux qu'on leur a fait trop long temps subir. Vive les républiques où l'on prise le Savoir et les vertus. La France ne sera pas reconnoissable dans quelques années.' See Danielle Plan, *Un genevois d'autrefois: Henri-Albert Gosse (1753–1816). D'après des lettres et des documents inédits* (Paris and Geneva, 1909); Bruno Belhoste, *La formation d'une technocratie. L'Ecole Polytechnique et ses élèves, de la Révolution au Second Empire* (Paris, 2003).

7   Marc-Auguste Pictet, *Correspondance: science et technique*, ed. René Sigrist (4 vols, Geneva, 1996–), ii (1998), p. 344, Dolomieu to Pictet, 16 December 1796: 'Nous n'avons rien de nouveau dans les sciences; ceux qui les cultivent se ralentissent un peu cet hiver. On pourrait dire, *sine pecunia friget scientia*. Ce manque d'argent porte sur tout ce qui exige quelque activité un bien grand engourdissement'. Six months later, the situation had improved: 'Les sciences on repris ici une grande activité, et ceux qui les cultivent montrent une grande émulation. Le gouvernement ne fait pas encore des choses bien importantes pour elles et pour eux; mais la considération est indépendante

Though the economic situation improved over the following months, and publishing activity slowly regained momentum, the livelihoods of independent scientific practitioners remained under severe threat. Those who received regular salaries, albeit irregularly paid, did not receive hard currency, but paper money, the infamous and highly inflationary *assignats*. This forced them to compete for resources with colleagues left out of state employment, whose survival depended on their medical practice, the sale of specimens, or their pen. Waiting for a post that never came in the Directoire central administration, Louis-Augustin-Guillaume Bosc d'Antic (1759–1828) did not complain too loudly about his economic situation: 'I am quietly waiting for when it will please the Directoire to chase away those who are shadowing me. By working at Olivier's [Guillaume-Antoine, 1756–1814] entomology, I am gaining ten times more in real money, than my colleagues get in current *assignats*'.[8] Today's cliché 'publish or perish' was never truer. Getting into print meant to acquire visibility, money and friends, as well as the possibility of further employment. It also helped to slight enemies and competitors by making oblique reference to their dangerous past or by adopting a language that contemporaries were immediately capable of decoding for its political significance. Thus, for instance, when in 1802 Charles-Nicholas-Sigisbert Sonnini de Manoncourt (1751–1812), editor of a highly successful edition of Buffon's works, called Cuvier 'un homme nouveau', an authoritarian 'instituteur' who had had the good fortune of getting a job at the Muséum nationale d'histoire naturelle, readers well understood the innuendoes.[9] Cuvier was where he was thanks to the Revolution: he had lost the cap but not the manners of a hard-line Jacobin. The truth or falsehood of the allegation is of course beside the point. In Jean-Claude Delamétherie's (1743–1817) editorship of the *Journal de physique*, which recommenced publication in 1798, after a forced break of almost five years, political aims were not far from the surface. In his eyes, the new chemists, their arrogant proposal of a

---

de l'état de nos finances, et quoiqu'elle n'échauffe pas la cuisine, elle aide au moins à supporter les privations', in Alfred Lacroix, *Déodat Dolomieu* (2 vols, Paris, 1921), ii, p. 153, Dolomieu to the Ch. de Fay, 25 May 1797. See also Therése Charles-Vallin, *Les aventures du chevalier géologue Déodat de Dolomieu* (Grenoble, 2003).

8 Gosse, 'Lettres adressées à Henri-Albert Gosse', Geneva, Bibliothèque publique et universitaire, MS 2628, fol. 137v, Bosc to Gosse, 9 Germinal an IV (25 March 1796): 'J'attends en silence qu'il plaise enfin au Directoire de chasser les gens qui m'offusquent. Je gagne, en travaillant à l'entomologie d'Olivier, dix fois plus en numéraire, que n'en gagnent mes collègues en assignats au cours.'

9 Charles-Nicholas-Sigisbert Sonnini de Manoncourt, ed., *Histoire naturelle, générale et particulière, par Leclerc de Buffon* (127 vols, Paris, 1798–1808), lxv (an XI, 1802), p. 37. On Sonnini and the Buffonians after the Revolution, see Pietro Corsi, *Lamarck. Genèse et enjeux du transformisme, 1770–1830* (Paris, 2001), new expanded edition of *The Age of Lamarck. Evolutionary Theories in France, 1790–1830* (Berkeley, 1988). Sonnini was a protégé of Lacepède, rising star of the Napoleonic regime, a naturalist and politician who considered himself as Buffon's literary and scientific heir.

completely new language for their discipline, and their politics were one and the same thing. The *Journal de physique* was there to oppose them, even though Delamétherie was increasingly aware that the battle had been lost: 'This coalition of people, *fatigued by blood but not satiated*, will make sure that whatever is contrary to their opinion and could do harm to their self-respect will never enter our country. They have cut the throat of their boss, Lavoisier, as they have done with the chief of the Nation, because they wanted to become the masters'.[10]

A close reconstruction of the shifting political situations and alliances, and of the different and, at times, divergent meaning an epistemological standpoint could take in different political contexts, still remains a desideratum of studies on French science after 1794, up to the consolidation of the Napoleonic regime. To my knowledge, the only example is Chappey's study of the 'Société des Observateurs de l'Homme'. Attitudes towards Buffon, his work, his style of natural history and his literary style *tout court*, as well as the debate on the language of science are considered below in some detail. They constitute two interesting examples of the complex situation prevailing after 1794, and its equally complex interpretative framework.

Changing views of Buffon

Positively disliked by representatives of the Enlightenment such as d'Alembert and Condorcet, and subjected to an exercise in character assassination in the latter's academic eulogy, Buffon was seen as standing for everything natural history and science in general should not and could not be: rhetorical and moralistic, based on imagination rather than on reason, undertaken to please the readers rather than to convince the experts, better suited for the salon than for the academy. The famous naturalist was also portrayed as the prototype of the court savant, using his power to prevent criticism of his own works, distributing favours and jobs, relegating Linnaean taxonomical reform to the provinces or the margins of institutional science. Needless to say, not all the naturalists or the intellectuals undergoing the experience of the Revolution and its aftermath shared this attitude. And if it would be wrong to claim that everyone in favour of political and intellectual change was opposed to Buffon, it would be equally wrong to maintain that since Buffon was

---

10   Jean Senebier, 'Lettres adressées à Jean Senebier', Geneva, Bibliothèque publique et universitaire, MS Supp. 1039, fol. 253v, Jean-Claude de la Métherie à Senebier, 18 January 1796: 'et [cette] coalition de gens, *lassati sanguinis sed non satiati*, empêchera de pénétrer dans ce pays tout ce qui est contraire à leurs opinions et puisse choquer leur amour propre. Ils ont égorgé leur chef, Lavoisier, comme ils ont égorgé celui de la nation, parce qu'ils vouloient être les maîtres.' De la Métherie announced in 1793 his intention to adopt the more democratic 'Delamétherie' spelling of his name, with which he signed all his subsequent works. See also Riskin, his *Science in the Age of Sensibility*, pp. 269–79; Anderson, 'Scientific nomenclature and revolutionary rhetoric'.

highly respected by some influential representatives of the Enlightenment or the Assemblée nationale, he was immune from criticism from that quarter. It would also be wrong to assert, as it has been by some, that criticism of Buffon amounts to irrelevance. Once again, the key issue is that it remains difficult to generalize so far as to claim that there was a Jacobin natural history or science, one totally devoted to the theme of utility, and contrary to all forms of academic speculation and theorizing, that could accommodate Buffon's moral overtones and pedagogical objectives. Similarly, it is difficult to claim that the real issue was specialization versus encyclopaedic curiosity, a conflict settled once and for all in favour of better-defined and often rigid disciplinary boundaries. Those who proclaim 'the end of natural history' in its broadest sense have to explain why Buffonian 'natural history' survived well into the nineteenth century. One might assume it was to please millions of readers who were not informed of the death of the discipline or of the disrepute Buffon had supposedly fallen into. Reformulated in Humboldtian, romantic, Darwinian or Haeckelian terms, the idea (one that Buffon shared with many representatives of the 'histoire naturelle') that disciplinary specialization had to be subservient to the higher goal of understanding nature as a whole, remained a constant within western natural sciences during the nineteenth and for much of the twentieth centuries.[11]

To return to the issue of the political nature of many scientific or epistemological views expressed during the revolutionary decade, it should be emphasized that different individuals, at different times, expressed different views of Buffon, often very contradictory ones. To take only one case, and a very distinguished one, it would be difficult to summarize in a coherent framework Cuvier's attitude towards Buffon, as expressed throughout his career, from the cruelty of his youthful enthusiasm at the news of the death of the naturalist in 1787 ('The naturalists have finally lost their leader. This time, the Comte of Buffon is dead and buried') to his signing an edition of Buffon's works in 1830. In a patently self-contradictory and fascinating eulogy of Jean-Guillaume Bruguières (1750–1799), published in 1799, Cuvier declared that before the Revolution the only place where natural history had been taught in France at advanced (i.e., Linnaean) level was at Montpellier:

Through his lectures and his example, the respectable Gouan [Antoine, 1738–1821] disseminated Linnaeus' austere method, which in Paris and elsewhere was eclipsed by the success of Buffon's works: I do not mean to say that Buffon was

11 See the classic study by Charles C. Gillispie, 'The Encyclopédie and Jacobin philosophy of science: a study in ideas and consequences', in *Critical Problems in the History of Science*, ed. Marshall Clagett (Madison, 1959), pp. 255–89 and his *Science and Polity in France: the Revolutionary and Napoleonic Years* (Princeton, 2004). Emma C. Spary, *Utopia's Garden. French Natural History from Old Regime to Revolution* (Chicago, 2000), denies that Buffon was subjected to criticism during the period under discussion. Wolf Lepenis, *Das Ende der Naturgeschichte. Wandel kultureller Selbstverständlichkeiten in den Wissenschaften des 18. und 19. Jahrhunderts* (Munich, 1976).

not an accurate naturalist; on the contrary, I know that his works are even more true, factually more precise than those by Linnaeus: but in those times uneducated readers did not possess enough knowledge to be able to recognize this type of merit.[12]

In 1804, in the brochure announcing the launching of the still-born first edition of the *Dictionnaire des sciences naturelles* (1804–1805), under the editorship of his brother Frédéric (1773–1838), Cuvier blasted the highly successful rival *Nouveau Dictionnaire d'histoire naturelle* published in 24 volumes by a team of avowed hard-line Buffonians in the space of two years (1803–1804). By 1804, in the increasingly conservative political climate of the early Napoleonic regime, Buffon and Linnaeus were represented by Cuvier as sharing the merit of having taken natural history out of the chaos, which inconsiderate and ignorant Buffonians were now trying to recreate with their empty rhetorical exercises and their boundless thirst for speculation. No mercy for the Buffonians, then, but the master could regain his place in the pantheon of natural history.[13] It is worth mentioning that the complete edition of Buffon's work edited by Sonnini de Manoncourt, which Cuvier disliked so much, found a place in the library Napoleon took with him to the loneliness of St Helena. Finally, Cuvier's seemingly favourable biographical sketch of Buffon, published in 1812 in the highly popular *Biographie universelle* edited by Louis-Guillaume Michaud (1773–1858), reaches extraordinary levels of ambiguity. Every criticism or anecdote unfavourable to Buffon is related in sharp and concise detail. It culminates in a parting shot in the very last sentence of the article: a reference to the slanderous *Voyage à Montbard* by Marie-Jean Hérault de Séchelles (1759–1794), followed by the comment that Hérault had violated basic rules of hospitality by indulging in juicy scandalous remarks. An irresistible invitation to read the pamphlet, one might say.[14]

12   Georges Cuvier, 'Extrait d'une notice biographique sur Bruguières, lue à la Société Philomatique, dans sa séance générale du 30 nivôse an 7', *Magasin encyclopédique*, V année, 3 (an VII,1799), 42–57, p. 43: 'Le respectable Gouan y propagea, par ses leçons et par son exemple, la méthode sévère de Linné, qui se trouvait éclipsée à Paris et ailleurs par l'éclat des ouvrages de Buffon: non pas que je veuille dire par là que Buffon n'étoit pas un naturaliste exact; je sais, au contraire, que ses ouvrages sont même plus vrais, plus soignée sur les faits que celles de Linné: mais le vulgaire ne possédoit pas alors assez de connoissances pour y distinguer ce genre de mérite.'

13   For what I have called 'the war of dictionaries', see Corsi, *Lamarck*, pp. 37–9 and 270.

14   Georges Cuvier, 'Buffon', in Louis-Guillaume Michaud, ed., *Biographie universelle, ancienne et moderne* ([1812] 45 vols, Paris, 1843 edn), vi, pp. 117–21: p. 121: 'Il est fâcheux que les détails où il entre soient en partie calomnieux, ou doivent au moins être considérés comme une violation manifeste de l'hospitalité'; Marie-Jean Hérault de Séchelles, *Voyage à Montbard: contenant des détails très-intéressantes sur le caractère, la personne et les écrits de Buffon* (Paris, 1801), new edn, in Yann Gaillard, *Buffon. Biographie imaginaire et réelle* (Paris, 1977), pp. 141–74. The 1801 edition of the pamphlet, originally printed in 1787, had been edited by Aubin-Louis Millin. It is

Cuvier's scientific and methodological priorities were diametrically opposed to the concept of natural history that Buffon had advocated and promoted. The very idea of a systematic comparative anatomy was inconceivable to Buffon, for whom nature takes a step in every direction with every successive animate and inanimate being, whereas men can see only one thing at a time.[15] True, Buffon also argued that nature had probably created only one single animal or plant type, a concept Etienne Geoffroy Saint-Hilaire (1772–1844) took up and used against the idea, about which Cuvier became increasingly dogmatic, of well-defined structural plans characterizing different 'embranchements'. Yet, it was Geoffroy Saint-Hilaire who added comparative anatomy to a concept Buffon had hinted at in order to proclaim, using different words, the impossibility of any taxonomy and of Linnaean taxonomy in particular. Cuvier's insistence on the need to overcome the literary natural history Buffon and his followers cherished, and his repeated advocacy of a 'stile sevère' as an antidote to their excesses, could never be mistaken for a sign of respect, let alone sympathy, for the author of the *Histoire naturelle*. Thus, it is fair to conclude that Cuvier simply adapted his judgment to the current cultural and political climate, and to the behaviour of readers, who continued to buy edition after edition of Buffon's works, to the point that Cuvier himself, as already mentioned, decided to endorse yet another edition, nominally put under his care.[16]

The language of science: a public debate

The question of the rapid emergence of an intense public debate on the language of science around 1795 and its equally rapid disappearance from the pages of monographs, encyclopaedias and periodicals in 1802–4 will contribute to a deeper appreciation of the role of politics in contemporary scientific debates. As already pointed out, the issue was far from being a new one. To some extent, it was Buffon who had given the debate its polemical edge and public appeal with his repeated assaults on Linnaeus and his followers. He disparagingly labelled the latter 'nomenclateurs', and accused them of giving away the language of tradition, of trades and pleasure in favour of telegraphic Latin binomial definitions, pathetically (in his eyes) meant to exhaust all that had to be known of a plant or an animal. In turn, his own luxuriant, colourful digressions on the animal world were vulnerable to sarcastic comment, the most famous (related by Cuvier) being d'Alembert's

---

notable that Hérault even hinted that Buffon indulged in scandalous relationships with very young girls: a classic of anti-aristocratic rhetoric.

15 Thierry Hoquet, 'Buffon: histoire naturelle et philosophie', unpublished Université de Paris-X doctoral dissertation (2002).
16 The complex relationship between Lacepède and Cuvier, and the possibility that much of Cuvier's ambiguity with respect to Buffon was in part the effect of his desire not to antagonize Lacepède, is currently being investigated.

ironic remark that the horse had been defined by Buffon as 'man's noblest conquest'.[17]

Without doubt, the 1782 essay by Louis-Bernard Guyton de Morveau (1737–1816), 'Sur les dénominations chymiques', and the *Méthode de nomenclature chimique* (1787), had contributed powerfully to the idea, inspired by Condillac, that a science was 'a well-organized language', and that the degree of maturity of a discipline could be measured by the logical consistence and perspicuity of its language.[18] If Buffon had criticized Linnaean terminology for its betrayal of vernacular names, the new 'nomenclators' argued that vernacular names had to be abandoned altogether. Yet, before 1795, this debate did not appear to concern the educated public. Indeed, apart from the great popular success of Buffon's work, contemporaries such as the young Cuvier or the experienced Delamétherie did not consider France a country characterized by vigorous scientific production and debates. Before reading the anatomical treatise by Felix Vicq d'Azyr (1748–1794), the *Traité élémentaire de chimie* by Lavoisier, and the *Genera Plantarum* by Antoine-Laurent de Jussieu (1748–1836), which fired his enthusiasm, Cuvier, still writing in German (and Latin) to his friend Christoph Heinrich Pfaff (1773–1852), complained that 'the sciences possess today very few worthy priests in France, and this scarcity is all the more painful, when one recalls the brilliancy with which they once shone'.[19] In 1793, sketching in the *Journal de physique* a general view of the geographical distribution of intellectual pursuits in Europe, Delamétherie accorded to France the primacy in philosophical writings, whereas anatomy flourished in Italy, natural history, chemistry and mineralogy in Germany and Sweden, geometry and moral philosophy in England.[20]

17 Cuvier, 'Buffon', p. 118: 'Ne me parlez pas de votre Buffon, de ce comte de Tuffière, qui au lieu de nommer simplement le cheval, dit: La plus noble conquête que l'homme ait jamais faite est celle de ce fier et fougueux animal.'

18 Louis Bernard Guyton de Morveau, 'Sur les dénominations chymiques, la nécessité d'en perfectionner le système, et les règles pour y parvenir', *Observations et mémoires sur la physique*, 19 (1782), 370–82; Louis Bernard Guyton de Morveau, Antoine-François Lavoisier, Claude Louis Berthollet, Antoine-François Fourcroy, *Méthode de nomenclature chimique...on y a joint un nouveau système de caractères chimiques adaptés à cette nomenclature, par MM. Hassenfratz et Adet* (Paris, 1787). See Beretta, *The Enlightenment of Matter*, on the intense debate inside Lavoisier's circle, leading up to the writing of the *Méthode*.

19 Christoph Heinrich Pfaff, *Lettres de Georges Cuvier*, ed. L. Marchant (Paris, 1858), p. 78, 31 December 1788: 'Les sciences ont aujourd'hui peu de dignes prêtres en France, et cette pauvreté est d'autant plus pénible, que l'on se souvient encore de l'ancien éclat dont elles ont brillé.'

20 Jean-Claude Delamétherie, 'Discours préliminaire', *Journal de physique*, 42 (January 1793), 3–34: p. 7. The 'Discours préliminaires' Delamétherie contributed to the *Journal de physique* over a period of more than twenty years are available at the address http://www.crhst.cnrs.fr/i-corpus/science1800/ (ed. Pietro Corsi). They should be read as a partisan counterpoint to the equally partisan reports Cuvier wrote on the state of contemporary science.

For the reasons Roger Hahn has well illustrated and which we have alluded to, Cuvier's and Delamétherie's remarks would have sounded strange only a few years later, as, to some extent, they do sound strange today. Yet, it is undeniable that for a variety of reasons the debate on science, its foundations, public utility and prospects had become one of the key features of Parisian and French culture, high and low, only after the dark months of the Terror. Scientific proficiency helped those with connections to the previous administration to mark their distance from it, as was the case with Fourcroy, one of the first proponents of the charge of scientific 'vandalism' brought against a regime he himself had been part of. Though Fourcroy could quote his cautious interventions against 'patriotic' vandalism exercised against artistic or architectonic emblems of the monarchy in the early 1790s, opponents did not forget his role in the abolition of the Académie des sciences, or, as was also the case with Delamétherie, his lack of determination to save Lavoisier's life.[21] Young and ambitious provincial amateurs flocked to Paris in the hope of taking advantage of the temporary disruption of old networks and institutions, as well as of the need for trained personnel in the medical and pharmaceutical services of the growing republican army. Journals like the *Décade philosophique*, the *Annales des mines*, and, with systematic dedication, the *Magasin encyclopédique*, constantly reported on scientific publications, on private lecture courses being offered in natural history or mineralogy, and on the public meetings held at the Institut, the new form the ancient Académie had been given in late 1795.

The case of the *Magasin encyclopédique*

It is to periodicals that one has to turn in order to appreciate the extent, and the chronological limits of the post-1795 debate on science and language. We will once again focus on one single example, the *Magasin encyclopédique*, established (briefly) in 1792, and successfully re-launched in 1795. Its editor, Aubin-Louis Millin (1759–1818), who contributed scores of articles, reviews and short news on institutional and private science, made no mystery of his determination to introduce rigour and disciplinary specialization within traditional natural history. Personally linked to the Girondins and the Roland family, Millin had been one of the founders of the Société Linnéenne, and of the Société d'histoire naturelle. A polyglot, classicist and Germanist, archaeologist, lover of theatre and one of the first directors of the Bibliothèque nationale, Millin is a figure strangely overlooked by historians of the period.[22] He gathered around him an impressive cohort of contributors,

21   Edouard Pommier, *L'art de la liberté. Doctrines et débats de la Révolution française* (Paris, 1991), pp. 123–4 ; Joseph Fayet, *La Révolution française et la science, 1789–1795* (Paris, 1960), chap. 6.
22   Chappey, *Société des Observateurs de l'Homme*, deals with selected features of Millin's career.

ranging from Jean-Louis Alibert (1768–1837), Philippe Pinel (1745–1826), Cuvier, Charles-Louis Dumas (1765–1813), Antoine-Nicholas Duchesne (1747–1827) and the very young André-Marie Constant Duméril (1774–1860). They argued for the need of a radical reform of natural history, in order to transform a literary exercise into a well-founded, epistemologically rigorous, disciplinary domain. The road to follow was already well established by an illustrious philosophical and scientific tradition:

> After Locke and Condillac have reformed the theory of sensations and of ideas, after in particular the latter has demonstrated the need and advantages of analysis in the search for truth, the sciences of observation have improved with prodigious speed, and all obstacles subside under the efforts of human ingenuity.[23]

Linnaeus himself had employed the analytical method when he isolated the sexual organs as the foundation for a taxonomy that was logically, as well as ontologically, reliable. Analysis again was at the basis of the experimental work undertaken by Lavoisier and his collaborators; in the *Méthode de nomenclature chimique* they had publicly acknowledged their debt to Condillac, and proved that a mature science was, and ought to be, a well-organized language. Analysis, conducted through observation and experimentation, was seen as capable of reducing natural objects to their ultimate components, and of establishing their spatial and temporal relationships. The choice of appropriate names for each element identified through analysis opened the way to the possibility of reconstituting the structure and properties of the object under investigation through the very definition employed to describe it. In the well-ordered language of science, the sentence became the representation of an ontological structure. Thus, if names could and indeed often were by necessity arbitrary and conventional, the language of science, that is the succession of definitions and descriptions of space-temporal relationships, was not.[24] From these premises, Duméril deduced a conclusion he chose to express in the form of a rhetorical question: 'Is there a science more in urgent need of a methodical nomenclature than natural history? How to apply to the immense series

---

23   Jean-Louis Alibert, 'Compte-rendu de Philippe Pinel, *Nosographie philosophique, ou la méthode de l'analyse appliquée à la médecine*', *Magasin encyclopédique*, IV année, 3 (an VII, 1798), 1–21, p. 1: 'Depuis que Locke et Condillac ont refait la théorie des sensations et des idées, depuis que ce dernier sur-tout a démontré les avantages et la nécessité de l'analyse dans la recherche de la vérité, les sciences d'observations se perfectionnent avec une rapidité qui tient du prodige, et tous les obstacles s'aplanissent devant les efforts de l'esprit humain.' There is no need to stress that opinions expressed in the periodical literature often lacked philosophical discrimination. Thus, crucial differences between Locke and Condillac were almost regularly overlooked.

24   See Riskin, *Science in the Age of Sensibility*, for a discussion of conventionalist *versus* ontological views of the language of chemistry and of science in general.

of beings it embraces, names capable, in our judgment, of representing to us the objects they are meant to represent?'[25]

Duméril had no doubt that the chemical nomenclature first suggested by Guyton de Morveau, then perfected by Lavoisier and his collaborators, constituted the model to be followed. As far as the choice of words was concerned, Linnaeus's *Philosophia botanica* had taught naturalists to mistrust names handed down by custom and tradition: 'orphans of whim and prejudice, they are the adopted children of habit'. Linnaeus was therefore to be taken as an example of rigour and of verbal parsimony, though doubts were expressed as to the preference the Swedish naturalist had accorded to Latin. Duméril, referring again to the new chemical nomenclature, gave preference to Greek names, or, even better, to Greek roots, capable of being combined with prepositions, or entered into the composition of other names.

Young Cuvier, still an obscure 'instituteur' in Normandy, had preceded Duméril in this choice, as, with elegance and false modesty, he wrote to his friend Pfaff in the early summer of 1790: 'I have taken the new names for genera, in preference, from Greek rather than from Latin, not so much to make a show of vain erudition, since I consider myself less proficient than it is decent in the Greek language, but because the Latin expression dislikes composite names, as Horace once remarked'.[26]

In some extreme cases, innovation came to the point of dispensing with the new 'philosophical language' grounded on Greek roots, and made authors opt for algebraic formulae, thus ushering a discipline of natural history into the empire of applied mathematics. In the *Journal des mines*, Réné-Juste Haüy (1743–1822) announced:

the idea of translating in a very concise language, analogous to the language of algebraic analysis, the expression of the various laws determining secondary crystals, and to compose in this way some kind of formulae representing these very crystals. It will be sufficient, in order to achieve this, to indicate with letters the angles and the edges of the primitive form, and to accompany these letters with

25 André-Marie-Constant Duméril, 'Projet d'une nomenclature anatomique basée sur la terminaison', *Magasin encyclopédique*, II année, 2 (an IV, 1796), 452–63, p. 454: 'Étoit-il une science pour laquelle une nomenclature méthodique se trouvait plus indispensablement nécessaire que l'histoire naturelle? Comment appliquer à l'immense série des êtres qu'elle embrasse de noms qui rapportassent, à notre jugement, les objets qu'ils représentent? Où trouver cette langue nouvelle?'
26 Pfaff, *Lettres de Georges Cuvier*, p. 163, 25 June 1790: 'Nomina generica nova, e graeco potius desumpsi, quam e latino sermone, non ad vanam eruditionem ostentationem, nam me graecarum litterarum radiorem quam deceret esse fateor, sed quia voces compositae latini sermonis indoli repugnant, uti jamdudum observavit Horatius.'

numbers indicating the law of decrease this angle or that edge is subjected to, the result of which being that particular secondary form.[27]

Returning to the *Magasin encyclopédique*, several contributors expressed the view that Jussieu's *Genera Plantarum*, Vicq d'Azyr's comparative anatomy, Dumas' and Duméril's human anatomy, Haüy's crystallography, Pinel's philosophical nosography, or Alibert's dermatology represented the latest results obtained in the march of specialization so spectacularly under way.

As with objects or phenomena, disciplines too had to be submitted to a critical analysis capable of distinguishing the useful from the futile, the rhetorical turn of phrase from the well-established fact. Analysis and new nomenclature would dissipate the declamatory haze characterizing traditional natural history, ever more ready to expand lyrically upon its objects than carefully to dissect them, logically and physically. Disciplines, like objects, were given new names, to indicate their emancipation from the all-encompassing 'histoire naturelle': crystallography and crystallotechnics, ichthyology and herpetology, nosography and pasigraphy, biology and hydrogeology, technology and biotechnology, organology and phrenology: and, last but not least, ideology, a term which first appeared in 1797, and rarely to be pronounced in public after 1803.[28]

It is, of course, an essential part of our thesis to stress the danger of drawing general conclusions from this rapid excursus of positions defended in the *Magasin encyclopédique*, as if this periodical was unanimously consecrated to the cause of reform, or that the word 'reform' did not admit of a plurality of often contradictory meanings. Thus, for instance, Jacques-Louis Moreau de la Sarthe (1771–1826) could not agree on the superiority of Linnaeus over Buffon:

> I only knew parts of his [Linnaeus'] works, those where, though admiring the width and variety of his knowledge, the precision of his language and the exactness of his distributions, one could search in vain for that warmth of style,

27   René-Just Haüy, 'Exposé d'une méthode simple et facile pour représenter les différentes formes cristallines par des signes très-abrégés, qui expriment les lois de décroissement auxquelles est soumise la structure', *Journal des mines*, 4 (1796), 15–36, pp. 15–16 : '[l']idée de traduire, dans une langue très-abrégée, analogue à celle de l'analyse algébrique, l'énoncé des diverses lois qui déterminent les cristaux secondaires, et de composer ainsi des espèces de formules représentatives de ces mêmes cristaux. Il suffit, pour y parvenir, de désigner, par des lettres, les angles et les arêtes de la forme primitive, et d'accompagner ces lettres de chiffres qui indiqueront les lois de décroissement qui subit tel angle ou telle arête, et dont le résultat est telle forme secondaire.' See Peter J. Stevens, 'Hauy and A. P. de Candolle: crystallography in the development of botanical systematics and comparative morphology, 1780–1840', *Journal of the History of Biology*, 17 (1984), 49–82.

28   For a critical discussion of the introduction of the term 'idéologie', see Chappey, *Société des Observateurs de l'Homme*, p. 61. As mentioned below, 1803 was the year in which the First Consul Bonaparte disbanded the Moral and Political Sciences Class of the Institut dominated by the *idéologues*.

that eloquent and picturesque turn so typical with Buffon, which are in my view inseparable from the art of observing the phenomena of nature, more inspiring than the wonders of fables.[29]

Moreover, even naturalists who were fiercely opposed to the new chemistry, and deeply disliked the upper hand the 'nomenclators' had gained in contemporary institutions, made their own terminological proposals. Thus, Lamarck, an author the *Magasin encyclopédique* repeatedly invited not to meddle with matters outside his botanical expertise, announced in 1802 his intention to launch an ambitious research programme centred on three new disciplines: meteorology (certainly not a newcomer), hydrogeology and biology. Slightly too late, as we shall argue below.

Fading enthusiasm

The Parisian scientific and philosophical scene between 1795 and 1800–1802 was characterized by the simultaneous presence of a plurality of actors and of theoretical standpoints, of styles of research and of scientific writing, and of individuals in need of patrons and allies. Some were intent on renewing old friendships, especially if they had emerged from prison or re-emerged from hiding and returned from exile. Those new to Paris were often in search of good contacts, as was the case with the Cuvier brothers, Duméril, Duvernoy, Julien-Joseph Viery (1775–1847) or Pierre-André Latreille (1762–1833) and Sonnini de Manoncourt, to name just a few. The effect of living in uncertain times, which explains more or less sudden changes of views, and the plurality of actors and of positions to be considered, should not exempt us from hazarding an interpretative framework that might open new lines of research. It will be therefore our task to offer a convincing explanation for the fact that the self-assured proclamations identifying (new) science with the reform of language progressively lost momentum, and by 1803–1804 they had almost completely disappeared. Which did not imply, needless to say, that the question of botanical, anatomical, geological or mineralogical nomenclature had disappeared: what was gone was the announcement of the unbounded progress Duméril had promised, the programmatic – if not epiphanic – value attributed to the reform of scientific language.

Cuvier will once again help us illustrate this key change of emphasis. We have already heard the young 'instituteur' calling upon Horace to convince his friend

29 Jacques-Louis Moreau de la Sarthe, 'Considérations philosophiques sur l'histoire naturelle en général, et en particulier sur celle des Insectes, adressées au C. Millin', *Magasin encyclopédique*, IV année, 4 (an VII, 1798), 7–23, pp. 7–8 : 'Je ne connoissois qu'une partie de ses [Linné] ouvrages, ceux où, en admirant l'étendue et la variété des connoissances, la précision du langage et l'exactitude des distributions, on cherche en vain cette chaleur de style, cette manière éloquente et pittoresque qui caractérisent Buffon, et qui me paroissent inséparables de l'art d'observer les phénomènes de la nature, plus inspirans que les merveilleux des fables.'

Pfaff that Latin was not as flexible as Greek, as far as compound names were concerned: the names, that is, useful in science. In his early days, still under the influence of his German mentors, Carl Friedrich Kielmeyer (1765–1844) in particular, Cuvier dreamt of a science of everything, which would move from the study of chemical elements in order to ascend, law after law, to life, man and intelligence; a project Lamarck, Delamétherie or Bernard-Germain-Etienne de la Ville, Count Lacepède (1756–1825) would have found appealing, if the one they had already developed had not been, in their eyes, clearly the better.[30]

Upon his arrival in Paris, in 1795, Cuvier was admired and feared for his proficiency in comparative anatomy; the death of Vicq d'Azyr in 1794 left him free scope, and a wealth of notes his predecessor had accumulated. Not without a certain degree of arrogance and aggressiveness, he advocated the adoption of a 'stile sévère' in natural history, criticized the followers of Buffon with devastating irony, denied legitimacy to all forms of 'roman philosophique', including the then fashionable 'theories of the earth', and unfavourably compared France with Germany, where, he claimed, there were specialized natural history periodicals in every major town. Yet, despite all his accomplishments Cuvier needed help from other sources to further his career. He had to turn to bribery to get the post of assistant to Mertrud at the Muséum, and then all the political support he could muster to secure a permanent position. It was only in 1802, when his position was politically established, that he finally got his full chair at the Muséum. With the help, it should be added, of the ultra-Buffonian Lacepède.

In the meantime, his youthful sympathy for Bernardin de Saint-Pierre, and the Germanic dream of an all-encompassing science, had gone. His ardour for the Greek language and the new nomenclature cooled down increasingly from one text to the next. Many terms in science, he wrote in 1796, were indeed 'children of habit', but habits were difficult to change. To impose a brand new language to domains of knowledge embedded in the culture of the country meant to sacrifice the national idiom, and names familiar to tradesmen, amateurs, and artisans. The compromise he proposed was to adopt new terms, possibly based on Greek roots, to indicate species newly discovered or new taxonomical propositions. For instance, 'gastropods' was a good descriptive term for the class of molluscs he had established, within which old species could continue to be indicated as tradition had chosen.

In 1800, at the end of the preface to the first volume of his *Leçons d'anatomie comparée*, Cuvier, not known for his generosity, generously acknowledged that the new anatomical nomenclature proposed in the book had been elaborated by Duméril, the editor of the first two volumes of his five-volume course. Generosity, then, or a way to mark a distance?[31] A few years later, with a full chair at the

30   Robert J. Richards, *The Romantic Conception of Life. Science and Philosophy in the Age of Goethe* (Chicago, 2002).

31   André-Marie-Constant Duméril, ed., *Leçons d'anatomie comparée de G. Cuvier, recueillies et publiées sous ses yeux* (2 vols, Paris, 1800). Vols 3–5 were edited by

Muséum, the position of perpetual secretary of the first class of the Institut, the favour of Lacepède, Président of the Senate, and of Napoleon himself on his side, Cuvier came to the rescue of his friend Fourcroy, when he protested vigorously against the widespread notion that the chemical nomenclature represented the best example of what the reform of the language could do for a science, 'as a modern school had pretended'.[32] Contemporaries could not miss the political point: the new chemistry had nothing to do with the 'modern school' of the *idéologues*, who, on the contrary, had tried to exploit the experimental results of the chemists, their discovery and subsequent naming of new elements and compounds, for their own philosophical and 'ideological' ends.

How do we explain Cuvier's change of view concerning the relationship between science and language? Was it the result of an epistemological reflection or the consequence of the repeated attacks, scientific as well as political, that the proposal for a 'linguistic' reform of science was subjected to? I have discussed elsewhere the spectrum of positions concerning the reform of the 'histoire naturelle', the slow and difficult ascent of Cuvier in the Parisian scientific scene, and his strategy to maintain power in the event of a change of regime.[33] In fact, opposition to Cuvier's institutional as well as scientific leadership was constant and at times dangerously effective, in particular towards the end of his life. In the early 1800s, attacks concentrated on his opposition to geological theories, and on the neologisms he had introduced in natural history. Not surprisingly, the Buffonians gathered around Sonnini de Manoncourt, who had always condemned the linguistic novelties introduced by Linnaeus, Lavoisier, Haüy and their followers, did not miss a chance to remind readers that it was Cuvier who had dared to propose terms as barbarous as 'gastropods'.

By 1802, when Pierre Denys de Montfort (1768–1820) made fun of Cuvier for having proposed such a word, no one could mistake the political edge of the polemic.[34] Indeed, after the return of the political *émigrés* in 1799, and the promise

---

Georges-Louis Duvernoy (1777–1855). See vol. 1, p. xxi: 'Le citoyen Duméril a inséré presque partout sa nouvelle nomenclature, qui est analogue à celle qu'avoit proposée le citoyen Chaussier, et qu'ont modifiée, chacun à leur manière, les citoyens Dumas et Girard. Sans attacher à cet objet une grande importance, il sera cependant intéressant que les anatomistes conviennent de quelque fixation dans leur idiome'.

32 Georges Cuvier, 'Rapport', *Magasin encyclopédique*, IV année, 7 (an IV, 1796), 161–4. The report concerned a memoir by Antoine-Nicholas Duchesne, 'Sur l'établissement d'une nomenclature européenne d'histoire naturelle', *ibid.*, pp. 147–60; the expression 'nomenclature radicale', that is, established on Greek roots, was by Duchesne. See also Georges Cuvier, *Histoire des progrès des sciences naturelles depuis 1789 jusqu'à ce jour* (2 vols, Paris, 1827), i, pp. 13–16 and 71–9.

33 Corsi, *Lamarck*, and the English language edition, *The Age of Lamarck*, chap. 1.

34 Pierre Denys de Montfort, in Sonnini de Manoncourt, ed., *Histoire naturelle*, 87 (an X, 1802), p. 35: 'On ne voit chez Buffon ni mammaux, ni plantigrades, ni gasteropodes'; pp. 22–3: 'Quand on écrit pour la société, on doit lui parler son langage, et ne point affecter d'être étranger au milieu d'elle; on doit désirer se faire

of pacification made by Bonaparte, the project of disciplinary specialization so loudly extolled during the previous five years, and in particular the connection between analysis, language and specialization, posed serious problems.

The language of science and of politics

In a very direct, almost trivial way, the new language of science was embarrassingly similar to other linguistic reforms that the Jacobin republic and the Directoire had imposed, impinging upon the daily life of all French citizens, even the illiterates: the calendar, weights and measures, cities and streets, departments and festivities. As years later Chateaubriand reminded his conservative admirers, 'This habit of Latinizing and Hellenizing our language is not new... In our time it has been revived by science; our revolutionaries, great Greeks by nature, have compelled our merchants and farmers to calculate in hectares, hectolitres, kilometres, millimetres, decagrams'.[35]

After 1795, key protagonists of the reform of weights and measures, for the most part well-known scientists, had indeed to fight hard against the accusation of introducing barbarous terms into the French language, as has been well documented by Isabelle Laboulais-Lesage.[36] Not only were traditional forms of trade going to be disrupted, critics argued, but the basic form of national identity the common language represented was also demolished. Political vandals, the Jacobins, had proposed to change the names of days, months, weights and measures; they had found powerful allies in the scientific barbarians wishing to change every word the French people used to describe nature and its wonders; they even tried to dispense with traditional philosophical reflections on man's intellectual and

entendre de tous et abandonner une nomenclature greco-gothique qui ne peut qu'embrouiller toute chose.' Cf. Corsi, *Lamarck*, pp. 207–8.

35 René de Chateaubriand, *The Memoirs of François René vicomte de Chateaubriand sometime Ambassador to England, being a Translation by Alexander Teixeira de Mattos of the Mémoires d'outre-tombe* (6 vols, London, 1902), i, p. 133; R. de Chateaubriand, *Mémoires d'outre-tombe* (2 vols, Paris, [1951] 2000), i, p. 142: 'Cette manie de gréciser et de latiniser notre langue n'est pas nouvelle...De nos jours elle a ressuscité par la science; nos révolutionnaires grands Grecs par nature, ont obligé nos marchands et nos paysans à apprendre les hectares, les hectolitres, les kilomètres, les millimètres, les décagrammes'.

36 Isabelle Laboulais-Lesage, *Lectures et pratiques de l'espace. L'itinéraire de Coquebert de Montbret, savant et commis d'Etat (1755–1831)* (Paris, 1999), pp. 288–96 ; Witold Kula, *Les mesures et les hommes* (Paris, 1984); Bernard Garnier and Jean Claude Hocquet, eds, *Genèse et diffusion du système métrique, Actes du Colloque 'La naissance du système métrique'* (Caen, 1990); Denis Guedj, *Le mètre du monde* (Paris, 2000); Ken Adler, 'A revolution to measure: the political economy of the metric system in France', in *The Values of Precision*, ed. M. Norton Wise (Princeton, 1995), pp. 39–71 and Adler, *The Measure of All Things: The Seven Years Odyssey that Transformed the World* (London, 2002).

moral attributes by establishing 'idéologie'. More than that, it was the scientists who had suggested the reforms and the bizarre names to be adopted. They were key members of the various agencies and commissions that had formulated and tried without much success to implement the new system. In the sentence by Chateaubriand – a biased witness, no doubt, but an influential and representative one – we have quoted, revolutionaries and scientists were one and the same thing. It is not irrelevant to our argument to point out that in November 1800 the First Consul Napoleon decided to allow people to go back to traditional names, though preserving the decimal norm, and that in February 1812 old measures were reintroduced for commerce and local trade. The metric system was finally abolished at the Restoration, in February 1816.[37] Furthermore it need only be recalled that General Bonaparte considered the '*idéologues*' – a term he used with sarcasm – as the only intellectual opposition to his monarchic ambitions. Between December 1802 and January 1803 he dissolved the Moral and Political Sciences Class of the Institut, dominated by his philosophical opponents, after having suppressed in May 1802 the 'Ecoles Centrales' the *idéologues* hoped would have reformed the cultural climate of the country. Last but not least, contemporaries commented on the First Consul's deep dislike for the Greek language: a linguistic, or a political idiosyncrasy?[38] For different reasons, Chateaubriand and, as we have seen, Delamétherie, agreed with Bonaparte: scientists and philosophers radically innovating the language of their discipline were hard-line revolutionaries. To the eyes of Catholics and monarchists, of moderates of all political factions, vandals and barbarians in general had destroyed the language of commerce and exchange, the names of towns, days and months, the names of plants and animals. They had almost drowned the country in a bath of words – and of blood.

It was a difficult task, then, to use science to acquire wealth and power as Cuvier had managed to do, when the word 'science' could constantly evoke dramatic and dangerous memories. For Cuvier, the task remained difficult throughout his career, having first to justify himself for his substantial as well as linguistic contributions to comparative anatomy and taxonomy, and in later life for his conservative standpoint regarding philosophical anatomy, embryology, and evolutionary theories. Cuvier had to fight off criticisms from the practitioners of traditional natural history – verbose and moralistic lovers of systems of the universe and all-encompassing theories, from old-fashioned chemists opposing the new chemical nomenclature and the new 'nomenklatur' running institutional chemistry, and from mineralogists and geologists debating theories of the earth. In

37 For the chronology, legislation and debates concerning the metric system see the website http://smdsi.quartier-rural.org/.
38 Johann-Friedrich Reichardt, *Un hiver à Paris sous le Consulat (1802–1803)*, ed. Thierry Lentz (Paris, 2003), p. 198. Commenting on the curriculum for the newly created Lycées, Reichardt pointed out that the study of Greek had been omitted at Napoleon's request. Even private institutions offering classes in Greek were told to conform to the rule: 'Bonaparte paraît, en effet, avoir une antipathie décidée contre ce qui vient de la Grèce.'

addition, Cuvier had to take measures to counteract the successful editorial enterprises launched by his enemies. Specialization and austerity of style could be presented as a good antidote against literary natural history only if one could persuade contemporaries to forget the arguments used for the intellectual justification of specialization in the years following the fall of Robespierre. After 1800, the rhetoric justifying specialization concentrated on the anti-materialistic and anti-atheistic virtues of well-defined fields of investigation, respectful of the division of intellectual labour, incapable of invading territories of higher generality and importance to man. In a popular course given in 1805 to a fashionable audience, Cuvier went so far as to suggest that the book of Genesis was always in agreement with the findings of geology. Palaeontology was a rigorous science, well aware of its limits, whereas current geological speculations on the antiquity of the earth and on the history of life were not.[39]

Conclusion: scientists at Napoleon's court

More generally, the reasons of public and ideological order that made science useful to the Directoire authorities disappeared when order was finally assured by Napoleon, and traditional religious values were once again called upon to provide their support to the throne. Scientists, who had gained posts, influence and relative wealth thanks to the political uncertainties of the 1790s, had to demonstrate their usefulness to the new ruler, in order to receive much-needed protection. The reasons they had advanced earlier on to forward their interests could be turned against them, as indeed they were. This line of interpretation is suggested by a fascinating passage in Stendhal's autobiographical sketch, where he denounced the role of scientists in the rise of Napoleon:

> The Emperor then [1797] began to raise up the throne of the Bourbons and was seconded by the extreme and boundless baseness of M. de Laplace. It's a strange thing that poets are courageous, and learned people, so-called, are base and servile. What servility, what abasement towards authority did M. Cuvier display! It horrified even the sensible Sutton Sharpe. At the Council of State M. le Baron Cuvier always supported the meanest policy.
>
> When the order of the Reunion was instituted, I was in the innermost Court circles; he came *weeping*, there's no other word, to try and get it. I'll tell the Emperor's reply in due course. Bacon, Laplace, Cuvier, all sold themselves out of cowardice... Secure of glory through their writings, these gentlemen hope their scientific reputations will cover up their political conduct; whether it's a question of money or of favours, they rush to feather their own nests. The celebrated Legendre, a geometrician of the first rank, on receiving the Cross of the Legion of Honour, fastened it to his coat, looked at himself in the glass and jumped for joy. The room was low, he hit the ceiling with his head and fell down half dead. What

39   Corsi, *Lamarck*, pp. 221–5.

a worthy death for this successor of Archimedes! What despicable things have they not done in the Academy of Sciences from 1815 to 1830 and since then, to get themselves decorated![40]

Stendhal's caricature contains an important hint: scientists who retained their political power after 1800 did so because they had become political figures performing political functions. As far as the others were concerned – those who had not acquired political power, or were not capable of maintaining it in the difficult environment of an imperial court – they had to face the hard consequences of an increasingly conservative political and intellectual climate in which scientific prominence was, if anything, a source of danger. Between 1796 and 1802, engaging in science, publishing scientific works, attending lectures at the Muséum and at the Collège de France, or the meetings of scientific societies, attested one's moderate patriotism, one's aspiration to occupy the position justified by one's merits. It also meant actively opposing the revolutionary vandalism responsible for prosecuting science and scientists – even though those who took this line had often themselves been active members of the 'vandalistic' administration. Bonaparte's election to the Institut in 1797, favoured by Laplace, his former teacher, illustrates his political shrewdness, more than his scientific accomplishments. After 1800–1802, politics did not need science any more, and conservatives could question the reliability of scientists who claimed they had been persecuted, but had in fact emerged from the storm with jobs and increased influence. At all events, public scientific activities decreased dramatically. Scientific publishing, it has rightly been argued, suffered the general crisis of publishing, and the vagaries of a protracted war economy. True, but why did attendance at free science lectures decrease as well? Data emerging from the study of the audiences attending Lamarck's lectures from 1795 to 1823 show a sharp decline in numbers after the record year 1802 (131

---

40 Stendhal, *The Life of Henry Brulard*, translated and with an introduction by Jean Stewart and Bert C.J.G. Knight (London, 1958), p. 180; Stendhal, *Vie de Henry Brulard* (Paris, [1973] 2002), p. 237: 'L'Empereur commença alors [1797] à élever le trône des Bourbons et fut secondé par la lâcheté sans bornes ni mesure de M. de Laplace. Chose singulière, les poètes ont du cœur, les savants proprement dits sont serviles et lâches. Quelle n'a pas été la servilité et la bassesse envers le pouvoir de M. Cuvier! Elle faisait horreur même au sage Sutton Sharpe. Au Conseil d'État M. le baron Cuvier était toujours de l'avis le plus lâche. Lors de la création de l'ordre de la Réunion j'étais dans le plus intime de la cour, il vint *pleurer*, c'est le mot, pour l'avoir. Je rapporterai en son temps la réponse de l'Empereur. Rentés pour la lâcheté: Bacon, Laplace, Cuvier. M. Lagrange fut moins plat, ça me semble. Sûrs de leur gloire par leurs écrits, ces Messieurs espèrent que le savant couvrira l'homme d'État ; en affaires d'argent, comme en faveurs, ils courent à l'utile. Le célèbre Legendre, géomètre de premier ordre, recevant la croix de la Légion d'Honneur, l'attacha à son habit, se regarda au miroir et sauta de joie. L'appartement était bas, sa tête heurta le plafond, il tomba à moitié assommé. Digne mort c'eût été pour ce successeur d'Archimède! Que de bassesses n'ont ils pas faites à l'Académie des sciences de 1815 à 1830 et depuis, pour s'escamoter des croix!'

subscriptions); politicians, military men, bureaucrats and senior members of the public had already deserted his classroom as from 1798.[41] Notably, 1802 was the year in which Lamarck announced his ambitious plan to establish a new terrestrial physics, articulated in three main disciplines: meteorology, hydrogeology and biology. This was also the year in which Chaptal, a fellow scientist and Minister of the Interior, decided to help Lamarck in setting up a meteorological correspondence involving scores of provincial amateurs, with the support of '*préfets*' and local authorities. From 1803 to 1809, no more mention was made of this ambitious research and institutional programme. No more mention was made of hydrogeology either, and as far as biology was concerned, Lamarck stated in 1809 that for his part the project would not be undertaken. Lamarck's main publications were limited to a series of memoirs on the fossil shells of the Parisian basin, published in the *Annales du Muséum*, and to his successful meteorological almanacs. Used to having to print books at his own expense, Lamarck was probably discouraged by having to talk to an audience of only 7 members in 1805, not a very promising basis for sales.

Examples could be multiplied, attesting the sharp decline in publishing by authors as diverse as Gaspard Monge and Geoffroy Saint-Hilaire, Fourcroy and Laplace (among the two most powerful scientist-politicians of the time).[42]

As from 1800–1802, the pretence that science was going to contribute to the happiness of mankind was increasingly put in question, in Europe as well as in France, where Chateaubriand led a powerful counter-attack with his *Génie du Christianisme* (1802). The idea that nature, man, society and politics could be amenable to final scientific assessment and managed scientifically was seen as one of the main intellectual components (if not the most important) of the arrogance that had lead to the revolutionary drama. Thus, scientists who had risen to power during the Revolution, the Directoire and the Consulate, needed all the political support they could get in order to preserve and possibly expand their privileges: in the highly partisan words of Chateaubriand, 'the Laplaces, the Lagranges, the Monges, the Chaptals, the Berthollets, all the prodigies, once haughty democrats, became Napoleon's most obsequious servants'. This was the case, he might have

---

41   For the prosopographic database concerning the 973 pupils attending Lamarck's lectures from 1795 to 1823, see Pietro Corsi, ed., www.Lamarck.net, and the statistical evaluation given there by Raphaèl Bange. See also Pietro Corsi, 'Les élèves de Lamarck: un projet de recherche', in *Jean-Baptiste Lamarck 1744–1829*, ed. Goulven Laurent (Paris, 1997), pp. 515–26. The website contains all the theoretical works by Lamarck, in word format and searchable by word, for a total of 7200 pages.

42   Jérôme Laurentin, 'Fidelités et reconstructions, l'exemple de l'école géometrique française de Gaspard Monge (1771–1816)', Paris, E.H.E.S.S., unpublished doctoral dissertation (3 vols, 2000), offers interesting statistics on the decline of mathematical publications after 1800, and their resumption after the fall of Napoleon. The decline in publications has been called in question by historians of the period: a crucial distinction to be kept in mind is between journal articles – which did not decrease – and books and pamphlets – which did.

added, with Cuvier and Lacepède as well, who had never been ultra-democrats, but needed Napoleon all the same. And had to mark their distance from the intellectual and epistemological values that had characterized the aggressive reform proposals put forward during and immediately after the Jacobin Republic.[43]

The new republican calendar did not survive long after the consolidation of the Empire, nor did the new weights and measures; some new scientific terms or the names of new disciplines were kept, though it would be interesting to draw up a list of those that were not. What was abandoned, as we have already seen, was the epistemological foundation of the radical linguistic programme that had been argued about in periodicals, dictionary articles and books during the crucial years following the Terror.

43   Chateaubriand, *Memoirs*, ii, pp. 187–8 ; French edition, i, p. 467: 'Les La Place, les Lagrange, les Monge, les Chaptal, les Berthollet, tous ces prodiges, jadis fiers démocrates, devinrent les plus obséquieux serviteurs de Napoléon. Il faut le dire à l'honneur des lettres: la littérature nouvelle fut libre, la science servile; le caractère ne répondit point au génie, et ceux dont la pensée était montée au plus haut du ciel, ne purent élever leur âme au-dessus des pieds de Bonaparte: ils prétendaient n'avoir pas besoin de Dieu, c'est pourquoi ils avaient besoin d'un tyran.' Chateaubriand's strictures against Lacepède were particularly severe.

Chapter 13

'Babies of the Empire': The Evolution of Infant Welfare Services in New Zealand and Britain in the First Half of the Twentieth Century

Linda Bryder

In 1939 New Zealand's Director-General of Health, Dr Michael Watt, described New Zealand's infant nursing services as 'wasteful of time, money and effort'. He wished to see them absorbed into general public health nursing.[1] The trend in Britain, which he had just visited, was to combine home visiting for maternal and infant welfare with other forms of health visiting.[2] The Plunket Society, a voluntary organization which ran the infant nursing services in New Zealand, received about half of its funding from the state, and yet the state's health agency, the Health Department, had no control over how that money was spent. Moreover, the nursing services operated with little medical supervision. In 1938 the paediatrician Dr Ian Ewart complained that 'New Zealand was the only country where nurses prescribed for babies'.[3] Twenty years later Dr Harold Turbott, shortly to be New Zealand's Director-General of Health, maintained that 'it is this virtual exclusion of the medical profession from well-baby care and its provision mainly through a voluntary organised nursing service, which is anomalous in our land'.[4]

I wish to acknowledge the support of a Wellcome Trust Short-term Travel Grant in 2002, which enabled me to complete research on British services.

1   M.H. Watt, 'The rest of the day to myself', unpublished autobiography (held by New Zealand Health Department), pp. 124–5; M.H. Watt, *Report of the Director-General of Health Reviewing Public-Health Administration in North America, the UK and Scandinavia, with Consequent Proposals for the Development of the New Zealand System* (Wellington, 1940), pp. 30–1.
2   Annual Conference of Women Public Health Officers, London, 1934, p. 4: Wellcome Library Archives (hereafter WLA), SA/HVA Box 71, D1/3.
3   Vida Jowett to Daisy Begg, 6 September 1938: Plunket Society Archives, Hocken Library, Dunedin (hereafter PSA), 239.
4   M.W. Raffel, 'A consultative committee on infant and pre-school health services', *New Zealand Journal of Public Administration*, 28, 1 (1965), 48. For further details on the

While the absence of medical input was being lamented by some in New Zealand, in Britain the maternal and infant welfare services were subjected to the criticism of being 'over-doctored'. Reviewing those services in 1938, Dr J. Greenwood Wilson, Medical Officer of Health (MOH) for Cardiff, argued that the medical officer of any large city was becoming 'more and more a director of medical services and having less and less to do with the maintenance of health... The maternity and child welfare centre of today, when it is not chiefly a milk depot, is too much like a hospital outpatient department or dispensary and too little like a school for mothers'.[5] This article examines how and why these two countries followed such divergent paths.

'Babies of the Empire'

The Plunket Society arose out of the early twentieth-century Western concern with maternal and infant welfare for the sake of future military and economic strength. A 1904 memorandum by New Zealand's Prime Minister Richard Seddon on infant life preservation, which stated, 'Babies are our best immigrants', echoed the conclusion of a recent report from New South Wales.[6] Given their geographical position these young British colonies were particularly worried about a potential influx of Asians. For Seddon:

> In the younger colonies of the Empire population is essential and if increased from British stock the self-governing colonies will still further strengthen and buttress our great Empire. In British interests it is clearly undesirable that the colonies should be populated by the inferior surplus of people of older and alien countries.[7]

Immigration policies were restricted accordingly and there were also attempts to foster the local white population. As in Britain, it was hoped to build up the local population by educating women in mothercraft. New Zealand was well aware of British trends. In parliamentary debates on infant life protection, two members, Dr William Collins and Attorney-General John Findlay, cited *Infant Mortality. A Social Problem*, written in 1906 by George Newman, then a public health officer and later Chief Medical Officer of the Ministry of Health for England and Wales.[8]

The Plunket Society, initially called the Society for the Protection of the Health of Women and Children, was founded in Dunedin in 1907 as a voluntary

history of the Plunket Society, see Linda Bryder, *A Voice for Mothers: The Plunket Society and Infant Welfare 1907–2000* (Auckland, 2003).

5   *Mother and Child (M&C)*, 9, 9 (1938), 330.
6   Reported in *New Zealand Yearbook 1905* (Wellington, 1906), p. 253.
7   'Early Plunket', PSA, AG7–27. For a similar scenario in the USA see Alisa Klaus, *Every Child a Lion: The Origins of Maternal and Infant Health Policy in the US and France, 1890–1920* (Ithaca, 1993), p. 12.
8   *New Zealand Parliamentary Debates*, vol. 140 (1907), p. 655.

organization which employed nurses to advise mothers on infant care. As a prelude to the setting up of the Auckland branch in 1908, the wife of New Zealand's governor, Lady Plunket, who became the Society's patron, explained the scheme to the local press. She claimed, 'The scheme which I have placed before your readers is not an untried novelty; it is working successfully at Home [i.e. Britain] and abroad'.[9] Dr Frederic Truby King, who provided medical backing for the new infant welfare movement, was also inspired by events in Britain. A New Zealander by birth, he had trained as a doctor at Edinburgh University, and was the first student to be awarded the new Bachelor of Science in Public Health in 1888. Once back in New Zealand, as medical superintendent of Seacliff Asylum near Dunedin, he had his attention drawn to the British infant welfare movement by his assistant, Dr Alexander Falconer. The latter had undertaken a public health course at University College London. His teacher, Professor H.R. Kenwood, was keenly interested in infant mortality and had taken the class to see Dr George McCleary's milk depot for infants at Battersea, London, in 1903. Falconer later claimed that McCleary's work in Battersea had a direct influence on the infant welfare movement in New Zealand.[10]

Thus New Zealand was directly inspired by Britain but the links worked both ways. The infant welfare movement based on concerns of 'national efficiency' gained added poignancy during the First World War. In 1917 Lord and Lady Plunket, who had returned to Britain in 1910, helped found the Babies of the Empire Society as a voluntary effort to 'solve one of the great problems of national reconstruction'.[11] Truby King was invited to Britain to set up a Mothercraft Training Centre on the New Zealand model, and the Mothercraft Training Centre at Earl's Court was formally opened by New Zealand's Prime Minister William Massey in 1918. Truby King was appointed medical director and another New Zealander, Anne Pattrick, was appointed matron.

This was no insignificant organization. Vice-presidents included a selection of eminent people such as Dame Margaret Lloyd George. It also included some well known in the field of public health such as Benjamin Broadbent, who had pioneered an infant welfare service in Huddersfield, and Sir Arthur Newsholme, Chief Medical Officer to the Local Government Board from 1908 to 1918. The executive committee, as in New Zealand, was largely made up of women, including Lady Plunket (now Lady Victoria Braithwaite), Lady Dawson of Penn, Lady Galway, Lady Mond and Lady Sydenham among others. Its medical advisory board included Sir Bertrand Dawson, Sir John Byers of Belfast, Sir William Smyly, Professor Kenwood, and doctors involved in infant welfare initiatives such as A.K. Chalmers, MOH of Glasgow and a founder of the National Conference on Infant Mortality in 1906, E.W. Hope of Liverpool, Janet Lane Claypon, and Marie

9   *New Zealand Herald* (*NZH*) (29 January 1908).
10   Letter from Alex R. Falconer to Watt, 3 February 1936, PSA, AG7 5–27.
11   Babies of the Empire Society, *Annual Report 1918–19*, p. 1: Highgate Literary and Scientific Institution, London (hereafter HLSI).

Scharlieb of London. The Duchess of York, later the wife of King George VI and Queen Mother, became president in 1923 and showed a real interest in the work by frequent visits. The matron after the first year was Mabel Liddiard who was in post for many years and later became President of the Royal College of Midwives. She was awarded the CBE in 1951. She wrote a manual which went through several editions, and has recently been described by a historian as 'the major source of orthodoxy on infant care and management [in Britain] for... 30 years'.[12] The first bound volume was presented to and accepted graciously by the Duchess of York.[13]

The new centre and the Mothercraft Training Society (MTS), as it was now called, had as their major goal the promotion of breastfeeding. This followed closely the Plunket Society of New Zealand. Despite his efforts to create a safe form of infant feeding from cow's milk, Truby King never wavered in his promotion of breastfeeding. Indeed, he advocated breastfeeding to such an extent that following his death in 1938 the British journal *Mother and Child* maintained that he had 'hypnotise[d] thousands of mothers into the belief that breast feeding [was] *the* important factor in infant care'.[14] While many of the infant welfare centres in Britain stressed breastfeeding, the MTS became particularly well known for it, and its magazine was full of success stories of establishing or re-establishing breast-feeding or, as it described it, 'complete motherhood'.[15] Dr John Fairbairn, Consulting Obstetric Physician at St Thomas's Hospital, London, who became medical consultant to the MTS, was a strong advocate of breastfeeding.

In 1925 the MTS moved to larger premises at Highgate, called Cromwell House, where it was based until the Society folded in 1951. Branches were set up in London – at Earl's Court, Kensington, and Chelsea (the Violet Melchett Infant Welfare Centre, affiliated in 1931) – and a Cardiff clinic, opened in 1928, became affiliated in 1931. In the 1930s branches were also opened in Newport, Cambridge, Brighton and Hove, Kingston-upon Thames, Oxford, and Glasgow.[16]

Throughout its history the MTS retained close links with New Zealand. When New Zealand politicians and businessmen moved to Britain, their wives, who had been active in the Plunket Society, became involved in the MTS. It also acted as a centre for New Zealand's Plunket and Karitane nurses; the MTS helped them find

12 Cathy Urwin and Elaine Sharland, 'From bodies to minds in childcare literature', in Roger Cooter, ed., *In the Name of the Child: Health and Welfare 1880–1940* (London, 1992), pp. 174–99: p. 177. See also Christina Hardyment, *Dream Babies: Three Centuries of Good Advice on Child Care* (New York, 1983), p. 179. Mabel Liddiard, *Mothercraft Manual* (London, 1924; 6th edn, London, 1954). Visitors to the Centre included Truby King and Anne Pattrick, and Liddiard visited New Zealand in 1926 to study Plunket methods further. The contacts were close: Mothercraft Training Society (MTS), *Annual Reports*, HLSI.
13 Obituary, Liddiard, *The League of Mothercraft Nurses, Newsletter 1962*, pp. 10–11.
14 *M&C*, 8, 12 (1938), 454.
15 Babies of the Empire Society under the auspices of the Over-seas Club and Patriotic League, *Report for 6 Months Ending 31 August 1918*, p. 6.
16 *Mothercraft Training Society Magazine*, August 1946, p. 530.

employment in Britain.[17] However, when Cromwell House closed in 1951 it was given almost no publicity in New Zealand. The local press office in New Zealand wrote to the Minister of Health about the closure and he forwarded the letter to the Director-General of Health, Dr Harold Turbott. Although Turbott had had little personal experience of the British situation, he pronounced:

> The fact is that the principles of infant feeding and welfare as advocated and practised by the Plunket Society in New Zealand have never found any wide acceptance in Great Britain and over recent years at least the Mothercraft Training Society has made little progress in enlisting public sympathy or financial support. While one may regret the passing of a link with our own New Zealand system, there is really little more that can be said.[18]

The closing of Cromwell House had little to do with whether the methods of infant feeding and welfare found favour, and more to do with the way in which public health services in Britain had evolved. In 1917, 321 voluntary societies known to the Local Government Board were operating 446 infant welfare centres in England and Wales, and a further 396 centres were run by local authorities.[19] The 1918 Maternity and Child Welfare Act gave local authorities in England and Wales statutory responsibility for welfare services for mothers and infants. During the interwar period local authorities created large numbers of ante-natal and infant welfare clinics, totalling 4,700 by 1948.[20] While there was nothing to stop local authorities from supporting voluntary initiatives, the trend was to combine infant and maternal health visiting with other public health services, such as visiting tuberculosis patients, geriatrics, school health, and convalescence from hospital treatment. This made it uneconomical to support specialized services. The move to combine services culminated in the National Health Service Act of 1946 which defined health visiting under Section 24. This required local health authorities to make provision 'for the visiting of persons in their homes by visitors, to be called "Health Visitors", for the purpose of giving advice as to the care of young children, persons suffering from illness and expectant or nursing mothers, and as to the measures necessary to prevent the spread of infection'.[21] Local authorities no longer could, or would, invest money in centres specializing only in infant and maternal welfare. Nor was fundraising possible when the local authorities were

17 Karitane nurses were not registered nurses but trained as nannies at the Society's hospitals, while Plunket nurses were registered general or maternity nurses.
18 Turbott to Minister of Health, 13 July 1951, 'Plunket Society overseas': National Archives, Wellington (hereafter NA), H1 37996 127/5/5.
19 Jane Lewis, *The Politics of Motherhood: Child and Maternal Welfare in England, 1900–1939* (London, 1980), p. 96.
20 Charles Webster, *The Health Services since the War. Volume 1, Problems of Health Care: the British National Health Service before 1957* (London, 1988), pp. 7, 378.
21 'Health visiting in the seventies and the staffing of the health visiting and school nursing services', WLA, D2/11 1975.

setting up their own centres with their own health visitors. The New Zealand Health Department would have dearly loved to follow the same course. However, the New Zealand system had evolved in such a way, and with such powerful support from women, that this was not possible.

A universal free infant nursing service

From the beginning about a third of the funding of the Plunket Society came from the state. In return it was agreed that the Health Department should approve the appointment of additional Plunket nurses. When Westport's Plunket committee sought approval in 1914, it was told the appointment would only be sanctioned if Plunket work were combined with that of a district nurse. The response of Plunket's president, Amy Carr, 'emphatically protest[ed] against any such interference with the plan of the work of the Society'.[22] The Chief Health Officer, Dr Thomas Valintine, retorted that if the Department paid a subsidy it had a right to see that the money was well spent, and 'you will pardon me for saying that I do not regard you as being in a position to say how the Government subsidies can be best devoted and the Nurses' services best utilised. A certain amount of training and technical knowledge is required before anyone can give an opinion on that subject'.[23] Not to be cowed by a male bureaucrat, the women who ran Plunket felt perfectly competent to make such decisions; they believed that their womanly instincts and training as mothers put them in good stead to do so. As part of a movement which historians of early twentieth-century America have dubbed 'maternalism', they believed that it was their right and duty to become publicly involved in infant welfare.[24] They saw their organization as a women's mutual aid society, with women helping other women. They were determined to dissociate the movement from charity, explaining that while the functions of the Society were 'broadly humanitarian', they were not 'patronising or charitable', or even in the ordinary sense philanthropic, but essentially 'patriotic and educational'.[25] Truby King explained to Valintine that district nurses visited 'the sick poor of the indigent class, who receive it as a charity', and that 'the self-reliant class' would regard it as an 'absolute humiliation' to see a district nurse. As a mark of Plunket's difference, he noted that Plunket nurses were invited into the homes of the medical profession,

22   Plunket Society correspondence, 26 May 1914, PSA, AG 7, 3/174, items 13–16, 22, 23.
23   *Ibid.*
24   For general discussions of maternalism, see Theda Skocpol, *Protecting Soldiers and Mothers: The Political Origins of Social Policy in the United States* (Cambridge, Mass., 1992); Seth Koven and Sonya Michel, eds, *Mothers of a New World: Maternalist Politics and the Origins of Welfare States* (London and New York, 1993), introduction; Lynn Weiner, 'International trends: maternalism as a paradigm', *Journal of Women's History*, 5, 2 (1993), 96–8; Molly Ladd-Taylor, *Mother-Work: Women, Child Welfare and the State, 1890–1930* (Urbana, 1994).
25   Plunket Society, *Annual Report, 1912–13*, p. 8.

which pointed to their acceptance among 'the higher professional classes'.[26] This was indeed to be a feature which distinguished Plunket from many schemes overseas, including Britain. Neville Mayman, commissioned by the New South Wales Legislative Assembly in 1918 to conduct an inquiry into the welfare of mothers and babies in New Zealand, explained that the Plunket Society had 'taken the rather unusual course of appealing primarily to the better-to-do and more intelligent women of the community'.[27]

The infant welfare clinics in Britain, which had been set up from the first decade of the twentieth century, targeted working-class mothers. As Lara Marks has shown, they operated on particular assumptions about the poor and their ignorance. While many medical professionals argued that wealthy mothers needed just as much instruction as poor mothers, it was assumed that these mothers could not be imposed upon in the same way as their poorer sisters, for fear of causing offence.[28] One of the subjects discussed in the first issue of *Mother and Child*, the official mouthpiece of the National Council for Maternity and Child Welfare, in 1930, was the fact that middle-class women missed out on the benefits of the infant welfare centres. The editor commented that:

> Though theoretically the maternity and child welfare services established under the Maternity and Child Welfare Act, 1918, are available for any children and their mothers irrespective of class, as a matter of actual practice it is found that the more or less well-to-do parents do not avail themselves of the services of the health visitor or the infant welfare centre.[29]

The chairman of a small urban welfare centre suggested a paying day once a week for better-off mothers, who 'for obvious reasons' would not care to attend the ordinary welfare meetings.[30] Dr Eric Pritchard, a leader in Britain's infant welfare movement, saw this as an obvious gap in welfare services, as did Sir Arthur Stanley, chair of the National Council for Maternity and Child Welfare and vice-president of the National Baby Week Council.[31]

The result was the Babies' Club movement, a subscribers' club for mothers, which started in Chelsea and Kensington in 1927 and which was intended 'to give the middle-class mother the same advantages as the poorer mother, who was able

---

26 Conference between Valintine and Plunket Society sub-committee, March 1913, PSA, AG7 5–27.
27 Report of the Commissioner, Mr Neville Mayman, on the Inquiry into the Welfare of Mothers and Children in New Zealand, *New South Wales Parliamentary Papers*, vol. 5, 291 (1918), p. 10.
28 Lara Marks, *Metropolitan Maternity: Maternal and Infant Welfare Services in Early Twentieth Century London* (Amsterdam, 1996), p. 168.
29 *M&C*, 1, 1 (1930), 17.
30 *M&C*, 1, 1 (1930), 19.
31 *M&C*, 1, 4 (1930), 123.

to take her child to a welfare centre'.[32] By the 1930s there were three babies' clubs in London, with varying subscriptions according to locality and circumstances. The advantages of membership included a weekly clinic, home visits by a fully qualified nurse, and classes for expectant mothers. Vera Brittain, the well known feminist and pacifist, and one of the founders of the Chelsea Babies' Club, stressed that the clubs were not in any way centres for treatment and there was, therefore, no interference with family doctors, with whom they co-operated.[33] However, this was not the view of the British Medical Association. The BMA considered that the Babies' Club movement 'embodied an objectionable method' and 'rejected the whole thing'. It argued that mothers should be taught to consult their doctors 'when advice was necessary and not only when the child was ill', and that the financial aspects could easily be sorted: 'there was not one doctor in a thousand who would not modify his fees in cases of need'.[34] This totally missed the point about middle-class women not wanting to ask for charity.

In the early twentieth century the New Zealand Branch of the BMA (NZBMA) had similarly objected to the nurses providing free services to middle-class mothers. However, this opposition occurred at a time when Plunket was newly formed, when infant welfare was regarded as a matter of great national importance, and when many influential people were backing the new movement. In June 1910 a resolution was put forward by the Hawke's Bay division of the NZBMA, stating that there should be a restriction placed on the 'unlimited use' of Plunket nurses. The South Canterbury division objected that this would 'arouse hostility to the medical profession on the part of the public' and it was abandoned.[35] Yet Plunket nurses had their job descriptions and these did not include medical treatment. It was agreed in 1910 that the doctor was to be called 'in cases of serious illness only'. The words 'serious illness... are not intended to include mere infantile ailments, e.g. simple diarrhoea, indigestion or colic, such as would ordinarily be dealt with by the mother or grandmother, without calling in a doctor'.[36]

Despite attempts to specify divisions of responsibility, Plunket nurses were sometimes in effective competition with doctors, particularly in the early days. Nurses were explicitly instructed to delete references to babies' ailments (other than dietetic) and to deaths in their annual reports. As Plunket's secretary Gwen Hoddinott explained in 1934, 'it is not considered advisable, in view of the criticism sometimes made by the medical profession in regard to the treatment of disease by Plunket nurses, for such references to be published in the reports of Plunket Nurses presented to the public by Committees'. Nurses were advised that

32   *M&C*, 3, 5 (1932), 158.
33   *Ibid*. See also Lewis, *Politics of Motherhood*, p. 102. Vera Brittain had married (Sir) George Catlin in 1925, and by 1932 had a two-year-old daughter (her daughter, Shirley Williams, was later to become a Social Democrat leader).
34   *M&C*, 1, 1 (1930), 18.
35   *New Zealand Medical Journal*, 8 (August 1910), 78, 80.
36   Honorary Secretary NZBMA Otago Branch, to Plunket Society, 29 August 1910, PSA, AG7 11–5.

they were only to include the references to deaths in their confidential reports to the committees.[37] An outright admission of competition came in 1922, when the Auckland branch secretary, Eileen Partridge, claimed it would be 'fatal' to move a 'weaker' nurse to the Remuera or Epsom districts: 'These mothers would be away to Dr Sweet at once', she explained.[38] Dr Bruton Sweet, New Zealand's first paediatrician, complained to the Auckland committee about the nurses' interference with the treatment of babies under his care. He discovered that his feeding advice had been frequently criticized and that mothers were being warned that their infants would be injured if they followed it.[39] Paediatrician F. Montgomery Spencer similarly complained in the 1930s that it was 'not at all uncommon for mothers to be told by Plunket nurses that my methods of feeding will prove harmful to their babies'.[40]

Disputes with the medical profession reached a height in the 1930s when a new breed of paediatricians, some with postgraduate training from Britain or America, argued that Plunket's feeding schedules were causing gross malnutrition. During the discussions, Plunket's acting medical adviser, Dr Ernest Williams, pointed out that one justifiable criticism levelled at the Plunket nurses was that they kept in contact with sick children 'for an unnecessarily long time'.[41] He believed this to be at the heart of medical criticisms.[42] Dr Herbert Robertson, a paediatrician from Wanganui, added that, 'the biggest grouse in the profession is that they are not getting the cases referred back to them, and are losing pounds, shillings and pence'.[43]

Some doctors, however, thrived under Plunket. The Society operated six hospitals for mothers and infants with feeding problems, and paediatricians were appointed as consultants. Even those not attached to the hospitals could find Plunket useful. In 1938 Dr Marie Stringer Buchler claimed that many doctors 'pander[ed] to the P.N. [Plunket nurse] as it's good for business'.[44] Dr Edna Birkenshaw, who specialized in the health of women and children in her private practice, admitted in 1950 that the Plunket Society was her 'largest source of consultations'.[45] Yet others did not have a close relationship, as was discovered by a medical student undertaking research into Plunket nursing services in 1951. She found that the family doctors of the mothers she interviewed had not encouraged them to call on Plunket. However, she added that, 'it must be realised that the Plunket

37   Hoddinott to Tweed, 30 April 1934, PSA, 231.
38   Partridge to Pattrick, 16 November 1922, PSA, 722.
39   Bruton Sweet to Partridge, 22 November 1928, PSA, 1186.
40   Spencer to Begg, 18 December 1937, PSA, 239. For further discussion see chapter 4 of Bryder, *A Voice for Mothers*.
41   Bryder, *A Voice for Mothers*.
42   Spencer to Begg, 18 December 1937, PSA, 239.
43   *Ibid.*
44   M.P. Buchler to Spencer, 22 March 1938, cited in Christine Daniell, *A Doctor at War: A Life in Letters, 1914–43* (Masterton, 2001), p. 171.
45   Edna Birkenshaw to Helen Deem, 31 May 1950, PSA, 581.

Society is quite adequate in itself in recruiting new mothers to give service to'.[46] From 1922 registrars notified Plunket of all non-Maori births and the Society wrote to new mothers inviting them to make contact with the Plunket nurse. Sometimes Plunket nurses visited maternity homes. By the 1950s Plunket nurses were seeing almost 90 per cent of all new non-Maori mothers.[47]

The fact that Plunket provided free and non-targeted child health services helped to enlist to the Society the support of a large number of women who had a stake in the system. When Truby King suggested in 1932 that middle-class women should be charged for the services, this was flatly rejected as against the Society's principles.[48] Its strength lay in its universality.

Public and political support

In 1930, following Plunket's request for additional state funding, Director-General of Health Thomas Valintine argued that, 'stripping the question of the mere senti-mentalism', Plunket could not take credit for the declining infant death rate. Moreover, as the Society had 'on repeated occasions steadfastly opposed anything in the nature of Departmental oversight or supervision of its work I do not see that we can justify the grants asked for'.[49] Valintine and his Department, however, enjoyed little political support in this matter, and Plunket subsidies continued to increase. The Treasury lamented in 1958:

> the basic fact remains that for over forty years the State has paid increasingly heavy subsidies for this purpose. On each occasion in the past when the matter has been considered, the Government of the day has decided to provide increased subsidies rather than face the upheaval that a change of policy, such as withdrawal or curtailment of State financial aid, would inevitably bring in its train.[50]

The Treasury recognized Plunket's wide support, as did former Director-General Michael Watt, who wrote in his unpublished autobiography, 'I hope I will not be misunderstood if I say that Governments in their approach to the matter [Plunket] were in no sense deterred from proffering financial aid by knowledge of the

46 Margaret Woods, 'Plunket nursing in the Invercargill area', University of Otago Public Health thesis (1951), p. 21.
47 *Report of the Consultative Committee on Infant and Pre-school Health Services* (Wellington, 1960), p. 6. Maori mothers and babies were the charge of the Health Department: see L. Bryder, 'New Zealand's infant welfare services and Maori, 1907–60', *Health and History*, 3, 1 (2001), 65–86.
48 Plunket Society, Central Council minutes, 25 October 1932, PSA.
49 Valintine to Hoddinott, 16 June 1930, 'Plunket Society General 1929–33', NA, H.127.
50 D.J. Sheppard, Chief Accountant, Department of Health, 'Report and recommendations on the Plunket Society's application for an increase in the rate of hospital benefit for Karitane hospitals', 1 October 1958, p. 7, NA, H1 127/5/9/1 37999.

fact that the Society had very wide membership and if so inclined could have exercised considerable political pressure'.[51] The wives of many politicians, businessmen and mayors served on Plunket's local committees. During the dispute with the paediatricians over feeding practices in 1938 one doctor complained that her local press would not publish her views on Plunket: '*The Press* in Christchurch refused publication – it is practically owned by very powerful Plunket sympathisers', she claimed.[52]

Plunket enjoyed support across the political spectrum. The more conservative governments of the 1920s and 1930s supported Plunket with its principles of self-help, but so too did the first Labour Government which came to office in 1935 promising social security from the cradle to the grave, paid for out of general taxation, and a national health service. Dr David McMillan, the architect of Labour's 1935 blueprint for health, commented upon the 'great benefits which have accrued from our one health experiment along national lines', the Plunket Society. Sceptical of Valintine's assessment of mortality trends, he described Plunket as having 'made New Zealand the doyen of the world in matters of infantile mortality'. In his view, 'a national health service would utilise the Plunket Society, building and strengthening it by financial and administrative assistance'.[53] In 1937 Plunket's president, Daisy Begg, wrote to Health Minister Peter Fraser asking for a public statement of reassurance to refute the 'fairly widespread' idea that the Government intended to take over the Society's work under the new State National Health Service. This belief, she said, was having an adverse effect on fundraising.[54] Fraser, whose wife Janet was involved with Plunket,[55] had no hesitation in providing that reassurance. He did so privately to Begg by letter, adding 'You are at liberty to give whatever publicity to this letter you think necessary', and publicly at the annual meeting of the Wellington Plunket branch one month later.[56] In his address he noted that Finance Minister Walter Nash had found that even in Russia doctors were familiar with the system.[57] He also paid tribute to the work of the Society in the foreword to the sixth edition of Plunket's handbook, *The Expectant Mother and Baby's First Months* (1939). Nash, who sat on Wellington Plunket's Advisory Board, opened the 1938 national Plunket conference, explaining that he was convinced that there was 'no society doing work of more value than the Plunket Society in New Zealand'.[58] Arnold Nordmeyer, Minister of Health once Fraser became Prime Minister, wrote

51 Watt, 'The rest of the day to myself', pp. 56–7.
52 Daniell, *A Doctor at War*, p. 186.
53 D.G. McMillan, *A National Health Service, New Zealand of Tomorrow* (Wellington, 1935), pp. 6, 11.
54 Begg to Fraser, 22 June 1937, NA, H1 127 9251 127.
55 Hilary Stace, 'Fraser, Janet', *Dictionary of New Zealand Biography, Vol.4, 1921–1940* (Auckland, 1998), p. 182.
56 Plunket Society, Wellington branch minutes, letter from Fraser to Begg, 8 June 1937, read at meeting 3 September 1937, PSA; *Evening Post* (22 July 1937).
57 *Evening Post* (22 July 1937).
58 Plunket Society, *Report of Twenty-fifth General Conference 1938*, p. 6.

the foreword to Plunket's 1945 official handbook, *Modern Mothercraft*, pointing out that the service had become indispensable and had no equal in the field of maternal and child welfare.[59]

Thus Plunket enjoyed the support of Labour, which held office from 1935 to 1949 and duly increased its subsidies. Some historians have argued that maternalism flourished in weak welfare states.[60] However, as Philippa Mein Smith has also argued, the New Zealand and Australian cases show that maternalism could co-exist with a pronounced paternalist welfare system.[61] Labour's welfare policies, which included free maternity care, family allowances and housing for families, and gender-differentiated minimum wages, were premised on the view of women as wives and mothers rather than as equal citizens. Maternalists appeared comfortable with that interpretation of welfare. Just as Anne Digby found in relation to the earlier maternalist movement in Britain, Plunket appealed successfully to male policy-makers precisely because they were able to ground their policies in sexual difference, and in the perpetuation of traditionalist roles for women; the body politic remained paternalistic.[62] The women who ran Plunket, embued with the same ideology which underlay Labour Party policies, believed that they were entitled to state support for their services (though to them this did not involve relinquishing any control).

One trend within the maternal and infant welfare movement in Britain in the 1930s, which attracted favourable comment in *Mother and Child*, was a new fathers' movement. Fathers' councils were set up as part of the infant welfare centres in Britain from the 1920s.[63] In 1932 the Central Union of Fathers' Councils was formed,[64] followed in 1939 by a National Fathercraft Advisory Council. The initiative for this movement, which was described as 'a new phase of the maternity and child welfare movement',[65] came primarily from the medical officers of health, and it was hoped that before long every infant welfare centre would have a fathers' council attached to it. The movement had several aims. One was to influence working-class wives through their husbands. Medical officers claimed to find that

59 H. Deem and N. Fitzgibbon, *Modern Mothercraft: A Guide to Parents, The Official Handbook of the Royal New Zealand Society for the Health of Women and Children (Inc.) Plunket Society* (Dunedin, 1945), p. 7.

60 Anne Digby, 'Poverty, health and the politics of gender in Britain, 1870–1948', in A. Digby and J. Stewart, eds, *Gender, Health and Welfare* (London, 1996), p. 67; Koven and Michel, *Mothers of a New World*, p. 21; Skocpol, *Protecting Soldiers and Mothers*, p. 522; Klaus, *Every Child a Lion*, p. 92.

61 See also Philippa Mein Smith, *Mothers and King Baby: Infant Survival and Welfare in an Imperial World: Australia 1880–1950* (London, 1997), p. 5.

62 Digby, 'Poverty, health and politics', p. 84. See also Jane Lewis, 'Women's agency, maternalism and welfare', *Gender and History*, 6, 1 (1994), 117–23, and Mein Smith, *Mothers and King Baby*, p. 246.

63 *M&C*, 3, 8 (1932), 302.

64 *M&C*, 3, 7 (1932), 246.

65 *M&C*, 10, 4 (1939), 118.

the obstructionist husband was a myth behind which many women hid.[66] It was also hoped that the Councils would attract more funding and support for infant welfare; the medical officers wanted to get the support of men as ratepayers and taxpayers and because they claimed husbands had more influence in the public sphere than did their wives.[67] Finally, the Councils aimed to teach the 'science of fathercraft', which admittedly appeared to consist primarily of making nursery furniture, shoe repairs and gardening.[68]

New Zealand was looked to as a model. In 1939 one medical officer of health wrote that, 'In New Zealand many a he-man is not ashamed to confess that he can, and does, cook the Sunday dinner and can turn the heel of a sock. Need this be confined to the Antipodes?' He went on to point out, as an encouraging sign, that shortly before the war broke out a National Advisory Fathercraft Council had been set up in Britain.[69] However, women in New Zealand might let their husbands cook dinner but they did not give them any voice within the Plunket Society. In 1951 Plunket Society president Elizabeth Bodkin commented that, while the Society had always sought the help and advice of prominent commercial and professional men, the 'burden of administration [fell] on the shoulders of women'.[70] Women continued to control policy decisions. Moreover the women of Plunket had no trouble in gaining access to the corridors of power. Nor did they need to seek to influence women through their husbands; they appeared to have no trouble in reaching the women of New Zealand.

Plunket nurses and mothers

An explanation for the overwhelming support by New Zealand women for the Plunket Society must be sought largely in the relationship between the nurses and mothers. Without any involvement from medical officers of health and without any statutory or other responsibility to inspect and report upon conditions found in the homes, Plunket nurses could build up an intimate and unthreatening relationship with mothers. This rapport was built up through regular home visits in the first three months of the baby's life. Health visitors in Britain, on the other hand, were responsible to the medical officer of health, and were required to report any insanitary conditions or other problems to that officer.[71] Repeat visits were generally to those regarded as more ignorant and inexperienced and whose homes were seen to be more dirty and neglected.[72] Judgements therefore had to be made, which was not the case in New Zealand.

66 *M&C*, 6, 5 (1935), 210.
67 *M&C*, 9, 9 (1938), 331.
68 *M&C*, 9, 9 (1938), 339.
69 *M&C*, 10, 9 (1939), 329.
70 Deputation to J.T. Watts, 17 April 1951, p. 1, NA, H1 127 26040.
71 Marks, *Metropolitan Maternity*, p. 173.
72 *Ibid.*, p. 177.

It does appear that New Zealand women were, as noted by Valintine, 'senti-mentally' attached to Plunket. Local committees, who supported the nurses, had been set up around the country, and in their reports they spoke highly of the nurses. As one Plunket nurse, who qualified in 1947, reflected, 'The best thing about Plunket was the friendships I made with the mothers. They were wonderful to me. Mothers I knew stop me today and talk to me.... Plunket was my life'.[73] Another Auckland Plunket nurse, who worked from 1925 to 1946, 'had made herself avail-able to mothers and their babies during the day, at night and during holidays'.[74] Nurse Ruby Pierson recalled an occasion when she stayed all night with a baby suffering from pneumonia.[75] Another Plunket nurse, Joan Meyer, remembered occasionally taking children home for the weekend if the family was not coping.[76]

Much depended, of course, on the personality of the individual nurse. Two 'country women' complained, when consulted in 1934, that though they were educated, 'the Plunket nurse would not credit them with an ounce of brain between them, so they ceased calling on her'.[77] Local committees were well aware of the need to attract nurses who were approved by mothers, and kept a close eye on them. These women were both employers and clients.

The fact that the nurses did not have to report to a medical officer meant that Plunket staff assumed less of an inspectorial role. Although Plunket nurse Ruby Pierson had been taught that she should look over mothers' homes in order to check that they were providing everything needed by the child, she believed that nurses should not do this. She said she did not like walking through people's houses as if on an inspection, and so would always wash her hands at the kitchen sink, in order to avoid having to walk through the entire house to the bathroom. She also said that she taught her young nurses to do the same thing.[78]

If the 1934 comment by Dr Henry Mess, an English medical officer of health, was at all typical, then the absence of medical officer input possibly made Plunket nurses more attractive than their British counterparts. He urged frequent super-vision, claiming 'the health visitor must say "Scrub this floor – Wash that bedding – Clean Susan's head – Take baby to the Centre – Cut Lancelot's finger nails – Did you comb all the girls' heads last night? – Clean the windows – Swill the yard"'. Nothing less than this, he said, would keep these families in a reasonably

---

73		'Joan', in Joyce Powell, 'Keep pumping those brakes nurse', interview transcript, c.1997 unpublished manuscript.
74		*NZH* (11 August 1962).
75		Ruby Pierson, Plunket Society Oral History Project, 1992: Alexander Turnbull Library, Wellington, OHColl 0314.
76		Oral History Project, 1992, cited in Elizabeth Cox, 'Plunket plus commonsense: women and the Plunket Society, 1940–1960', Victoria University of Wellington MA thesis (1996), p. 100.
77		*Dominion* (10 February 1934).
78		Cox, 'Plunket plus commonsense', p. 97.

satisfactory condition.[79] Certainly Plunket's medical adviser from 1939 to 1955, Dr Helen Deem, had reservations about some medical officers she had observed during her visit to Britain and the United States in 1948. She came to the post hoping to strengthen medical control of Plunket clinics, but after her trip abroad she told a colleague that, 'in kindness to the medical profession I did not state that my overseas observations of the conduct of infant welfare clinics by paediatricians convinced me that much more than their presence was required to make the sessions wholly successful in so far as the interests of the mothers and babies were concerned'.[80] She described some American clinics as 'more office-like than... our Plunket rooms', with the sessions 'conducted in a business-like manner'.[81] Later she explained, 'I have toyed with the idea of using paediatricians or paediatrically minded general practitioners at the Plunket rooms, but after weighing the pros and cons have thrown the idea overboard'.[82] Instead she strengthened the nursing services by appointing nurse supervisors from 1952.

Conclusion

The Plunket Society arose out of the early twentieth-century maternalist movement, but developed into a unique organization, controlled by women and serviced by nurses. Because of their public and political support, maternalists in New Zealand continued to wield power much longer than many of their overseas counterparts. To reinforce their position they could point to New Zealand's international status in infant welfare. Watt may have considered the Plunket nursing services wasteful, others did not agree. The 1940 issue of *Mother and Child* noted New Zealand's 'astonishingly low' infant death rate of 31 per 1,000 live births, remarking that it was the lowest in the world and that the credit for this low rate was 'largely due to the splendid work carried on by the Plunket Society'.[83] Plunket was given formal recognition when the National Baby Welfare Council awarded it the British Commonwealth Challenge Shield for the best record of child welfare work in the British Commonwealth during 1939–1944.[84] In 1952 Dr Jean Mackintosh, Director of Maternal and Child Welfare for Birmingham, England, told delegates at a Plunket Society conference in New Zealand that she had needed little persuasion to visit New Zealand because for more years than she could remember, New Zealand – and specifically the Plunket Society – had been held up

79 Henry Mess, 'The health visitor', Fourth Annual Conference of Women Public Health Officers, p. 9, WLA, D1/4.
80 Deem to S. Ludbrook, 16 May 1950, PSA, 595.
81 Plunket Society, *Annual Report 1947–8*, pp. 15, 16.
82 Deem to Ludbrook, 20 December 1952, PSA, 581.
83 *M&C*, 11, 1 (1940), 11. Maori infant death rates were, however, much higher than non-Maori; for Plunket involvement among this sector, see Bryder, *A Voice for Mothers*, and Bryder, 'New Zealand's infant welfare services and Maori', pp. 65–86.
84 Plunket Society, Auckland Branch, *Thirty-ninth Annual Report 1947*, p. 9.

to the rest of the world as an example of what could be done in maternal and child health.[85]

While they could draw on these favourable impressions of visitors and others, New Zealand women were determined to retain a service which many personally found valuable. In London the MTS received (and published) many appreciative letters, and maintained in 1929 that the 10,000 attendances at Cromwell House that year 'is clearly the best evidence that the help and advice given to mothers is appreciated'.[86] Yet a specialized maternal and infant welfare service was one that the National Health Service did not think it could afford. It was a 'luxury' which New Zealand women fought hard to retain.

85 Plunket Society, *Report of Thirty-first General Conference 1952*, p. 7.
86 MTS, *Annual Report 1928–29*, p. 13.

Chapter 14

Hospitals, Regions, and Central Authority: Issues in Scottish Hospital Planning, 1947–1974

John Stewart

In the early summer of 1947 Scotland gained a socialized health care system by way of a separate piece of legislation, the National Health Service (Scotland) Act, from that covering England and Wales.[1] In November the same year the inaugural meeting of the South-Eastern Regional Hospital Board (SERHB), centred in Edinburgh, was addressed by Sir George Henderson, Secretary to the Department of Health for Scotland (DHS). Sir George's message was rather mixed. The Board's function, he suggested, was to 'weld together...a heterogeneous collection of hospital systems'. It was, though, 'unfortunate that, at this time, new building or large-scale alterations to existing premises was impossible'. In administrative terms the Board was directly responsible to the Secretary of State for Scotland but there was 'no intention of administering the hospital service from St Andrew's House'.[2] Four days later, Sir George spoke to the Western Regional Hospital Board (WRHB), centred in Glasgow and Scotland's largest by some way. As in Edinburgh, he pointed out that the Board was directly responsible to the Scottish Secretary and that the hospital system 'would not be run by bureaucratic methods from St Andrew's House'. Nonetheless the Secretary of State had statutory responsibilities, most notably 'his responsibility to the National Exchequer', and this would necessitate the Board submitting its annual budget for his approval. More

I am grateful to the Scouloudi Foundation for its support of my research on the National Health Service in Scotland. John Welshman kindly commented on an earlier draft.

1 For Scottish twentieth-century health policy prior to 1948 see Jacqueline Jenkinson, *Scotland's Health 1919–1948* (Bern, 2002). For a chronologically wide-ranging discussion of Scottish medicine and health policy see Helen M. Dingwall, *A History of Scottish Medicine* (Edinburgh, 2003).

2 Edinburgh, University of Edinburgh, Lothian Health Services Archive, Records of the South-Eastern Regional Hospital Board (hereafter LHB), LHB 38/1/1, Minutes of the Board, 10 November 1947.

generally, the DHS 'would also wish to know what the Board was doing and would be only too glad to advise in all matters about which it was consulted'.[3] As we shall see, the relationship between the Boards and the Department, ambiguously dealt with in these remarks, was to be a recurring issue in Scottish health service administration, as was the more obvious problem of the volume and allocation of resources.

A quarter of a century later we again find concerns being expressed about future planning and administrative relationships in the broader context of structural change. Scottish reorganization in 1974 saw, *inter alia*, the creation of a single-tier structure and the demise of the Regional Hospital Boards. Negotiations prior to 1974 took place, it was claimed, in a more relaxed and consensual manner than south of the border. Only one Green Paper was issued in Scotland – two for England – and the Scottish Act was passed one year before its English counterpart. The new Scottish system was, its proponents claimed, highly integrated and centralized – a marked contrast, in the event, to the cumbersome, two-tier structure introduced in England.[4] The SERHB certainly agreed that the proposed new system was highly centralized. However from the late 1960s until 1974 it consistently complained about centralizing tendencies on the part of the DHS's successor from 1962, the Scottish Home and Health Department (SHHD). So, for example, in 1971 it argued that 'it is implicit in the White Paper that the National Health Service in Scotland will be dominated and run by the Scottish Home and Health Department...[The Board] agree that the new Health Boards should be the hub of the service, but they do not think that this will be so'.[5] This therefore suggests a lesser degree of consensus than previously ascribed to Scottish reorganization.

In the financial sphere the resources desired in the late 1940s were clearly found, most obviously by way of the Hospital Plan for Scotland. Published in 1962 this stressed both the regional organization of hospital services and the concept of – implicitly, centralized – planning.[6] As we shall see, under the NHS the SERHB's capital expenditure increased dramatically, as indeed it did for Scotland as a whole. But this did not resolve the Board's problems or aspirations. So, for example, the need for the Board to employ resources in a particular way had resulted in a number of unwelcome, if unintended, outcomes. Its own 'strategy of planning', it was noted in 1969, had previously rested on 'the early and concurrent replacement

3   Glasgow, University of Glasgow, Greater Glasgow NHS Board Archive, Records of the Western Regional Hospital Board (hereafter HB), HB 28/2/1, Minutes of the Board, 14 November 1947.

4   Charles Webster, *The National Health Service: A Political History* (2nd edn, Oxford, 2002), pp. 90ff; John Stewart, 'The National Health Service in Scotland, 1947–1974: Scottish or British?', *Historical Research*, 76 (2003), 389–410.

5   LHB 38/1/24, Minutes of the Board, 5 October 1971, Appendix – Comments on the White Paper.

6   DHS, *Hospital Plan for Scotland* (Edinburgh, 1962); for a recent critique of the Hospital Plan in England see John Mohan, *Planning, Markets and Hospitals* (London, 2002), chaps 6 and 7.

of the major teaching hospitals in Edinburgh' and much capital expenditure had been directed to that end. However this had meant that 'investment in accommodation for geriatric, psychiatric and mentally subnormal patients' had been inadequate 'to place these aspects of the service on a firm footing'. Further prioritizing of the teaching hospitals would thus be at the expense of other aspects of the service. It was consequently proposed, in a way that nonetheless continued, no doubt unwittingly, to seek the best of all worlds, to gain a 'considerable improvement in the services available to psychiatry, mental deficiency, geriatrics and obstetrics' while simultaneously continuing to develop the major teaching hospitals and taking steps to 'provide some special regional units and rehabilitation facilities'. This was to cost some £20.25 million over an unspecified period.[7] In short, from a SERHB perspective, the promise of freedom from central direction contained in Sir George Henderson's 1947 speech remained problematic; and the greater resources acknowledged to be required in the late 1940s had been forthcoming, but not forthcoming enough.

This chapter seeks to further develop some of these issues. It complements analyses I have employed elsewhere where it is argued, *inter alia*, that both in its origins and development down until 1974 the NHS in Scotland had certain distinctive characteristics; and that these included a Scottish form of governance and relatively higher levels of expenditure than in England and Wales. Attention was also drawn to the definitional problems involved in deciding whether the service was indeed 'Scottish' or 'British'; and to the fact that different versions of 'Scottishness' could be used to argue both for and against particular policy initiatives. These arguments were, finally, placed in the context of a relatively weak existing historiography, a superficially surprising situation given, on the one hand, the importance of the NHS to the Scottish people; and, on the other, their poor health record.[8] In the space available it will not be possible to analyse the whole, complex period of the first quarter century of the Scottish NHS. So, for example, while their distinctive medical traditions were often cited as a reason for a separate Scottish Act, we can only note that at least in certain areas, such as geriatric medicine, the Scots remained in the vanguard of medical innovation. Nor will it be possible to discuss the broader context of the tension in Scottish social welfare history between its consciously separate identity and the integrative forces of the twentieth century.[9] Instead, the focus is upon the difficult relationship between the various bodies involved in hospital provision and planning, difficulties

7   LHB Regional Planning Committee, 17 July 1969, Appendix I.
8   Stewart, 'The National Health Service in Scotland'. For what might lie behind Scottish ill-health see Mary Shaw et al., *The Widening Gap: Health Inequalities and Policy in Britain* (Bristol, 1999). For comparative expenditure data see Charles Webster, *The Health Services since the War. Volume 2, Government and Health Care: The British National Health Service 1958–1979* (London, 1996), Appendix 3.13.
9   Pat Thane, *Old Age in English History: Past Experiences, Present Issues* (Oxford, 2000), pp. 3, 444ff. On Scottish welfare's 'relative autonomy' see Lindsay Paterson, *The Autonomy of Modern Scotland* (Edinburgh, 1994).

which revolved around matters of governance and were exacerbated by matters of finance. Evidence is derived from the records of the central Departments and from those of the two largest Regional Hospital Boards, the Western and the South-Eastern. These two devoured the bulk of Scottish hospital resources although it should also be noted that the SERHB was, like most of the Scottish Boards, smaller than even medium-sized English Boards such as that based on Oxford. The significance of this for central control will become apparent.[10]

The National Health Service in Scotland

Although in essence the same as its English counterpart the Scottish NHS was nonetheless under the supervision of the Secretary of State for Scotland by way of the DHS and then the SHHD; fully integrated its teaching hospitals into the new system; gave the Scottish Secretary responsibility for health centres and ambulance services, local authority responsibilities in England and Wales; and allowed for, or created, specifically Scottish administrative structures. From the outset the Scots also had, by way of the Secretary of State, permanent Cabinet representation. This was not the case for the period under discussion for England and Wales where, in these terms, the Ministry of Health had a chequered career, at least until the late 1960s. This had implications for the ability of those responsible for the respective health services to stand up to, in particular, Treasury pressure.[11] As Duncan McTavish suggests, this may in part account for the higher quality of civil servants enjoyed by the Scottish NHS. In Scotland the health department was viewed as an important staging post for ambitious career civil servants whereas it was not, again at least until the 1960s, in England and Wales. As he pithily puts it, if 'Health was the place for the most able to avoid in England, this was not so in Scotland'.[12] An earlier commentary, the Acton Society Trust's important survey carried out in the mid-1950s, further remarked that Scotland had not experienced the disruptive changes which had significantly altered Ministry of Health responsibilities.[13]

10   The Acton Society Trust, *Hospitals and the State I: Background and Blueprint* (London, 1955), p. 27; The Acton Society Trust, *Hospitals and the State IV: Groups, Regions and Committees Pt.2* (London, 1957), p. 3. I am grateful to Charles Webster for alerting me to this important source.

11   Charles Webster, *The Health Services since the War. Volume 1, Problems of Health Care: the National Health Service before 1957* (London, 1988), chap. 4; The Acton Society Trust, *Hospitals and the State I*, pp. 26–9.

12   Duncan McTavish, 'The NHS – is Scotland different? A case study of the management of health care in the hospital service in the West of Scotland 1947–1987', *Scottish Medical Journal*, 45 (2000), 155–8: pp. 155, 156.

13   The Acton Society Trust, *Hospitals and the State V: The Central Control of the Service* (London, 1958), p. 23.

Confirmation of a distinctive form of health service governance comes from a Treasury official who visited Scotland in the early 1960s. 'So far as control of hospitals generally is concerned', he reported:

> I was struck once more by how close a grip the Department [of Health for Scotland] have on what is going on. They have much closer knowledge of Scottish hospitals and activity there than one can expect from the Ministry [of Health]. When one talks to people from outside the Department, it is quite clear that their working relationships with the Department are of the closest.

The official continued that while the advantages of large-scale organization were often, and as far as he was concerned rightly, expounded, nonetheless 'in the Scottish hospital service, one is aware of what the advantages of the small-scale organization can be'. The size of the Scottish NHS permitted 'tight control'. Given that hospital Boards of Management were usually 'smaller and weaker' than their English equivalents this allowed the Regional Boards in virtually all the Scottish regions 'considerable authority'. These regions were thus 'probably well run because the calibre of control is high in relation to their size'. The one region which appeared to buck this trend, and with which the DHS was least satisfied, was the Western.[14] The power of the centre, further enhanced by the Scottish tradition of prioritizing hospital over local authority services, had apparently welcome outcomes. When the Hospital Plans were being formulated in the early 1960s the influential newspaper *The Glasgow Herald* was moved to remark that in this respect 'Scotland...seems to be ahead of the rest of the country'. This was a view shared by Scottish civil servants themselves, for example in a DHS memorandum of the same year.[15] For a slightly later period we might note Charles Webster's comments on the SHHD. Its health branch was, he suggests, 'well-integrated and its organization permitted greater coordination of activity at senior levels than was possible with the Ministry of Health'. Such organization, moreover, when combined with 'the more centralized structure of the NHS in Scotland, encouraged a more interventionist approach to health service policy than was found within the Ministry of Health'.[16] This in turn fitted closely with broader traditions of Scottish governance.[17]

It would be wrong to overemphasize Scottish autonomy and centralization. In the last resort the NHS in Scotland was funded by the Treasury and Scottish officials could not simply demand what they wanted – on the contrary, they

14 Public Record Office, Kew (hereafter PRO), T 227/1321, Memorandum 26 March 1962, 'Visit to Scotland'.
15 PRO T 227/1318, cutting from *The Glasgow Herald* (18 January 1961); Edinburgh, National Archives of Scotland (hereafter NAS), HH 101/3216, Memorandum 30 November 1961.
16 Webster, *Government and Health Care*, p. 41.
17 See Richard J. Finlay, 'Scotland in the twentieth century: in defence of oligarchy?', *The Scottish Historical Review*, 73 (1994), 103–12: pp. 110, 111.

remained highly sensitive to the disparities in Scottish and English and Welsh expenditure.[18] And, as we shall see, bodies such as the Regional Hospital Boards could be far from passive in the face of what they saw as overbearing central control. Nonetheless the Treasury official's astute observations, and the analyses of Scottish governance by historians such as Webster, give us a number of insights into the way in which the service was run in Scotland, and it is on these that we now focus by way of a discussion of the tensions inherent in hospital planning, administrative organization, and expenditure.

Hospital planning in Scotland

The intention of the central department to keep Regional Boards under close supervision and scrutiny was evident from the outset. In late 1949 a meeting took place between DHS officials and a SERHB committee over the latter's proposal for a new 500-bed general hospital. The lead civil servant suggested that as 'long-term policy' such a proposal 'must not be ignored'. Nonetheless, the Board could not expect there to be sufficient funds available in the near future, not least when other hospital projects were to be undertaken. Planning would have to be restricted to a very limited number of projects in the coming ten years and it was unlikely that building works on any of them could be well advanced until at least 1953. The official further suggested that the local authority, Edinburgh Corporation, might be hostile to the proposed scheme.[19] We shall see that local authorities were, at various points, to give the Regional Board considerable criticism and thus might speculate on the matter being raised in this way. Two months later the Board again met with Department officials, this time to ask for 'special consideration in respect of new hospital provision' as a result of a shortage of beds and an anticipated influx of population. Once again the DHS made sympathetic noises about the 'special needs' of the region but the lead civil servant, when asked if he could indicate 'when the Board might be authorised to build new hospitals', replied firmly in the negative. Although there was further, rather desultory, debate the Department's intention not to budge comes through clearly.[20] The sense that the DHS was determined to keep a tight grip on its health service, and that in this it could be differentiated from practice in England and Wales, is further witnessed by its evidence to the Royal Commission on Scottish Affairs which reported in the early 1950s. Noting that administrative responsibility was 'centred in the Department's headquarters in Edinburgh' it was then suggested that there was no demand in Scotland for 'anything equivalent to the regional organization of the corresponding English Departments' whereby 'authority to take decisions within a

18   Stewart, 'The National Health Service in Scotland'.
19   LHB 38/1/2, General Purposes and Establishment Committee, Meeting between the General Purposes and Establishment Committee and Representatives of the DHS, 11 November 1949.
20   LHB 38/1/3, Hospital and Specialist Service Committee, 5 January 1950.

specified field is delegated to out-stationed administrative officers'.[21] From a different, but complementary, angle the Acton Society Trust noted that the integration of the teaching hospitals and the match up between Scottish regional and local authority boundaries (a highly problematic issue elsewhere) meant that 'consultation between different branches of the Health Service' was 'a much less complex business than in England'.[22] Such relative simplicity of structure almost certainly aided the DHS in its desire to maintain control.

In the 1960s we find further evidence of the particularities of Scottish health service governance in the Hospital Plan for Scotland. The Plan was, unsurprisingly, initially met with considerable enthusiasm. In his retirement letter of July 1961 the SERHB Secretary noted that earlier that year, at its hundredth meeting, 'the Board came of age and was confronted with a formidable ten-year development programme offering a supreme challenge to its early maturity. That challenge has been expeditiously and confidently accepted'.[23] The scale of what was being proposed is captured in a DHS memorandum earlier the same year which asserted that it was now possible 'to contemplate building the Ninewells Hospital at Dundee, the new Edinburgh Royal Infirmary and the reconstructed Glasgow Western Infirmary each in a single operation, carried straight through in four or five years'. Here we are again reminded of the confidence that Scottish planning was in advance of its southern counterpart.[24] Only a few years later, however, the SHHD noted that in both the Western and the South-Eastern Regions, albeit for different reasons, 'major changes in the later stages of the original ten-year plan have to be introduced' in 1964. This had brought 'serious planning and public difficulties for the various hospital and other authorities concerned' and had involved thereby a 'considerable amount of abortive planning and administrative work by the officers and members of the Boards concerned with the building programme'.[25] Such problems had, in fact, been indicated from spring 1964 onwards. In May the SERHB discussed correspondence from the SHHD on the revised Hospital Plan published a few weeks earlier. The Department had suggested that since the original plan 'there had been, in almost every case, considerable increases in the scope of the schemes included'. These had to be finished and in the meantime it was 'quite unable for the present to accept additional major schemes until after the period of the present review of the Plan'. Some of the Board's major projects, for example additional maternity accommodation in Fife and Edinburgh, were thus not currently included in SHHD plans. The Board had responded that it was 'gravely concerned' with this revision to the Hospital Plan which had been undertaken *'without proper consultation, and* [the Board] *could not be regarded as having*

21   *Royal Commission on Scottish Affairs: Volume 1, Memoranda Submitted to the Royal Commission by the Scottish Departments* (Edinburgh, 1953), p. 45.
22   The Acton Society Trust, *Hospitals and the State IV*, p. 3.
23   LHB 38/1/14, Minutes of the Board, 31 July 1961, Appendix.
24   NAS HH 101/2043, Memorandum 'Hospital Building Programme', 23 March 1961.
25   SHHD, *Review of the Hospital Plan for Scotland* (Edinburgh, 1966), p. 6.

agreed to the exclusion from the Revised Plan of the several important projects put forward by them' (my emphasis).[26]

What is important here is the way in which the Board felt it was being treated rather than the detail of the proposed cuts. This would have been reinforced by the letter from the SHHD a few months later which stated that the Secretary of State had authorized a review of the whole building programme to examine its scale; its guiding principles; and how building priorities had been established. This letter also explained that the Regional Board 'would be consulted *in due course* about this review of the programme' (my emphasis).[27] In this context it is instructive to note that in 1965 a committee of the Scottish Health Services Council commented that Regional Boards were responsible 'for planning and co-ordinating the development of the hospital and specialist services in their regions and for generally supervising the administration of these services (particularly in relation to expenditure)'. All this took place under the 'general guidance' of the SHHD on behalf of the Secretary of State. The careful choice of language here might result from precisely the sort of strained relationships which could emerge between the central authority and the Regional Boards. The committee then concluded, optimistically in the light of what was shortly to follow, that relations and communications between the SHHD and the Boards were 'good and call for no major change in existing arrangements'.[28]

Administrative reorganization

By the late 1960s administrative reorganization had moved to the top of the health service agenda, ironically because of what was increasingly being perceived as the 'failure' of the Hospital Plans. In the case of England John Mohan conjectures whether 'a more dirigiste state apparatus, with stronger strategic capacities, would have done a better job'.[29] If we view Scotland as from the outset more 'dirigiste' then important comparative work remains to be done on the Scottish *versus* the English experience. In any event the 1968 Green Paper for Scotland was openly critical of the existing tripartite structure and, in seeking to explain this, noted *inter alia* that 'the 1947 Act was not as radical as may sometimes be thought'. There were divisions not only between the three branches of the service – hospital, general practice, and local authority – but also within, in particular, the hospital service. The allocation of responsibility between Regional Boards and Hospital Boards of Management was potentially problematical and could not be 'embodied without question in an administrative framework which aims at greater integration'. The key word here was 'integration'. Administrative integration was not only

26   LHB 38/1/17, Regional Planning Committee, 21 May 1964.
27   LHB 38/1/17, Regional Planning Committee, 19 November 1964.
28   SHHD Scottish Health Services Council, *Administrative Practices of Hospital Boards in Scotland* (Edinburgh, 1966), pp. 10, 99.
29   Mohan, *Planning, Markets and Hospitals*, p. 129.

an end in itself but also 'a means towards better functional integration' for the benefit of the whole community. As to the role of the SHHD, it would be unacceptable under the proposed new scheme, as it was now, for it 'to intervene regularly in the detailed administration of the service or to concern itself only with the largest questions of policy. It would have to continue to pursue a middle course between these extremes'.[30] One way of construing this is as, in reality, a blank cheque for the central department. This was acknowledged in a 1971 SHHD paper which claimed that a 'fundamental part of the case for single tier structure in Scotland' – as opposed, that is, to the two-tier structure proposed for England – 'is the establishment of a strong central organization for the health service'.[31]

Regional Boards were conscious of such centralizing tendencies. In February 1968 the Secretary of the Eastern Regional Board, based in Dundee, wrote to his Glasgow counterpart about a recent SHHD discussion paper. The latter was, it was claimed, 'clearly slanted against a two tier structure with regional authorities'. Boards would have to make a clear and 'objective' case for regional organization, its previous successes notwithstanding. As to the future role of the SHHD itself, the Eastern Board felt that what was being proposed was obviously 'an expansion in depth of the functions of the central department, which may be seen as no more than a continuation of the trend of recent years', hence the necessity of regional organization to resist, it was strongly implied, any further such encroachment.[32] Commenting on the Green Paper the SERHB agreed the need for administrative changes, and that control not be handed over to the local authorities. But it was sceptical of the proposed one-tier structures based on Health Boards. Consequently the Board argued, 'having regard to the geography and population distribution of Scotland', that a two-tier system was essential 'both for the planning and for the management of an integrated health service'.[33] The appeal to Scottish distinctiveness alongside a proposal for an administrative structure not unlike that being put forward for England is notable here, not least because such distinctiveness had often been used to *justify* differences with England and Wales and was shortly to be so again. So, as the 1971 White Paper put it, its proposals represented 'a structure for a unified health service that will be acceptable and will work, taking account of special Scottish needs and circumstances'.[34]

The SERHB further addressed reorganization on the eve of the White Paper's publication. Again arguing for a two-tier structure, it made two key points – first, that the public would not 'readily understand a one-tier structure in Scotland and a

30   SHHD, *Administrative Reorganization of the Scottish Health Services* (Edinburgh, 1968), pp. 7, 11, 13, 8, 22.
31   NAS HH 101/2473, SHHD paper 'Reorganization of National Health Service Structure: Central Organization', January 1971.
32   HB 28/5/105, Letter, 13 February 1968, from the Secretary of the Eastern Regional Hospital Board to the Secretary of the Western Regional Hospital Board.
33   LHB 38/1/22, Minutes of the Board, 1 April 1969, Appendix.
34   SHHD, *Reorganization of the Scottish Health Services* (Edinburgh, 1971), p. 5; Stewart, 'The National Health Service in Scotland'.

two-tier structure in England'. Furthermore, they would be confused by the creation of two specifically Scottish bodies, the Common Services Agency and the Scottish Health Service Planning Council, and their proposed relation to the SHHD and the new Health Boards. Second, the SERHB claimed that the proposed different structures – the Scottish 'one-tier system' as against the English 'two-tier system with strong regional authorities' – would have the effect of 'reducing Scotland as a whole to a regional status with, in practice, direct government control'. This was in the best interests neither of Scotland nor of 'government'. The Board acknowledged that this was not intentional. Nonetheless such would be the perception, possibly by the public but 'more certainly in the eyes of the health service professions, with obvious repercussions on morale' that it foresaw 'a tendency for a drift of the most able administrative staff to England'.[35] These concerns can be seen as both understandable and self-serving – the Board had, presumably, no desire to acquiesce in its own demise and so mustered what arguments it could in opposition to reorganization.

In the event, the consequences of reorganization in England and Wales proved much more traumatic than in Scotland, the Regional Hospital Boards' objections notwithstanding. Nonetheless, some of their concerns appear to have been realized. In a study undertaken shortly after reorganization David Hunter pointed out that the relationship between the SHHD and the new Health Boards was highly complex and not simply top-down. But he also suggested that there were 'indications of a shift in the relationship between the SHHD and health boards, with greater interest by the centre in health priorities becoming a feature of it'. This he attributed to reorganization itself and, just as importantly, to 'resource constraints and related political pressures', a clear reference to the economic and political upheavals of the 1970s.[36] However for present purposes what is important is less the accuracy of the SERHB's analysis than that it was made in the first place. It is notable, first, that the Board countered one version of Scottish distinctiveness – as put forward by the 1971 White Paper, for example – with another wherein reorganization would reduce Scotland to a mere region. The broader context here is the rise of Scottish nationalism which had clearly raised questions about the very nature of Scottish identity. More generally, the Board's evident unhappiness over reorganization means that, as noted, we need to qualify the view of this process in Scotland as largely consensual. Second, a further undesired outcome of reorganization, by this account, would be the diminished quality of Health Service administrative staff. That this implied threat was made – whether it was an accurate assessment of future developments or not – reinforces, unwittingly, the points made earlier whereby both contemporary observers and subsequent commentators saw in the Scottish NHS bureaucracy high levels of administrative ability. Third, the Hospital Board's comments highlight an ongoing

35   LHB 38/1/24, Minutes of the Board, 8 June 1971, Appendix.
36   David J. Hunter, *Coping with Uncertainty: Policy and Politics in the National Health Service* (Chichester, 1980), p. 161.

tension between what it saw as its own status and relative autonomy against the centralizing tendencies of the DHS/SHHD.

The problems which the SERHB felt it faced with the central authority were, as we have seen, longstanding. Furthermore, Boards might be subject to pressure not just from the interventionist tendencies of the central department, but also from other organizations. This could take two forms. First, bodies outside the NHS, most obviously local authorities, had their own agenda. In spring 1962 Midlothian County Council wrote 'expressing concern that a new general hospital for Midlothian was not included in the Hospital Building Plan for Scotland for 1961/71'. The Council, rather imperiously, sought a meeting 'together with a full history of the Board's deliberations on this matter since 1950 and on their discussions with the County Council and other bodies'. Such a meeting duly took place with Council representatives being told by the Board that there was 'no possibility' of providing a new hospital in the County under the current Plan 'but that planning for the post-1971 period would take cognisance of the situation'.[37] Second, the Hospital Board might also be pressurized by its own 'subordinate' bodies, the Boards of Management. So in the autumn of 1964 the SERHB received letters of complaint about the Hospital Plan not only from local authorities but also from the West Fife Board of Management.[38] From the Hospital Boards' point of view, although pressure clearly came from both above and below, it was almost certainly easier to resist the latter than the former. However the nature of the complaints cited from the Board of Management and the local authorities, coming as they do from the era of the Hospital Plans, suggests that resources – their allocation and deployment – were a perennially important issue not only in themselves but in shaping the relationship between the various bodies with interests in the formation or implementation of hospital policy.

Income and expenditure

In October 1965 the Scottish Secretary wrote to the WRHB's Chairman in response to a communication from the latter regarding revisions to the Hospital Plan and the needs of his Region. The Secretary of State counselled caution, pointing out that for some time Scotland had had 'a disproportionately large share of the hospital capital programme'. It was further the case that 'forward programmes on which the two Hospital Plans, published in 1962, were based were planned to bring the programme for England and Wales up to the Scottish level' and so, in principle if not necessarily in practice, a 'substantially higher rate of increase was provided for England and Wales than for Scotland'. In such circumstances, the Scottish Secretary concluded, the Chairman would 'readily appreciate…that in the next three or four years only limited additions to the total programme are likely to

37 LHB 38/1/15, Medical Service Committee, 9 April and 18 June 1962.
38 LHB 38/1/17, Regional Planning Committee, 22 October and 19 November 1964.

be possible'.[39] In the first instance, of course, this letter indicates the constraints, economic and political, under which the highest echelons of the Scottish NHS had to operate. Treasury officials felt they had to be constantly vigilant over claims from Scotland: as one remarked in 1961, discussing the capital expenditure programme, 'I would counsel caution vis-à-vis the Scots'.[40] Caution or not, a considerable amount of bargaining clearly took place. Only two months later the Treasury agreed, albeit extremely reluctantly, to raise the hospital spending allocation for 1965/6 from the original £6.4 million to £7.8 million. In the event, Scottish hospital capital expenditure for that year was to exceed £10 million.[41] Nor was this a debate carried on simply behind closed doors. *The Glasgow Herald* remarked at the beginning of the Hospital Plans era that the question was now 'whether the noble intentions of the hospital administrators are to be matched by equal foresight from the Treasury. Restrictions on capital expenditure have been at the expense of progress which should no longer be delayed'.[42] Evident here are the rising expectations engendered by the Hospital Plan; the desire of the Regions – undoubtedly also pressurized from below – to get as large a share of the cake as possible; and, implicitly, the SHHD's perceived need not only to conciliate the Treasury but also to keep a significant measure of control over the planning process.

Resource allocation was hardly a new problem. As early as September 1948 the SERHB had to accept that while it had a building programme for the following year costed at just under one million pounds, the DHS intended to allocate around one third of this sum. A similar ratio emerged the following year. Significantly, this came in the wake of a DHS circular which – in addition to pointing to labour and material constraints on capital projects – had intimated that while initial financial allocations had been done on the basis of population, this would not necessarily always be the case.[43] Nonetheless the resources issue became particularly pronounced as a result of the aspirations engendered by the Hospital Plans. In December 1962 a special meeting was convened between the Western Region's Hospital Services Committee and SHHD officials. Recorded in the minutes under the heading 'Shortage of Capital Funds', this started with the Committee Chairman asking the civil servants to comment on the provisional ten-year building programme submitted to them by the Regional Board 'and on the considerable list of important schemes necessarily excluded from that programme'. The Committee

---

39 NAS HH 101/3461, draft letter from the Secretary of State for Scotland to the Chairman of the Western Regional Hospital Board, October 1965.
40 PRO T 227/1318, Treasury Memorandum 31 January 1961. For further instances, Stewart, 'The National Health Service in Scotland'.
41 NAS HH 101/2043, Memorandum 'Hospital Building Programme', 23 March 1961; SHHD, *Scottish Health Statistics 1968* (Edinburgh, HMSO, 1970), Section X, Table 3.
42 PRO T 227/1318, cutting from *The Glasgow Herald* (18 January 1961).
43 LHB 38/1/1 Works and Buildings Committee, 16 September 1948; and 38/1/2 Works and Buildings Committee, 4 October 1949; HB 28/2/1, copy of DHS Circular RHB (S) 48 (22), 'Hospital Building Programme 1949', 13 August 1948.

further claimed that the Board was facing an increasing number of requests from Hospital Boards of Management, the majority of which were 'completely justified'. Again showing the sort of 'pressure from below' to which Regional Boards were subject, it was suggested that great upset would be felt when the ten-year plan was announced and that this could be a source of embarrassment to the Secretary of State himself. Grievances were also aired about the balance between the major and the ordinary building programmes with the Secretary of the Board claiming that, overall, the hospital service 'was not progressing as it should'. The lead SHHD official, Mr Graham, claimed that the Scottish Secretary was indeed fully aware of the facts, and that in addition to the financial situation there was 'little skilled labour reserve available in the country', hence the 'limit to the number of schemes which could be undertaken'. The meeting drew to a rather desultory close.[44]

A probably more abrasive encounter took place five years later between the Secretary of State, William Ross, and the Regional Board Chairmen. The former made it clear that while the volume of resources would continue to expand, these had to be used more efficiently; and that controls were to be tightened at all levels. Ross conceded that part of the problem was that Boards put forward plans more quickly than had been thought possible and agreed that the Chairmen's assessment of future need was valid. Nonetheless as matters currently stood there was 'little prospect of the Chancellor providing more' for the Scottish hospital service. It thus had to be accepted that there would be no additional funds available 'and the programme to be prepared for the next five years would have to be fitted to the sums forecast'. Mr Stevenson, Chairman of the Western Board and of this meeting, responded that he and his colleagues understood the need for corrective actions and appreciated the decision not to reduce total funding. Nonetheless, and echoing his Board's tactics of five years earlier, he felt it 'likely that there would be a very strong reaction from Boards of Management, medical staff and the public when the measures finally agreed were announced'. Stevenson also noted that the Western Region would suffer most by current proposals, as indeed Ross had acknowledged. Summing up, he expressed his conviction that 'if the hospital service was not to suffer permanent damage, a very strong case indeed would have to be made for additional funds' and that he and his colleagues desired a forward programme extending to at least 1977.[45]

In his report for 1971/2 the SERHB's Treasurer commented that while the capital expenditure allowance from the SHHD had risen by more than £0.75 million over the previous year, nonetheless 'expenditure still falls well below that of three to four years ago'. It was thus insufficient to upgrade existing wards and

44   HB 28/2/15, Minutes of a Special Meeting of the Hospital Services Committee, 19 December 1962.

45   HB 28/5/106, Regional Hospital Boards, Scotland: Minutes of a Special Meeting between the Chairmen of the Scottish Regional Hospital Boards and the Secretary of State for Scotland, 13 October 1967.

replace outworn equipment. Furthermore, no major schemes had been completed or commissioned. The following year the Board itself, following a meeting with SHHD officials, noted that this had 'not resulted in the Board's receiving the substantial increase' essential for the development of 'urgent' projects, a situation which it viewed with 'concern and regret'.[46] The SERHB, at least from its own point of view, had cause for grievance. Its capital expenditure allocation rose fairly consistently between the founding of the NHS and the late 1960s, peaking in absolute terms in 1969 when it received £3.3 million. This constituted between one fifth and one third of total Scottish health service capital expenditure. In the last few years of the Board's existence, however, this fell to around 10 per cent. The Western Board's story was somewhat different. It too had experienced an almost consistent rise in capital expenditure but its peak came rather later, in 1973, when it received over £14 million. Initially the WRHB had consumed less than 50 per cent of total Scottish NHS capital expenditure, but by the early 1970s this had risen to around 60 per cent.[47] Nonetheless, this did not necessarily mean that the Board was satisfied. Commenting on the 1973 accounts the Finance Committee's convenor acknowledged that the 'scope and scale of the Hospital Service in the Western Region has changed since 1948 out of all recognition and the vast increase in moneys spent, and continuing to be spent, is evidence of a great improvement in the Service. Much, however, remains to be done'.[48] What this starkly reveals is that not only did the SHHD have to negotiate with the Treasury over the size of the cake, but also that it then had to make tough decisions about how that cake was divided in an atmosphere where expectations remained both frustrated and high. What such data also show, of course, is the preponderance of the Western Board; and that when it and the SERHB are taken together they consumed around two-thirds to three-quarters of Scottish hospital capital expenditure.

Furthermore, by this point the SHHD was clearly determined to keep a tight rein on capital expenditure and explicitly linked this with reorganization. In Scotland as elsewhere in Great Britain reorganization was not being carried out merely for its own sake. Rather, the 'failure' of the Hospital Plans, which had been created at least in part to make expenditure savings through increased efficiency, signalled a shift to a different strategy for controlling costs – administrative

46   LHB 38/9/16, Financial Review 1971/2, p. 1; LHB 38/1/25, Minutes of the Board, 4 April 1972.
47   Calculated from LHB 38/10/28, SERHB Capital Expenditure 5 July 1948 to 31 March 1973; HB 28/2/15, WRHB Memorandum, 'Running Costs of Hospital Service', July 1962; HB 28/1/25, 'The Western Regional Hospital Board and Constituent Boards of Management Statement of Accounts for year ended 31 March 1971'; DHS, *Scottish Health Statistics 1958* (Edinburgh, 1959), Section XI, Table 3; SHHD, *Scottish Health Statistics 1968* (Edinburgh, HMSO, 1970), Section X, Table 3; and Common Services Agency: Information Services Division, *Scottish Health Statistics 1974* (Edinburgh, 1976), Table 10.3.
48   HB 28/2/26, Statement on Accounts to 31 March 1973, by D.W. Mitchell, Esq., Convener of the Finance Committee.

efficiency. A 1972 memorandum, 'NHS Reorganization: Control of Capital Expenditure', by its very title illustrates this point; emphasized that any public expenditure was subject to parliamentary accountability; and observed that the Treasury had delegated to the SHHD the responsibility for 'the efficiency with which [the Department] does its work and, in this sphere, for the efficient management overall of the NHS building programme'. It was therefore suggested that post-reorganization limits be placed on the volume of money delegated to subordinate bodies.[49] Implicit here is the idea, the opposite of the viewpoint of the Regional Boards, that the latter had previously been allowed too much leeway and that reorganization presented the opportunity to enhance the central authority's position.

Conclusion

This chapter has sought to show how issues of governance and expenditure were complex and contested in the first quarter of a century of the NHS in Scotland. Tensions were evident not only between the Treasury and the central Scottish health department but also within the Scottish NHS itself. Regional Hospital Boards had both their own agenda and were subject to 'pressure from below'. Broadly speaking, the two main areas of dispute were, first, the control exerted by the central department over its subordinate bodies. It is apparent that Regional Boards sought to carve out their own autonomous fields of action but that the DHS/SHHD was equally determined to maintain control, notwithstanding the initial rhetoric around the health service's formation. In this struggle it is equally clear that the central departments were, on balance, the winners. This was attributable not only to Scotland's relatively small size – and the associated relatively small size of its Hospital Boards – but also to Scottish traditions of governance. The second broad cause of tension was, unsurprisingly, over resource allocation. Just as the Scottish central departments had to negotiate with the Treasury so too did Regional Boards have to negotiate with central departments. As might be expected, this resulted in the DHS/SHHD having to make decisions which, on occasions, advantaged one Regional Hospital Board at the 'expense' of another. Nonetheless, it should also be noted that capital expenditure on Scottish hospitals rose rapidly and apparently inexorably in the period under discussion. That it did so reflected not only the general British trend of the time but also the particular Scottish prioritizing of hospital care. Equally evident is the impact of, especially, the Hospital Plan for Scotland in raising expectations. The implications of all this need to be more fully teased out both in terms of Scotland itself and how it fared compared to the rest of the United Kingdom. For present purposes, however, it is apparent that the Scottish hospital planning in the period 1947 to 1974 has much to tell us both about modern

---

49   NAS 101/2429, SHHD Memorandum 'NHS Reorganization: Control of Capital Expenditure', 7 March 1972.

John Stewart

Scotland and about the problems – problems which were often unintended consequences of well-meaning policy decisions – of running a large, complex organization such as the National Health Service where 'goals' are difficult to determine with any clarity or accuracy.

Chapter 15

Hospital Provision, Resource Allocation, and the Early National Health Service: The Sheffield Regional Hospital Board, 1947–1974

John Welshman

Inequalities in health, and variations in resource allocation, are among the most important themes in contemporary health policy. Yet while historians are increasingly aware of geographical variations in health provision in Britain before the Second World War, less attention has been paid to resource allocation under the early National Health Service (NHS). This chapter takes up this theme through a case study of the Sheffield Regional Hospital Board (RHB), from its creation in 1947 to the health service reorganization of 1974. Sheffield was one of 14 RHBs in England and Wales, and an area that has been persistently singled out as being at the bottom of the resource allocation league table. The perspective of the chapter is not primarily quantitative and comparative, though this is one possible approach to the issues under consideration. Its approach is more qualitative, examining how the issue of resource allocation was perceived in one case study. The chapter thus tries to raise important issues in the regional implementation of health policy, thereby producing a useful antidote to broad national studies of policy formation.

The issue of resource allocation, and the choice of this particular region, are appropriate given that Charles Webster has stressed both this theme, and the usefulness of the Sheffield example, in the official history of the NHS. His own distinctive Nottingham accent will be what many students will remember best from his seminar papers. But some earlier commentators on the NHS made passing reference to the issue of resource allocation, and to the experience of individual regions. Harry Eckstein for example, an American observer writing in 1959, noted the uneven geographical distribution of services before 1948, and argued that

For their help, I would like to thank Sir George Godber; Charles Webster; John Stewart; the staff of Sheffield Archives; and those present at the Verona Conference of the International Network for the History of Hospitals, 19–21 April 2001, where an earlier version was given as a paper.

despite improvements in the distribution of general practitioners, 'an appointment in Manchester or Sheffield is still tantamount to self-imposed exile for all too many budding consultants'.[1] Similar points were made by Sir John Jewkes, an Oxford University academic, writing in 1962. Jewkes noted that there had been little change in the number and distribution of hospitals since 1939, and in the distribution of dentists and doctors, and many of the pre-war weaknesses were still evident.[2]

Nevertheless these were exceptions, and it is fair to say that much of the early secondary literature on the NHS made little reference to geographical variations in provision, or to the issue of resource allocation in general. Writing of devolution in 1975, George Godber, the former Chief Medical Officer, noted the disparity in the amount spent in Scotland and Wales, compared to England. Godber made the important point that stronger RHBs had pressed for an increase in their central allocation. In his view, the Sheffield region went short, partly due to less forceful personnel, but also because of the deficient resources it began with, and the rapid increase in population that occurred there.[3] But it was only after the creation of the Resource Allocation Working Party (RAWP) (1975) that this issue was highlighted in the 1980s. Alan Maynard and Anne Ludbrook have observed, for instance, that the NHS inherited a hospital stock characterized by a lack of co-ordination and by geographical differences in the distribution of beds. But there was little discussion of regional resource inequality since the main concern of policy-makers was containing the size of the NHS budget. Maynard and Ludbrook characterized the division of the budget as 'what you got last year, plus an allowance for growth, plus an allowance for scandals'. In their view, incremental increases in resources went to the 'noisiest rather than the neediest'.[4]

In surveying the background to RAWP, Nicholas Mays and Gwyn Bevan have argued that in the 1950s there was little interest in access to services, and the notion of normative planning to provide desirable provision for the population gained ground in the 1960s, to be replaced in the 1970s by a policy of rationing in response to financial stringency. Before 1962, the concern was to contain the increasing cost of the NHS, planning and funding were incremental and *ad hoc*, and resource inequalities were not perceived as an important policy problem. From 1962 to 1970, there was an attempt to link planning to resource allocation in the 1962 Hospital Plan, but resource allocation remained essentially an interesting idea. Mays and Bevan argue that given the context in which it evolved, it was not surprising the RAWP formula was aimed at geographical inequality rather than

1   Harry Eckstein, *The English Health Service: Its Origins, Structure and Achievements* (Cambridge, Mass., 1959), pp. 41–3, 233–5.
2   John Jewkes and Sylvia Jewkes, *The Genesis of the British National Health Service* (Oxford, 1962), pp. 11–18, 19–23.
3   George Godber, *The Health Service: Past, Present and Future* (London, 1975), pp. 47, 59, 78, 84.
4   Alan Maynard and Anne Ludbrook, 'Budget allocation in the National Health Service', *Journal of Social Policy*, 9 (1980), 290–312.

tackling the more controversial social class inequalities in health and health care use. They concluded that RAWP was a public policy success, though observing that moves towards equality since have been relatively slow.[5]

The official history of the NHS, of course, has also drawn attention to resource allocation in the hospital service, and to the experience of individual RHBs. Charles Webster has argued that during the first years of the NHS, little attention was given to resource allocation, and regions that were better provided for retained their advantages. The most deprived regions in 1947 were East Anglia, Sheffield, Newcastle, and Wales, while the Metropolitan Boards, Oxford, and the South Western region, were the most affluent. Comparison is difficult, requiring the aggregation of different sources and different time periods. The Sheffield region had 8.96 per cent of the capital allocation (1948–49 to 1956–57) and 7.08 per cent (1950–51) and 7.44 per cent (1955–56) of the revenue allocation, despite having 9.5 per cent of the population (mid-1953).[6] Sheffield was also under-provided with consultants. It had 6.70 per cent (31 December 1949) and 6.66 per cent (31 December 1955) of the consultants, despite having 7.4 per cent of the beds (31 December 1953).[7] It was short of junior doctors, and reliant on migrant doctors from India and Pakistan.

However Webster argues that there was little real appreciation of resource allocation as a problem. The result was that in the first ten years of the NHS, the position of the poorer regions had only 'marginally improved'.[8] He has noted that because the NHS could only apply basic mechanisms of financial control, often taken from pre-NHS bodies, 'the new health service therefore ossified many of the inherited inequalities in health care, and there was no mechanism for preventing the perpetuation of such evils'.[9] It was only with the formation of RAWP in the early 1970s that differences between the regions were acknowledged. Charles Webster argues further that the formula adopted for RAWP was seriously flawed, since it was based heavily on mortality rates, and failed to take account of general practitioner services or the personal social services.[10] Despite RAWP, the more affluent regions and acute specialties continued to be efficient at obstructing shifts of resources. Overall Webster has claimed that the NHS 'tended to mirror and

5   Nicholas Mays and Gwyn Bevan, *Resource Allocation in the Health Service: A Review of the Methods of the Resource Allocation Working Party (RAWP)* (London, 1987), pp. 4, 6–21, 23–30, 160.

6   Charles Webster, *The Health Services Since the War. Volume 1, Problems of Health Care: The National Health Service Before 1957* (London, 1988), p. 293, table V.

7   *Ibid.*

8   *Ibid.*, pp. 292–6, 305–6, 325, 395–6.

9   Charles Webster, *The Health Services Since the War. Volume 2, Government and Health Care: The British National Health Service 1958–1979* (London, 1996), pp. 27–8.

10   *Ibid.*, pp. 606–10, 765–8.

perpetuate the accumulated idiosyncrasies and inequalities in health-care provision contained in the inherited system'.[11]

The most important recent contribution to this debate is John Mohan's account of the development of hospital services in the Newcastle region.[12] The fact that Sheffield was at the bottom of the resource allocation league table has been well documented. What is missing is a detailed account of what the implications of these inequalities were for individual regions, and the extent to which they were able to remedy them. This chapter uses the Sheffield case study to look more closely at how the issue of resource allocation played out at the regional level, making comparisons with the neighbouring Oxford region, and Mohan's work on Newcastle. Sheffield is worth looking at because it has acted as a prime example of inequalities in resource allocation, with evidence that these persisted after 1974 and have been perpetuated in the new Trent region.[13] The chapter considers the origins of the region, and what the wartime hospital survey reveals about the institutions and resources inherited from the earlier period. Capital expenditure, and hospital building, are central concerns of the chapter, as are revenue expenditure and staffing levels. We explore the role of office-holders, and assess the extent to which they were able to put the case of Sheffield's relative poverty. The final section traces increasing recognition of inter- and intra-regional variations in the early 1970s, and the lag between evidence and action. The chapter argues that in fact the disadvantaged position of the region was known from an early stage. However existing expenditure systems, allied to passivity by regional officials, meant that there was a failure to remedy these inequalities until the 1970s.

Inventing the region

It is instructive to look at how the Sheffield region was invented, since in many ways it was an artificial creation. The origins of the region lay in the earlier British Hospitals Association (BHA) region of 1939, and the Civil Defence Region of 1939–45. Furthermore, under the 1939 Cancer Act, Derby, Nottingham, and Leicester had devised the beginnings of a regional scheme. The BHA East Midland region had comprised South Derbyshire, South Nottinghamshire, South Lincolnshire, Leicestershire, Rutland, Northamptonshire, Warwickshire, and Staffordshire. Later, the Civil Defence North Midlands Region had included Derbyshire, Nottinghamshire, Lincolnshire, Leicestershire, Rutland, and Northamptonshire.[14]

The original statement of proposed RHB areas, drafted in November 1946, was drawn up on the basis of the recommendations of the wartime hospital

11   Charles Webster, *The National Health Service: A Political History* (Oxford, 1998, 2nd edn, 2002), p. 57.
12   John Mohan, *Planning, Markets and Hospitals* (London, 2002).
13   NHS Executive, *Illustrations of Health Inequalities in Trent Region* (Sheffield, 1998), pp. 1–20.
14   Webster, *Problems of Health Care*, p. 266, table IV.

surveys, the views of regional medical staff, and the results of informal discussions with professional bodies, municipal associations, and local authorities.[15] A Ministry of Health memo stated that the size and extent of areas should be determined by the needs for planning, co-ordination, and provision of hospital and specialist services. They could be large, and university medical centres should be a focal point. Boundaries should coincide with those of local health departments for administrative efficiency, but these should not prevent free passage of patients.[16]

But debates about the parameters of the RHB indicated how the idea that existing regions were 'natural' entities was a myth. In creating the region, Lincolnshire was one area of difficulty. There were debates about whether Holland and Kesteven should be in the Cambridge rather than the Sheffield region. There was a proposal that a Regional Committee of the RHB should administer Lincolnshire, parts of Kesteven, Lindsey, Holland and Boston, and the County Boroughs of Lincoln and Grimsby.[17] Some wanted Burton-on-Trent to be in the Birmingham rather than the Sheffield region. Others wanted Hinckley to be in the Sheffield and not in the Oxford region.[18] Some argued Leicester should be in the Birmingham region, and Goole in the Leeds region.[19] These disagreements had been resolved by December 1946, with only minor changes thereafter.

It was logical to base the region on Sheffield, which possessed the only teaching hospital. Even so, the East Midland cities of Derby, Leicester, and Nottingham feared being dominated by Sheffield. At the Ministry of Health, George Godber admitted in August 1947 that 'the region includes three large towns, Nottingham, Leicester, and Derby which compete with and are extremely jealous of Sheffield'.[20] Debates about the most suitable name for the region continued into the mid-1960s. There were recurring suggestions that 'East Midlands' would be more descriptive of the area than 'Sheffield'.[21] As time went on, the balance of power shifted away from Sheffield, with the opening of new medical schools at Nottingham (1965) and Leicester (1974). However it is revealing that a meeting of the RHB was held outside Sheffield for the first time only in February 1970, at Nottingham. The way its boundaries were drawn, and the extent to which the region centred on Sheffield, would remain sources of tension until the 1974 re-organization.[22]

15   Kew, Public Record Office (hereafter PRO), MH 90/1: J.E. Pater to A. Rucker, 9/11/46.

16   *Ibid.*: J.E. Pater, 'National Health Service Act: Areas of Regional Hospital Boards', 15/11/46.

17   PRO, MH 90/2: G.E. Godber to J. Pater, 16/12/46.

18   PRO, MH 90/6: D. Evan Davies to Ministry of Health, 20/12/46.

19   *Ibid.*: C.H. Coggrave to Ministry of Health, 12/12/46.

20   PRO, MH 90/45: G.E. Godber to M. Reed, 23/8/47.

21   Sheffield Archives (hereafter SA), minutes of the General Purposes Committee, 27/7/64.

22   Webster, *Government and Health Care*, pp. 477, 479, 532.

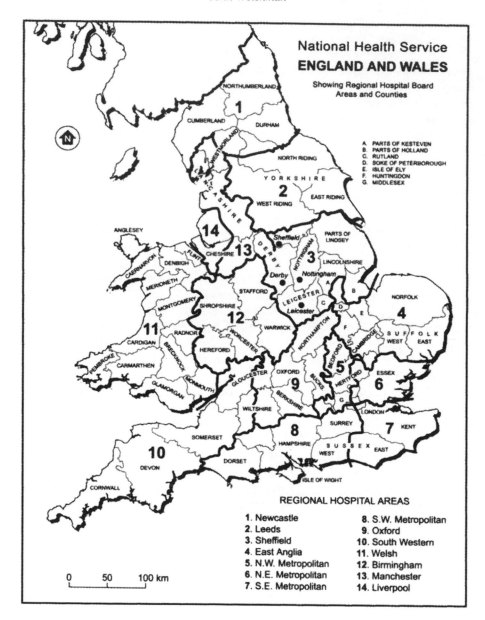

**National Health Service
ENGLAND AND WALES**

Showing Regional Hospital Board
Areas and Counties

A. PARTS OF KESTEVEN
B. PARTS OF HOLLAND
C. RUTLAND
D. SOKE OF PETERBOROUGH
E. ISLE OF ELY
F. HUNTINGDON
G. MIDDLESEX

REGIONAL HOSPITAL AREAS

1. Newcastle
2. Leeds
3. Sheffield
4. East Anglia
5. N.W. Metropolitan
6. N.E. Metropolitan
7. S.E. Metropolitan
8. S.W. Metropolitan
9. Oxford
10. South Western
11. Welsh
12. Birmingham
13. Manchester
14. Liverpool

**Map 1   National Health Service England and Wales: showing Regional
Hospital Board Areas and Counties**

The Sheffield region was one of the largest in England and Wales, covering some 5,688 square miles (Map 1). It included Leicestershire, Nottinghamshire, and parts of Derbyshire, Lincolnshire, Rutland, and the West Riding of Yorkshire. Its population was just over 4m, and there were extreme contrasts in population density, ranging from the highly industrialized areas of the north and west, to the more sparsely populated areas between the coast and the coalfields. The medical institutions within its boundaries included 201 hospitals with 35,800 beds. Originally there were 33 Hospital Management Committees (HMCs) in the Sheffield region, three of which, at Berry Hill Hall, Firbeck Hall, and Higham Grange, were Miners' Rehabilitation Centres.[23] Despite later debates about regrouping hospitals, the extent of regrouping was in reality quite limited, occurring only in Nottingham and Sheffield. The teaching hospitals in Sheffield included the Royal Hospital, Royal Infirmary, Jessop Hospital for Women, and Children's Hospital. They were administered by a separate Board of Governors, and were called the United Sheffield Hospitals.

The neighbouring Oxford region provides an interesting comparison. It comprised Oxfordshire and Northamptonshire, with parts of Berkshire, Buckinghamshire, Gloucestershire and Wiltshire. Its population was much smaller than that of the Sheffield region, at 1.3m. Included within its boundaries were 105 hospitals with 13,870 beds and 38 clinics, managed by 15 HMCs. The Oxford teaching hospitals comprised the Radcliffe Infirmary; the Churchill Hospital in Headington; the Oxford Eye Hospital; Cowley Road Hospital; and the Slade Isolation Hospital. The Oxford RHB was chaired by Dr Janet Vaughan in the early years, and its Senior Administrative Medical Officer (SAMO) was Dr J.O.F. Davies. This was an able team, and there was evidence that the need for new hospitals, for instance at Swindon, was recognized at an early stage.[24]

The inherited pattern of resources

What is clear from earlier work is the importance of the legacy of services and institutions that regions inherited from the pre-NHS era. An impressionistic but useful assessment of hospital services in the Sheffield region before the NHS is given by the hospital survey sponsored by the Nuffield Provincial Hospitals Trust (1945). The survey of Sheffield and the East Midlands, which was one of the most comprehensive, was conducted by Professor Leonard Parsons, Dean of the Medical Faculty at the University of Birmingham; S. Clayton Fryers, House Governor of the Leeds General Infirmary; and George Godber, then Regional Medical Officer at the Ministry of Health. The authors reported that this region was rhomboid in shape, comprising seven counties and part of an eighth. Geographically it was

23 Sheffield RHB, *Quinquennial Report Upon the Work of the Sheffield Regional Hospital Board From 1947 to 1952* (Sheffield, 1953), pp. 8–16.
24 Oxford RHB, *Annual Report 1950–51* (Oxford, 1951), pp. 3–7.

diverse, ranging from the sparsely-populated areas of north-west Derbyshire, to the rich agricultural fenland of south-east Lincolnshire. The main industries were coal-mining, agriculture, textiles, the manufacture of boots and shoes, and heavy industry, and the total population was 3.9m. John Mohan has drawn attention to the importance of the socio-economic landscape against which policies are implemented.[25] It was calculated that overall there were 20,385 hospital beds, and 32,521 were needed, especially in county areas where shortages were most severe.[26]

Institutions included voluntary, local authority, and chronic hospitals. The survey found 20 voluntary hospitals with 4,634 beds, ranging from the Leicester Royal Infirmary with some 500 beds, to the Newark and District hospital with only 66. In the most highly-developed hospitals, the honorary staff held higher qualifications and practised only as consultants, but many were staffed by general practitioners. Moreover there was a tendency to over-development, and lavish expenditure on equipment, especially in cottage hospitals which often had operating theatres and X-ray equipment.[27] This expensive equipment was rarely used. The local authority hospitals, on the other hand, catered for both acute and chronic cases. Some had developed acute services such as midwifery and orthopaedics. Here the County Boroughs generally had better provision than the County Councils, and there were other problems of co-ordination owing to administrative boundaries. Hospitals for infectious disease, for example, varied greatly, especially with regard to nursing – in one, the caretaker, an untrained woman, was the only nurse. The degree of co-operation between voluntary and municipal hospitals also varied greatly – although some transferred cases and shared consultant staffs, in others the co-operation envisaged in the 1929 Local Government Act was infrequent and ineffective.[28] On hospital building and design, very few large hospitals had been rebuilt on modern lines, and most were dark, overcrowded, and badly-equipped.

Chronic hospitals also varied greatly in size, ranging from 12 beds in the Lutterworth Institution, to 787 at Sheffield Firvale. The surveyors found that conditions in these institutions were particularly bad. Nurses were overworked and had little assistance, equipment was primitive and insufficient, and most of the buildings were appendages to Public Assistance Institutions (PAIs).[29] In terms of manpower, the number of consultants was inadequate, even in Sheffield, and, in fact, many consultants were still general practitioners. Specialisms were slow to develop – there was only one gynaecologist in Lincolnshire – while others such as paediatrics, orthopaedics, neurosurgery, and plastic surgery were either very under-developed or else limited only to the major urban centres. Some hospitals

25   Mohan, *Planning, Markets and Hospitals*, p. 16.
26   Ministry of Health, *Hospital Survey: The Hospital Services of the Sheffield and East Midlands Area* (London, 1945), pp. 2–4. Interview between Sir George Godber and the author, Cambridge, 13/2/98.
27   Ministry of Health, *Hospital Survey*, pp. 13–17.
28   *Ibid.*, pp. 6–8.
29   *Ibid.*, p. 6.

found it difficult to recruit nursing staff, particularly in the special and cottage hospitals, since there were few chances of promotion. The nursing problem was most acute in the smaller PAIs, and nursing the chronic sick was seen as one of the most urgent problems faced by the hospital authorities. Municipal hospitals did not usually maintain out-patient or casualty departments, and very few hospitals operated an appointments system. Other ancillary services, such as dentistry, social work, and transport, were either poorly-developed or subject to great variations.[30]

Arguably what comes through most strongly, in the diversity of hospital types, are the intra-regional variations in resources. The Doncaster PAI at Springwell House, for example, had not been taken over by the local authority because it was in such a poor state – there were 146 beds, and the surgeon visited three times a week. Smallpox hospitals at Worksop, Kirby-in-Ashfield, Hucknall, and Newark consisted of a few huts and were 'intended primarily for segregation rather than treatment'.[31] At the Burton Road PAI in Lincoln, children who were not ill were included in wards occupied by the chronically sick. The surveyors wrote of the Leicester and Leicestershire Maternity Hospital that 'no reconstruction could make these premises satisfactory and their replacement is an urgent and recognised need'.[32] On the other hand, the Nottingham Children's Hospital was an important consultant paediatric centre. The authors of the survey thought it should be considerably extended. Similarly the Newstead and Ransome Sanatorium near Mansfield was one of the best institutions for the treatment of tuberculosis. The City General Hospital in Leicester was regarded as one of the most advanced institutions of its kind, and there was reasonable co-operation with the Leicester Royal Infirmary in the transfer of cases. Elsewhere in Leicester, the City Isolation Hospital and Sanatorium had impressive operating and X-ray facilities – a thoracic surgeon visited once a week from London, and relations with the Leicester Royal Infirmary were excellent.[33]

Although an impressionistic rather than a comparative source, the wartime hospital survey gives a striking sense of the variable quality of the institutions in the Sheffield region, and spatial difficulties, inherited from the pre-NHS era. In fact similar issues were highlighted in the survey that covered much of the future Oxford region. An area that had a population of 867,140 in 1938, had some 75 hospitals with some 5,711 beds. Again, there were shortages of both hospital beds and medical personnel, particularly consultants. Public Assistance Institutions were singled out as being especially bad, and there were areas of special need, as at Aylesbury. Even Oxford, and the Radcliffe Infirmary, were seen as being unable to meet demands, while smaller centres like Slough and Windsor had no, or inadequate, hospitals.[34] Thus all regions had problems with the institutions that

30   *Ibid.*, pp. 8–12.
31   *Ibid.*, p. 40.
32   *Ibid.*, pp. 25, 32, 40, 42, 50.
33   *Ibid.*, pp. 36, 40, 49–50, 52–3.
34   E.C. Bevers, G.E. Cask, and R.H. Parry, *Hospital Survey: The Hospital Services of Berkshire, Buckinghamshire, and Oxfordshire* (London, 1945), pp. 1–49.

they inherited from the pre-NHS era. What was critical, arguably, was the size of the region; the level of resources it received; and the quality of its management team.

Hospital building and the Hospital Plan (1962)

One of the key questions in relation to inequalities in resource allocation is the extent to which the RHBs were able to make up their deficits through a hospital building programme. In evaluating hospital building, it is important to understand the system for capital expenditure under which the RHBs operated. Up to 1952–53, capital allocations reflected population distribution and bed complements weighted equally. This system was then changed, so that 95 per cent of the allocation was in relation to population, and the rest linked to low per capita bed provision in six of the RHBs.[35] The Acton Society Trust claimed there was some levelling up for regions with below-average resources, and evidence that the poorer regions increased their percentage share of the total revenue allocation.[36] In evidence to the Select Committee on Estimates in 1957, Treasury officials admitted 'the amounts available for hospital building...have been manifestly inadequate'.[37] Nevertheless inequalities in resource allocation were not a major source of concern. The Guillebaud Committee, for example, concluded in 1956 that 'the present system, though it has certain weaknesses, is probably the best that can be devised in present circumstances'.[38]

The key development, as far as building was concerned, was the Hospital Plan of 1962. David Allen suggests that the development of the Hospital Plan was very similar to that of the NHS – consensus allied to greater affluence and government expenditure produced it – and the only pressure group activity was by the BMA. This context was seized by three key individuals – Enoch Powell, the Minister for Health; Sir Bruce Fraser, Permanent Secretary at the Ministry of Health; and Sir George Godber, the Chief Medical Officer.[39] Nevertheless other judgements on the Hospital Plan have been more critical. Charles Webster claims that the Plan was vague, underestimating needs and overestimating the potential for economies. Even by 1964, it was realized that it would be more expensive than was originally thought. The Hospital Plan aimed for 90 new hospitals, 134 substantially-modernized hospitals, and 356 other big schemes. It envisaged capital expenditure on hospitals would rise steadily to reach £50m a year by 1964, and create a

35   Mohan, *Planning, Markets and Hospitals*, p. 100.
36   Acton Society Trust, *Hospitals and the State VI: Creative Leadership in a State Service* (London, 1959), pp. 10–15.
37   *Ibid.*, p. 12.
38   *Parliamentary Papers* 1955–56, XX (Cmnd. 9663), Report of the Committee of Enquiry into the Cost of the National Health Service, p. 104, paragraphs 282–3.
39   David E. Allen, *Hospital Planning: The Development of the 1962 Hospital Plan; A Case Study in Decision Making* (London, 1979), pp. 169–80.

network of District General Hospitals (DGHs). For the first time since 1914, new hospital facilities were part of the investment landscape. However Webster argues the Hospital Plan also fell well short of its objectives. By 1979, only a third of the 250 DGHs had been built, and many were obsolete by the time they opened. Overall Webster has concluded that 'even upon the most lenient interpretation... the Hospital Plan was little short of a disaster, the full ramifications of which are still largely unchronicled'.[40]

John Mohan's recent work represents an attempt to chronicle the ramifications of the Hospital Plan in the Newcastle region. Unlike Allen, he relates the origins of the Plan more to wider policy on economic planning, including the Plowden Report.[41] He argues that the Hospital Plan represented a positive attempt to maximize resources and respond to changing circumstances. It was at least a starting point, in trying to steer resources towards areas of greatest need, and the 1960s did see a steady rise in hospital capital expenditure. However Mohan argues it rested on insecure foundations and had technical weaknesses, so that a 'plan' became a 'building programme'. In this respect, the Hospital Plan was both a 'milestone and a millstone'.[42]

It is clear that the 1950s were marked by shortages of building materials and by severe restrictions on capital expenditure. Recent work suggests relationships between the Ministry of Health and Treasury were also crucial, with the Treasury regarding expenditure on health as consumption rather than investment, and with the Ministry being sceptical of the planning abilities of individual RHBs. In this context, funds tended to flow to the 'well-organised and vociferous'.[43] In an early circular, for example, the Ministry of Health quickly warned that, owing to shortages of labour and materials, the regions should concentrate on small schemes, such as repairs, adapting existing institutions, and maintenance work. It emphasized that 'in particular it is doubtful whether it will be possible to start any completely new hospitals before 1951, and even then only a very small number'.[44] Rationing of important building materials was still in force, and procedures overly bureaucratic. The wartime survey indicated the Sheffield region inherited a very varied stock of institutions, many of which required immediate replacement. Moreover the region was one where rapid demographic growth occurred during the period, and medical breakthroughs demanded better equipment and facilities. The Sheffield region's priorities at this time were to expand hospitals in Barnsley, Chesterfield, Doncaster, Leicester, Nottingham, and Sheffield, and to build a new hospital at Boston.[45] But it was not in a position to do much about them. Instead attention was

40   Webster, *Government and Health Care*, pp. 92–109; Webster, *The National Health Service: A Political History*, pp. 45, 121–4.
41   Mohan, *Planning, Markets and Hospitals*, pp. 114–20.
42   *Ibid.*, pp. 129–31, 155.
43   *Ibid.*, pp. 12, 87–110.
44   PRO, MH 90/30: Ministry of Health, 'National Health Service: Hospital Building Work', 8/48, pp. 1, 3.
45   SA, minutes of the Planning Committee, 19/9/55.

focused on closing down redundant infectious diseases hospitals, and on formulating plans for when increased resources would be available.

A report published in 1955, in response to indications the Ministry of Health might begin an expansion of the hospital building programme, attempted to plan for the future. It estimated the population in the region would be 4.4m by 1971, and that 22,479 beds would be needed against the existing total of 16,330 – a deficit of 6,149. The report provided a graphic account of conditions in individual hospitals in the region. Of Moorgate General Hospital in Rotherham, the report noted that 'the buildings are of poor quality and though many improvements have been carried out during the last five years, the buildings remain grim and forbidding'. The City General Hospital in Sheffield required 'complete alteration and reconstruction', while the Victoria Hospital in Mansfield was 'an old Public Assistance Institution of forbidding aspect'. The report noted of the Oakdene Institution in Lincoln that 'the amenities are primitive and the place should be evacuated as soon as possible'. Nevertheless the authors of the report were cautious in the face of unfavourable economic conditions. They concluded the RHB would have to 'cut its coat according to the cloth and to spend its money with care and discrimination like a modest and thrifty house-keeper'.[46]

Table 1   Capital Expenditure in the Sheffield Region, 1948–49 to 1967–68

1948–49	£0.3m
1951–52	£0.6m
1953–54	£0.6m
1956–57	£1.3m
1964–65	£4.2m
1967–68	£9.0m

Source: Sheffield RHB, *Quinquennial Reports*, 1947-52, 1952-57, 1962-67.

What is certain is that in the 1950s at least, this recognition of the difficulties did not translate into improved provision. Capital expenditure in the 1950s was very limited indeed (Table 1), and more importantly, no new hospital had been built in the region for over 20 years.[47] The background work leading up to the Hospital Plan did create some impetus at the regional level. In February 1961, the Ministry announced new methods for planning and executing the hospital building programme, including a ten-year programme. The Sheffield region's Planning Committee re-examined the planning proposals made in 1955, and produced an updated document. Planning procedures were revised, so that the region was

46   Sheffield RHB, *Hospital Planning Proposals of the Sheffield Regional Hospital Board 1955* (Sheffield, 1955), pp. 12–15, 24, 26, 29, 37, 52.
47   Sheffield RHB, *Quinquennial Report Upon the Work of the Sheffield Regional Hospital Board From 1952 to 1957* (Sheffield, 1958), pp. 26–7, 77–81.

organized into areas, and it tried to reconcile the desire for consultation with the need to avoid delay.[48] Overall, it was anticipated that capital expenditure would rise from about £2m in 1961–62, to about £9m in 1966–67, and that total expenditure would be in the region of £67m. Two-thirds of the proposed expenditure would be on 14 completely new hospitals or very substantial rebuilding and alterations. Small and uneconomic hospitals would be closed – the aim was to provide 'an integrated and efficient hospital service in the Sheffield region'.[49] But Ministry officials were critical of the plans that Sheffield put forward in advance of the Hospital Plan, commenting of them that 'it is difficult to get a comprehensive picture and one has to discover the "philosophy" in what is said about the various hospitals'.[50]

When published in January 1962, the Hospital Plan noted that the Sheffield region had fewer beds in relation to population than any other. Many were in old buildings, and diagnostic facilities were, in many places, out of date. In rural areas, notably in Lincolnshire, many of the hospitals were too small to provide the range of facilities that were needed.[51] Sheffield's share of the £500m capital expenditure was £56.5m. Interestingly, the Hospital Plan claimed that Sheffield had not done terribly badly. In the period 1948–61, Sheffield had spent £14.2m on its capital programme, more than any other region apart from Newcastle (excluding the London teaching hospitals). It had also provided the greatest number of additional beds (4,563 or 13 per cent) in England and Wales.[52] But while some levelling up of resources had occurred, this was not extensive enough to overcome the problems inherent in the inherited pattern of resources.

Some progress was made in the field of hospital design. A research group set up at the Ministry of Health produced publications that helped popularize the application of industrialized techniques to hospital and local authority buildings. After 1955, designs reflected the influence of Scandinavian post-war design, and research by the Nuffield Provincial Hospitals Trust and the University of Bristol. Systems of building based on standardized and rationalized techniques were applied to the Derby Royal Infirmary and a new maternity unit at the Nether Edge Hospital in Sheffield. The Sheffield and Oxford regions co-operated in a joint venture for the purchasing of building components.[53] Nevertheless, standardization did not get very far, and the emphasis on hospital design was rather ironic since the region had still not managed to build a completely new hospital. There was little long-term planning, and the need was to alleviate immediate problems. The region's Planning Committee concluded that 'by and large, the spectacle is still of

48   SA, minutes of the Planning Committee, 16/10/61.
49   *Ibid.*, 20/2/61, 12/6/61.
50   Cited in Mohan, *Planning, Markets and Hospitals*, p. 124.
51   *Parliamentary Papers* 1961–62, XXXI (Cmnd. 1604), A Hospital Plan for England and Wales, p. 59.
52   SA, minutes of Sheffield RHB, 12/2/62.
53   SA, minutes of the Planning Committee, 20/1/64–15/3/65. See also Mohan, *Planning, Markets and Hospitals*, p. 127.

hospitals which were built several decades ago having to adapt themselves not only
to dealing with large numbers of out-patients and in-patients, but to rapid changes
in techniques'.[54] Capital expenditure certainly did increase in the 1960s. However
analysis indicates that about half was used to improve ward and treatment areas in
existing hospitals, a quarter went on basic engineering services, and only a small
proportion went into building completely new hospitals.[55]

The experience of the region with respect to hospital building is perhaps best
illustrated by the case of Boston. The needs of both Boston, and Lincolnshire, had
been recognized by the wartime hospital survey, and this was discussed as early as
April 1950, when the Ministry advised a hospital might be built in stages.[56] In 1955
the Board noted that the four existing hospitals there were 'really unsuitable for
hospital purposes; they have varying degrees of bad ancillary services which make
nursing difficult, and they are uneconomic to maintain'.[57] Similarly one of the
Ministry's civil servants observed that 'the case for the new hospital is that the
present hospitals are old, badly sited and incapable of modernisation, or expansion'.[58] However work on the new hospital only began in 1966, with the new DGH,
the Pilgrim Hospital, being opened in June 1968. In the Oxford region, on the other
hand, the first stage of a new hospital at Swindon had been completed in 1958.[59]
Boston was perhaps the most dramatic example, but the delays in implementing the
Hospital Plan were evident elsewhere in the region, including at Leicester and
Doncaster.[60]

The Sheffield case study contributes to attempts to chart the impact of the
restrictions on capital expenditure that characterized the 1950s, and to chronicle the
ramifications of the Hospital Plan. Capital expenditure in the Sheffield region
compared well to that of RHBs in general, but was also insufficient to make up the
deficiencies the region had inherited from the pre-1948 era. In the 1950s in
particular, much capital expenditure went on small projects, and engineering and
maintenance work, in part due to shortages of resources. In the Sheffield region,
there was a clear change of pace following the publication of the Plan, with dramatic rises in capital expenditure. Even so, it is clear that hospital building made only
limited progress in this period. Very few new hospitals were constructed in the
region, even, as at Boston, where the inadequacy of provision had been noted by
the wartime hospital survey. Many of these restrictions on expenditure were

---

54   SA, minutes of the Planning Committee, 20/1/64 – 15/3/65.
55   Sheffield RHB, *Quinquennial Report Upon the Work of the Sheffield Regional
      Hospital Board From 1962 to 1967* (Sheffield, 1968), pp. 14, 71, 85–7, tables 37, 43.
56   PRO, MH 88/273: L. Faulkner to S.H. Findlay, 25/4/56.
57   Sheffield RHB, *Hospital Planning Proposals*, pp. 49–50.
58   PRO, MH 88/273: memo by E.A. Arnold.
59   Oxford RHB, *Commissioning a New Hospital: A Report on the Commissioning of the
      First Stage of the Princess Margaret Hospital Swindon* (Oxford, 1961), pp. 1–100.
60   SA, minutes of the Planning Committee, 16/7/56. See also Garry Swann, *The
      Doncaster Royal Infirmary, 1792–1972* (Doncaster, 1973), pp. 135–49.

imposed from the centre. However it is arguable that the region might have done more to publicize and address the inequalities it laboured under.

Revenue expenditure and staffing levels

As with capital allocations, it is important to understand how the system for revenue expenditure operated. Estimates for revenue expenditure were prepared by the HMCs, passed on to the RHB which discussed and collated them, and added its own; and were then passed to the Ministry of Health. The Ministry in turn discussed and collated these, and added its own estimates, and in December of each year passed them on to the Treasury. The Ministry and Treasury then agreed a total on the basis of an estimate of requirements for keeping the service running at its existing level. In addition to current activities, the Ministry could also put in a bid for any new 'developments', such as hospital extensions, additional staff, and capital works completed in the previous year. The Acton Society Trust claimed it used its discretionary power to use the 'development' element to try to effect some levelling up between the regions. It was claimed evidence showed that the poorer regions did increase their percentage share of the total in the 1950s.[61] In evidence to the Select Committee on Estimates, on the other hand, Treasury officials had conceded in 1957 that expenditure followed an 'inherited pattern', but did not appear overly concerned about its implications.[62]

Table 2   Revenue Expenditure in the Sheffield RHB, 1948-49 to 1967-68

1948–49	£6.5m
1951–52	£13.6m
1953–54	£15.0m
1956–57	£19.5m
1964–65	£36.5m
1967–68	£48.0m

Source: Sheffield RHB, *Quinquennial Reports*, 1947–52, 1952–57, 1962–67.

The Trust asked perceptive questions about how important it was that inequalities should be corrected; what had been done to correct them; and how could inequalities, or success in addressing them, be calculated. Nevertheless it also argued the Ministry had acted 'sensibly and fairly', and that attempts to apply more egalitarian policies would have been 'very dangerous'.[63] It seemed more concerned

---

61   Acton Society Trust, *Hospitals and the State V: The Central Control of the Service* (London, 1958), pp. 45–6; Acton Society Trust, *Hospitals and the State VI*, pp. 5–10.

62   *Parliamentary Papers* 1956–57, VI, Sixth Report of the Select Committee on Estimates, p. 54, q. 529.

63   Acton Society Trust, *Hospitals and the State VI*, pp. 5–7.

about hospital efficiency than resource allocation. In the Sheffield region, as shown in Table 2, net expenditure increased over the period, but Sheffield still fared badly compared to England and Wales as a whole. In September 1956, the Finance Committee observed that the amount spent per head of population was the lowest in the country.[64] Revenue allocations inevitably varied greatly between different HMCs.

Obviously these HMCs had differing numbers of institutions and levels of demand. Nevertheless it seems likely that allocation was made on a historic basis rather than on a systematic analysis of need. The effect of inequalities in revenue expenditure was reflected in staffing levels, for there was evidence that Sheffield had fewer consultants compared to other regions despite having one of the largest populations. As Charles Webster has pointed out, not only was Sheffield poorly provided for, in terms of consultants, but the quality of those consultants was inferior, as measured by the awards system. The Oxford and Sheffield regions illustrate some of these differences, as seen in Table 3, particularly since the population of the Sheffield region was three times greater than that of Oxford.

Table 3   Number of Consultants in the Sheffield and Oxford Regions, 1951

	Sheffield	Oxford
Consultants in general medicine	5.0 (5.9)	3.1 (3.5)
Consultants in mental health	7.0 (3.5)	2.9 (6.5)
Consultants in anaesthetics	5.9 (3.7)	3.8 (5.0)

The figures are shown as a percentage of the national total consultants,
with percentage of national awards in brackets.

Source: Webster, *Problems of Health Care*, p. 294.

As the official history points out, Oxford was ahead of Sheffield in respect of its staff relative to population, in the various specialties, and with regard to the numbers of consultants receiving awards. Sheffield was in marked deficit in both respects. Sheffield began in 1949 with 332 consultants (96 distinction awards), and in 1959 had 465 consultants (140 awards). This represented a 40 per cent increase, which compared poorly with other regions, such as Newcastle.[65]

Research at the regional level sheds light on these inequalities, and on the reasons for their persistence. Increases in consultant services were controlled in a Ministry of Health circular issued in December 1952 – budgetary limitations meant proposals had to be approved by the Ministry and based on a statement of need. Sheffield's Board argued, for example, that the suggestions made in early Ministry of Health circulars for building up the consultant services were impracticable, since

64   SA, minutes of the Finance Committee, 28/4/58.
65   Webster, *Problems of Health Care*, p. 295.

more consultants could not be employed unless more beds, out-patients space, operating theatres, laboratories, X-ray rooms, and other resources were provided. It adopted a pragmatic attitude, concluding in 1953 that 'a more practical approach had to be made and the consultant service could only be increased here and there whenever the necessary facilities could be made available'.[66] In 1958 the Sheffield RHB conceded that more consultants were needed, since the region had the lowest consultant to population ratio in the country. This was seen as in large part due to the relatively low proportion of beds per thousand population in the Sheffield region. Candidates of the right calibre were not always available in specialties such as radiotherapy, radiology, anaesthetics, and psychiatry. These problems continued to be taken philosophically in the region, where it was concluded that 'it is often wise to hasten slowly and also to insist upon quality'.[67]

More general problems of staffing in the Sheffield region were demonstrated well by the case of radiographers. In the early 1950s, the Sheffield RHB reached an agreement with the Society of Radiographers over payments for 'on call' duty, since the number of 'on call' duties was increasing due to the shortage of technicians. From April 1950, the Board agreed interim agreements for the payment of 'on call' duty that infringed Whitley Council negotiations. The Ministry of Health noted that this agreement was 'seriously embarrassing' for radiographers and other grades, and it had been 'flooded with enquiries' from other parts of the country.[68] Although this problem was resolved, and training allowances for student radiographers were introduced in the late 1950s, there remained a shortage of radiographers.

Despite increases in the number of nurses, the largest increases were in untrained staff, such as nursing auxiliaries and ward orderlies. Recruitment was difficult, especially in the mental health field, and there were also shortages of midwives, who preferred to work 'on the district' rather than in hospitals.[69] These problems were further exacerbated by the rise in the birth rate and increasing proportion of hospital confinements. Many of these staffing problems were solved through the recruitment of doctors and nurses from overseas. By the 1960s, the region's hospitals employed large numbers of nurses and midwives from the Commonwealth and other countries. The reliance on staff from overseas was particularly marked in the case of registrars. In 1958 it was estimated that less than 40 per cent of these posts in the region were occupied by doctors from the UK – 30 per cent were from India and Pakistan, 10 per cent from Australia and New Zealand, and 7 per cent from the Republic of Ireland.[70] If anything this increased in the early 1960s, since in 1961 it was estimated that 61 per cent of registrars were from overseas. Virtually all the Senior House Officer posts were occupied by

66   Sheffield RHB, *Quinquennial Report 1947–52*, pp. 58–9.
67   Sheffield RHB, *Quinquennial Report 1952–57*, p. 27.
68   PRO, MH 90/55: W. Douglas to B. Gibson, 27/6/50.
69   SA, minutes of the Nursing Committee, 20/10/58.
70   Sheffield RHB, *Quinquennial Report 1952–57*, p. 68.

overseas doctors, although this was true also of the Leeds, Manchester, and Newcastle regions.[71] Overall there was much evidence that patterns of revenue expenditure had failed to solve the particular problems of the Sheffield region.

The potential role of personalities

Many aspects of the resource allocation question were determined outside the region, in the revenue and capital expenditure systems operated in Whitehall by the Ministry of Health and Treasury. But an important aspect of the question of why Sheffield remained at the bottom of the league table of RHBs relates to its personnel and officers. It has been suggested that while inherited resources were a key factor, those areas that shouted loudest also tended to receive the most, and this issue seems underplayed in John Mohan's study of the Newcastle region. The key posts were those of Chairman and Senior Administrative Medical Officer (SAMO). Did the Chairmen, or the Boards that they chaired, have the power to reallocate resources within the region? To what extent were they able to argue that Sheffield deserved greater resources? Was there a national forum on which they could have put the case of Sheffield's relative poverty?

The region's first Chairman was Sir Basil Gibson. Born in York, Gibson was a solicitor by background who had served as Town Clerk of Sheffield, 1931–1942.[72] Initially appointed as Chairman until April 1950, he served a further two terms, until March 1956. Gibson was aged 70 when first appointed, and 79 when he retired. While Gibson was active at meetings of RHB Chairmen, he was less effective in demonstrating the particular problems faced by Sheffield. A civil servant at the Ministry of Health observed in December 1953 of the planned new hospital at Boston that 'things hang fire terribly once the Chairman of the Board takes them under his wing'.[73] Sir George Godber, who knew the region and its personnel well, has recalled that while an able man, and good manager of people, Gibson was not deeply informed about hospital services before his appointment.[74] There is little evidence in RHB minutes that Gibson took up the issue of resource allocation. Gibson was succeeded as Chairman by Albert Martin. Aged 57 at the time of his appointment as Chairman, Martin was a wealthy textiles manufacturer and experienced hospital administrator.[75] In the assessment of Sir George, Martin was a more effective Chairman than Gibson, and 'gingered the Region up quite a bit'.[76] He was certainly both younger and more experienced in hospital administration. But Martin died tragically in a car crash in November 1968, and was succeeded as Chairman by a local alderman, S. P. King.

71   Sheffield RHB, *Quinquennial Report 1957–62*, p. 56.
72   *Sheffield Telegraph* (12 February 1962).
73   PRO, MH 88/273: L.R. Macbeth to M. Reed, 7/12/53.
74   Interview between Sir George Godber and the author.
75   *Sheffield Morning Telegraph* (26 November 1968).
76   Interview between Sir George Godber and the author.

The most important administrative post was that of the SAMO. His job was to advise the RHB on the planning, organization, and staffing of the hospital and specialist services, and to carry out other administrative and executive functions.[77] In the late 1940s, Sheffield faced particular difficulties in appointing its first SAMO at the advertised salary of £2,250 – the post attracted 46 candidates, but none were appointable. George Godber wrote in August 1947 that the Sheffield region had a population of about 4m; its hospital services were backward, with only East Anglia and Wales being inferior; and the fact that Sheffield dominated the region posed problems of organization and planning. He admitted the Sheffield SAMO:

> will have the most difficult job of all and it is imperative to attract a good man to it. It would not be reasonable to leave a region of this kind to accept some other region's second choice.[78]

Godber argued unsuccessfully that a higher salary was necessary if Sheffield was to attract strong candidates. Following a second round of interviews, the Board appointed as SAMO, Dr William Ramsay, Medical Superintendent of the Crumpsall Hospital in Manchester.[79] Ramsay had studied at Glasgow University, had been a house physician and Assistant Superintendent at Glasgow Royal Infirmary, and later worked in hospitals in Liverpool and Manchester. Ramsay held the post of SAMO until his retirement in 1962, when he was succeeded by his deputy, Dr Shone. The most successful SAMOs had previously been Medical Officers of Health (MOsH) who in some cases had had wide experience, in the 1930s, of running municipal hospitals. With hindsight, Sir George argues Ramsay lacked this breadth of understanding of the needs of a large region, and also had poorer back-up than some of his counterparts – Ramsay was 'not in the front rank of SAMOs by any means'.[80] There seems some truth, therefore, in the claim that the region's staff were not of the highest calibre. Certainly their longevity was striking – most of the key posts were occupied by the same personnel from the creation of the RHB to the early 1960s.

With regard to resources, in the 1950s the Sheffield region was not ready with suitable schemes when money did become available. Sir George argues that the region's personnel were 'slow on the up-take', and 'less than forceful about redevelopment'.[81] Whether this is fair is difficult to judge. It does seem to be true in the case of hospital building in the early 1960s, with Sir George again arguing that staff in the Sheffield region 'weren't nearly so well geared up for getting into the action with the 1962 Hospital Plan'.[82] It was certainly striking that the region's

77   PRO, MH 90/45: J.E. Pater to RHBs, 27/6/47.
78   *Ibid.*: G.E. Godber to M. Reed, 23/8/47.
79   *Ibid.*: L. Faulkner to Ministry of Health, 29/10/47.
80   Interview between Sir George Godber and the author.
81   *Ibid.*
82   *Ibid.*

management left lobbying Ministers until 1969, when there had been awareness by the mid-1950s that Sheffield had the lowest per capita allocations. In August 1969, a deputation went from Sheffield to Richard Crossman, Secretary for State for Social Services, to discuss the region's share of capital and revenue funds. RHB minutes record he was impressed by the case for a larger share of the total available resources, and conceded that Sheffield, Manchester, and Birmingham had not been given a fair share of the revenue funds for their hospitals. However Crossman argued that in the current financial situation, any substantial additional allocation would have to be at the expense of other RHBs.[83]

Neither the region's Chairmen nor SAMOs seemed able to exploit the sense of drift at the national level regarding resource allocation. There was some limited activity by groups representing consultants in the region. In December 1958, the Sheffield Area Consultants Committee and Medical Committee argued the rate of capital expenditure was inadequate, and the region had the lowest ratio of beds to population in the country.[84] Again, in June 1971, the local Medical Committee pointed out that the total net revenue for the Sheffield region had reduced from 6.63 per cent of the national total (1958–59) to 6.56 per cent (1968–69). It argued the level of expenditure per head of population must be raised at least to the national average.[85] But in general the consultants played a sporadic and generally unimpressive role in lobbying for greater resources for their region. If anything, it was organizations such as the Socialist Medical Association, prominent in arguing for better services for older people, that were more vocal and active earlier in support of vulnerable groups.[86]

Greater attention to inequalities in resource allocation

While the potential role of personalities was important, there is also a need to see the wider context in which the issue of variations in resource allocation came to the fore in the early 1970s. A.E. Bennett and Walter Holland have argued that RAWP marked a transition in the NHS from 'muddling through' to 'rational planning', where objectives were established and the best means of achieving them identified.[87] Originally appointed in May 1975, the Working Party's terms of reference were to review the arrangements for distributing NHS capital and revenue to Regional, Area, and District Health Authorities, with a view to establishing a pattern of distribution responsive to relative need. It found that the supply of health facilities was variable and very much influenced by history. The methods used to

83   SA, minutes of the Sheffield RHB, 8/12/69.
84   SA, minutes of the Planning Committee, 15/12/58.
85   SA, minutes of the Medical Committee, 14/6/71.
86   Sheffield Branch of the SMA, *A New Deal for Sheffield Old Folk* (Sheffield, 1951), pp. 5–6.
87   A.E. Bennett and W.W. Holland, 'Rational planning or muddling through? Resource allocation in the NHS', *Lancet*, 309 (1977), 464–6.

distribute financial resources to the NHS reflected 'the inertia built into the system by history' – they incremented the historic bases for the supply of resources, and also perpetuated them through responding slowly to changes in demography and morbidity. Of capital investment, the RAWP report noted that 'there are not only geographical inequalities in the quantity of stock available but also in its age and condition'. The aim was to secure, through resource allocation, equal opportunity of access to health care for people at equal risk. The report sought criteria to establish and quantify the differentials of need in different geographical locations – measuring relative need was regarded as a start in addressing the major issues of resource allocation that existed.[88] In its *Priorities* paper (1976), the Department of Health and Social Security (DHSS) conceded that there was a need 'progressively to remedy the large variations in standards between different regions, areas, and districts'.[89]

The implications of RAWP for the Sheffield region are beyond the scope of this chapter, although the RAWP methods raise the question of how best historians can measure inequalities in resource allocation, including taking into account measures of need. What we can say is that there were signs that greater attention was being drawn, in the late 1960s and early 1970s, to inequalities in both capital and revenue allocations, and also to intra-regional inequalities. Figures that compared capital expenditure in relation to population from 1948 showed that Sheffield was average for the provincial RHBs, but below average when teaching hospital expenditure was taken into account. The Board argued that greater than average capital resources were essential to provide the physical facilities necessary to remedy these inequalities. But while the DHSS recognized inequalities and had devised a formula for revenue expenditure, there was no formula for capital expenditure. The Department simply stated in 1972 that it realized the region's 'special problems'.[90]

There were signs in the early 1970s, that as in aspects of inequalities of resource allocation in general, Sheffield's particular needs in revenue expenditure were recognized. Between September 1962 and September 1967, the number of consultants in the Sheffield region increased from 430 (345 full-time equivalents) to 556 (460 full-time equivalents). The recommendation of the Platt Committee in 1963, that the appointment of an additional 120 consultants should be spread over five years, was implemented. Even so, Sheffield continued to have the lowest ratio of consultants to population in England and Wales.[91] The total revenue allocation for 1970–71 of £56.8m represented an increase of 5 per cent over previous years. In targets for the expansion of consultants, from April 1973, Sheffield had the highest target of all the RHBs. The programme had been formulated so that

88 DHSS, *Sharing Resources for Health in England: Report of the Resource Allocation Working Party* (London, 1976), pp. 5, 7–10, 12, paragraphs 1.2–1.14, 1.17.

89 DHSS, *Priorities for Health and Personal Social Services in England: A Consultative Document* (London, 1976), pp. 8–9, paragraph 1.5.

90 SA, minutes of the Planning Committee, 17/4/72.

91 Sheffield RHB, *Quinquennial Report 1962–67*, pp. 64–6.

hospital medical staff in the regions would become nearly equal, in relation to population, in approximately ten years.[92]

We have noted that the creation of new medical schools at Nottingham (1965) and Leicester (1974) altered the balance of power in the region, away from Sheffield. The recommendation for a new medical school at Leicester had been made by the Royal Commission on Medical Education, but also reflected a growing awareness in the region of the importance of intra-regional inequalities.[93] In early 1971, for example, the region's Medical Committee noted that new indices, including staffing rates based on catchment areas, and on a population-served basis, exposed important intra-regional inequalities between Sheffield, Nottingham, and Leicester.[94] It argued subsequently that the provision of medical schools at Nottingham and Leicester should not be at the expense of development elsewhere in the region.[95] It is unclear the extent to which these intra-regional inequalities were remedied in the period before 1974.

What is apparent is that for health economists the Sheffield region continued to provide evidence of inequalities in resource allocation into the 1970s. M.H. Cooper and A.J. Culyer, writing in 1972, found from 31 official indices that in almost every instance the Sheffield region remained less well-endowed than the neighbouring Oxford region. Sheffield scored poorly on such indices as population per consultant, expenditure in hospitals per capita per annum, anaesthetists per million population, and consultants treating mental illness per million population. Indeed, since 1962, relative inequalities appeared to have been increasing.[96] In a comparison of expenditure in the hospital sector, Executive Councils, and local authorities, researchers based in the Derbyshire County Council Health Department pointed out in 1974 that twice as much was spent in 1971–72 per 1,000 population in the South West Metropolitan region as by Sheffield RHB.[97] This research work formed part of the background to RAWP. Summing up the experience of the Sheffield region in this final period, there were therefore signs of greater awareness of inequalities in resource allocation, but limited attempts to remedy them.

92   SA, minutes of the Planning Committee, 11/9/72.
93   *Parliamentary Papers* 1967–68, XXV (Cmnd. 3569), Royal Commission on Medical Education 1965–68: Report, p. 158, paragraph 388.
94   SA, minutes of the Medical Committee, 8/2/71, 8/3/71.
95   *Ibid.*, 14/6/71.
96   M.H. Cooper and A.J. Culyer, 'Equality in the National Health Service: intentions, performance and problems in evaluation', in *The Economics of Health Care*, ed. M.M. Hauser (London, 1972), pp. 47, 51–3, 55–7.
97   J. Noyce, A.H. Snaith, and A.J. Trickey, 'Regional variations in the allocation of financial resources to the community health services', *Lancet*, 303 (1974), 554–7.

Conclusion

This chapter has illustrated some of the difficulties in getting to the bottom of the issue of regional variations in resource allocation. Some of the reasons for inequalities in resource allocation lay outside the region, in the systems of revenue and capital expenditure that were supervised by the Ministry of Health and the Treasury. Regional sources augmented with oral materials only tell part of the story, as can a case study. More of a comparative dimension is necessary, in order to compare the experience of Sheffield with that of more fortunate regions. Some of the sources tend to provide snapshots, at particular moments in time, when a more dynamic sense of Sheffield's place in the ranking order is needed. The relative importance of the inherited pattern; role of personalities; and existing expenditure systems is hard to estimate. And it remains unclear how inequalities in resource allocation may have translated into inequities in access to services, and ultimately to inequalities in the health of the population.

Nevertheless, these points notwithstanding, it is possible to put forward some tentative reasons for the striking continuities in Sheffield's position at the bottom of the resources league table. First, this chapter has confirmed the extent of the inequalities in resource allocation inherited from the pre-NHS era, and chronicled in the wartime hospital survey. Second, it is clear that capital and revenue allocation systems were insufficient to bring Sheffield up to the level of the more affluent RHBs, and that the Hospital Plan of 1962 only had a limited impact on hospital building in the region. In part, this was because it was not really thought through at either the national or regional levels. Third, there is also evidence that the region's early Chairmen and SAMO, Gibson, Martin, and Ramsay, were not as forceful as they might have been, in the various forums available to them. Plans were not ready when new funding became available, and progress was further retarded by rivalries within the region, chiefly between Sheffield and the smaller cities of Derby, Nottingham, and Leicester. Fourth, it was only in the early 1970s that serious efforts were made, in the background to the creation of the RAWP, to explore and document the 'inherited pattern' of resources. Even then, a gap between evidence and action meant serious inequalities in resource allocation have remained, as demonstrated by the continuities between the old Sheffield RHB and its successor, the Trent region.

Chapter 16

International Recruitment of Nurses to the UK: The History of the Present

Anne Marie Rafferty

The international recruitment of nurses to the UK has proved to be one of the most controversial aspects of workforce policy in recent years. Currently, the key feature of the UK nursing labour market is skill shortages. The UK Health Departments in 2001 have acknowledged that 'the biggest constraint on the NHS's capacity to deliver was the need to increase the number of staff'.[1] Shortages have occurred as a result of a combination of factors. Some are demographically driven, with increased demand for healthcare related to an ageing population. More patients are being treated, and patient care has become 'sicker and quicker'. Supply-side factors, including increased competition from the private sector for skilled nurses, and the ageing of the nursing profession, are also exacerbating short/mid-term recruitment difficulties.[2] Since 1998, the implementation of National Health Service (NHS) strategies for nursing and human resources, and NHS modernization plans ('The NHS Plan'[3]), have symbolized a fundamental policy shift in the NHS.[4]

Targeting nurses from other countries has been identified as a key focus of UK policy action in recent years. The Department of Health in England has indicated that international recruitment represents part of the solution to meeting its staffing targets.[5] The UK government has also initiated government-to-government 'concordats' on nurse recruitment with other national governments, such as those of Spain, India and the Philippines. The overall effect of these initiatives has been a

1   Department of Health, *Review for 2002. Written Evidence from the Health Departments for Great Britain, Review Body for Nursing Staff, Midwives, Health Visitors and Professions Allied to Medicine* (London, 2001).
2   J. Buchan and I. Seccombe, *Behind the Headlines: A Review of the UK Nursing Labour Market*, Royal College of Nursing/Queen Margaret University College (London, 2002).
3   NHS Executive (Department of Health), *The NHS Plan* (London, 2000).
4   J. Buchan, 'What's the connection? British nurse recruitment in an enlarged EU', *Eurohealth*, 8 (2002), 15–16.
5   Bridget M. Robertson, *Angels in Africa: A Memoir of Nursing with the Colonial Service* (London, 1993).

significant growth in the numbers of nurses recruited from other countries to work in the UK.

The purpose of this chapter is to explore some of the historical antecedents to current policy. In doing so it can only begin to scratch the surface of a vast and complex subject, and suggest some further questions for research. The aim of the chapter therefore is to provide an introduction to the historical background of the current debate on international recruitment of nurses in the UK. It focuses on the activities of the Colonial Nursing Association (CNA) as the main recruitment vehicle for British nurses to the colonies. It tracks those activities in the context of international recruitment patterns to Britain before and after the introduction of the NHS.

Much of the debate surrounding the international recruitment of nurses so far has relied upon polemical press commentary and anecdotal reports.[6] A recent report launched at the conference of the International Council of Nurses[7] provides a more sober analysis and reviews the evidential base. It reveals the increasing reliance of selected industrialized countries, notably England and the USA, on international recruitment as a solution to their short-term labour problems. In identifying trends in the recruitment of nurses, Buchan and others point to the Philippines, South Africa, and Australia as the key sources of international recruitment to the UK, while among 'source' countries the UK still features prominently as a destination for Caribbean and Ghanaian as well as South African and Filipino nurses.[8]

The Colonial Nursing Association

While there has been an explosion of interest among historians in colonial medicine, nursing, by contrast, has been relatively neglected. Very little research has been conducted into the CNA archives and little is known of its activities beyond a small clutch of memoirs or oral histories.[9] It nevertheless provides a rich resource for analysing the role of British nursing in colonial health care, albeit within the confines of the organization's role as a recruitment agency. British nurses were recruited by the CNA to work in different parts of the empire. Their role initially was to look after the European population, and to help to make the hostile environment of the tropics habitable for government officials and traders so that commercial interests might be protected. Gradually that role extended into providing care to the indigenous population, often to maintain the efficiency of the workforce. Ultimately, it evolved into training the local population in nursing

6   H.P. Dickson, *The Badge of Britannia: the History and Reminiscences of the Queen Elizabeth's Overseas Nursing Service, 1886–1966* (Edinburgh, 1990).
7   Department of Health, *Investment and Reform for NHS Staff – Taking Forward the NHS Plan* (London, 2001), para. 3.26.
8   J. Buchan, T. Parkin, and J. Sochalski, *International Nurse Mobility: Trends and Policy Implications*, World Health Organization (Geneva, 2003).
9   *Ibid.*, p.14.

techniques, and the creation of a workforce capable of contributing to the British NHS. As the National Advisory Council on Nurses and Midwives noted in 1948:

> The ultimate goal for all colonies is the development of local nurse training schools and nurses' registration to such a standard and in such a form that reciprocity with Great Britain can be obtained, and Colonial-trained nurses can take their full place as part of the British nursing profession.[10]

During the lifetime of the Association some 8,400 nurses were sent out to the colonies, of whom 6,416 were allocated to government hospitals, and 1,984 to other appointments.[11]

Origins and organization of the CNA

The CNA was the brainchild of Mrs Frances Piggott, wife of the Procurer General in Mauritius, who held that an association should be formed in England to help British communities in the colonies and elsewhere to provide trained nurses. 'Skilled' nursing, by which was meant European nursing, was unobtainable in many isolated parts of the empire. British officials, settlers, and their families were thought to suffer excessive ill-health and hardship as a consequence. Doctors in particular were irked at having to act as nurses themselves. Nursing was perceived as an important adjunct to the Colonial Medical Service and to the success of government hospitals throughout the empire. Joseph Chamberlain, Secretary of State for the Colonies, took a direct and personal interest in the Association which was launched in 1895.

Like many philanthropic organizations the CNA relied upon the patronage of social elites. Lady Piggott remained closely involved with the Association until her death in 1949. Mrs Joseph Chamberlain served on the committee for nearly 60 years. Lady Antrobus and her husband, Sir Reginald Antrobus, Under-Secretary of State for the Colonies 1896–1909, both played an active role in the Association. Mrs Charles Hobhouse, wife of the liberal politician, and witness before the Select Committee for the Registration of Nurses in England and Wales 1904–5, was also involved during the Association's formative phase.[12]

Members of the Association took the superiority of European nursing for granted. Mrs Charles Robinson, a member of the CNA Executive Committee,

---

10   Edinburgh, Scottish Record Office, HH103.348: National Advisory Council on Nurses and Midwives, 'Training of Colonial Student Nurses in the United Kingdom', 1948, para. 9(iii).
11   Oxford, Rhodes House (RH), MSS British Empire s.400, ONA, Box 131 item 52, Final Annual Report, 1966, p. 9.
12   RH, MSS Brit. Emp. s.400, Executive Committee, Minute Book, vol. 1, 1896–1903, 16/5/96.

Anne Marie Rafferty

extolled the virtues of the European nurse at the expense of her indigenous counterpart. She wrote of the European nurse, in a publicity pamphlet in 1909:

> One white nurse – that is always something [but]...A coloured 'garde-malade' eating curry and rice at the end of the bed is hardly a good substitute. And I doubt if the baby, could it speak, would have been grateful for having its head well rubbed with brandy and other compounds.[13]

Interestingly the distinction drawn between the 'white' nurse and 'coloured' *garde-malade* reworked in racial terms the familiar dichotomy between 'Sarah Gamp'[14] and her pristine reformed counterpart, the 'new nurse', in the latter part of the nineteenth century. Just as Sarah Gamp's greatest deficiency was her identification with working-class culture and home-spun remedies, so the indigenous nurse came to be seen as representing a set of cultural norms and practices in need of reform and reconstruction.

Recruitment rationales

The significance of the Association lay in its being the first recruitment route for single women by the Colonial Office (CO). Charles Jeffries, a senior official within the CO, notes in his history of the Colonial Office that between 1922 and 1943, 2,189 nursing sisters were recruited to work overseas.[15] The Association's recruitment propaganda was upbeat: 'Join the CNA and see the world...you too can become one of the women pioneers...blazing civilisation's trail in far corners of the world'.[16] The CNA had three separate but interlocking strands to its work: one was supporting the colonial service through the work of nurses in government hospitals; the second was work in private institutions; the third was in contributing to the development of so-called 'native' nursing services. As early as 1903 a matron was selected for the Colonial Hospital in Sierra Leone to supervise and train 'native' nurses.[17] By 1930 reference was being made to the employment of English nurses in the native wards of government hospitals and to the fact that the increase in the numbers of such hospitals meant that nurses were no longer looking after Europeans but local populations. Indeed, it was remarked that the demand for nursing was so great that the supply had to be met from local sources and that steps were being taken:

13   M. Robinson, *The Story of the Colonial Nursing Association by Mrs Charles Robinson* (London, 1909), p. 4.
14   A.M. Rafferty, *The Politics of Nursing Knowledge* (London, 1996), p. 10.
15   C. Jeffries, *Partners for Progress: The Men and Women of the Colonial Service* (London, 1949), p. 152.
16   'Nursing for the colonies', *Good Housekeeping* (January 1949), p. 33.
17   RH, MSS Brit. Emp. s.400, ONA, Box 131 item 52, Final Annual Report, 1966, p. 6.

to train native women as nurses on the spot and in some cases to send them to England to be trained. The role of the nursing sister became one of instruction and to provide tuition and tutoring in 'the traditions of her profession'.[18]

Dea Birkett, in her book *Spinsters Abroad*,[19] has written of the spirit of adventure and the desire to escape the social constraints of British society that motivated women travellers in the latter part of the nineteenth and early twentieth centuries. Much of the same spirit is evident in the testimony of the nurses who set sail for the far-flung corners of the empire. Freedom from the well-publicized restrictions of institutional life that featured so prominently in the official and semi-official reports on nursing during the inter-war period in Britain, plus the opportunity to travel, were incentives to work overseas.[20] Such nurses were given the title 'sister' which suggested there were status gains to be made by nursing in the colonies. Conditions could also be better than those they were used to at home, although highly variable. Sisters could also look forward to having their own house (or sharing with another sister), rather than enduring the confines of a nurses' home. As one nurse wrote from Kenya:

I am in a house by myself, with the Health Worker at the Hotel. We are having a new house built and then we shall live together. We shall both be glad to be settled in our new home. It will be awfully nice, three bedrooms, dining-room, sitting room, large front veranda.[21]

Some sisters may have been motivated by marriage prospects, as sisters were among the few single women in expatriate communities.[22] Early colonial communities tended to be male-dominated, and the provision of nursing can be seen as complementary to the gendered construction of male 'heroism' that characterized the colonial official's life. All this however could be undermined by sickness and disease. Nursing was portrayed as a source of succour and solace: 'skilful and kindly hands and that sympathy, that womanly attention, which will be found the best anodyne for their pain and perhaps the most effective cure for their disease'.[23]

18 *Ibid.*
19 Dea Birkett, *Spinsters Abroad: Victorian Lady Explorers* (Oxford, 1989).
20 'Nursing profession problem', *The Scotsman* (9 November 1937); 'Dragooned by petty rules', *Daily Sketch* (9 November 1937); 'Nurses' conditions', *Daily Worker* (18 September 1937); 'The shortage of nurses', *Nottingham Evening News* (15 December 1937); 'Ministering angels minus', *The Tribune* (27 August 1937); 'What the "life" of the probationer and training for the nurse in the average hospital is like', *Public Opinion* (10 December 1937).
21 'Overseas nursing as a career for the educated girl', *Journal of Careers* (February 1934), p. 108.
22 Cited by P. Holden, 'Nursing sisters in Tanganyika/Tanzania 1929–78: A report on the memoirs collected by Alison Smith for the Oxford Development Records Project on public health services in Africa' [typescript] (Oxford, Queen Elizabeth House, 1984), p. 4.
23 *Ibid.*, p. 13.

The role of the CNA was to screen candidates for the CO, for which service the Association received two guineas for every candidate recruited. Unlike its medical counterparts the CNA operated at arms-length from the CO. The lack of fully-fledged official sponsorship for the CNA, and its institutionalization within the CO, had a number of important consequences. First, there was never any investment in training for nurses working in the colonies equivalent to that provided for doctors.[24] Nurses were the lowest-paid of any colonial officer. Salary levels could nevertheless be attractive by voluntary hospital standards, although these varied enormously depending upon location and the relative wealth of the colony. Notwithstanding this, the archives reveal significant economic hardship suffered by colonial sisters, especially with respect to pensions. Penalties could also be high for breaking contracts, and applicants were asked to provide the name of a guarantor to cover the costs of passage (and presumably breach of contract). Salary levels could be especially disadvantageous for those who had responsibility for supporting elderly parents.[25]

Training for the tropics

While not all colonial nurses were sent to the tropics, few recruits underwent training or received any form of preparation for what they might encounter in the colonies. Recruitment patterns appear to have favoured the large teaching hospitals, whose courses were notoriously weak in public health, a feature much criticized during the interwar period.[26] While some nurses had post-registration qualifications such as health visiting, sick-children's nursing, dietetics, or domestic science, these were no substitute for training in tropical diseases, which was a routine requirement for doctors.[27] Linguistic competence was also noted but no demands or offers of training were made.

A number of recruits were attracted on account of previous missionary or family connections with the colonies.[28] Barbara Scofield, for example, was drawn towards the service through her brother who had been appointed to the Colonial Administrative Service in 1925. Equally it is possible that a number of women entered nursing with the objective of nursing abroad in mind.[29] Mary Watt's father had business interests in Nigeria and Sierra Leone. In 1929 she had visited her

24   M. Worboys, 'Science and British colonial imperialism, 1895–1940', University of Sussex D.Phil. thesis (1979), pp. 83–142.

25   *Ibid.*

26   A.M. Rafferty, 'Internationalising nursing education during the interwar period', in P. Weindling, ed., *International Health Organisations and Movements 1918–1939* (Cambridge, 1995), pp. 266–82; Rafferty, *Politics of Nursing Knowledge*.

27   PRO, Colonial Office (CO) 859/46/2, Training of Nurses: Committee on Training Nurses for Colonial Territories (Rushcliffe Committee, 1943–4), draft minutes, 24 2.44, p. 6.

28   Holden, 'Nursing sisters', p. 15.

29   *Ibid.*, pp. 15–16.

father, and entered nursing with the intention of returning to Africa. Elizabeth Wilson went to India in 1943, and had missionary connections there through her father. Elizabeth Elliott first visited Africa on a cruise with her parents, later returning to a post in Tanganyika.[30]

Recruitment practices were geared towards finding a fit between nurses and the social norms and routines of colonial life. Social activities were an important part of the colonial experience. Some sisters were asked questions at interviews solely concerned with sporting activities and hobbies.[31] Indeed such accomplishments were written into the Association's publicity material. Lady Wilson, in an article in the *Journal of Careers*, advised that in addition to professional qualifications applicants should be good players of at least tennis or golf, or be good riders – such activities would help applicants to keep fit in the tropics and to 'take their place in the social life of the community'.[32] Bridget Robertson's lively memoir of life in the colonial nursing service deals as much with ponies as it does with pellagra.[33] Elizabeth Elliott was asked whether she could light a primus stove and whether she realized that her patients would be black.[34]

Recruitment patterns

Recruitment patterns varied over time but demonstrate an almost linear increase up to and during World War Two (see Figure 1).

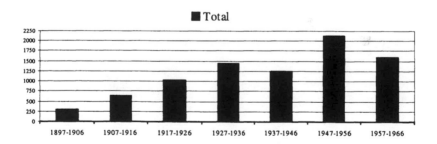

Source: Compiled from Annual Reports of Overseas Nursing Association, Rhodes House, Univ. of Oxford.

Figure 1   Numbers of Nurses Sent Overseas

30   *Ibid.*, p. 19.
31   *Ibid.*, p. 18.
32   'Overseas nursing', p. 103.
33   Robertson, *Angels in Africa*.
34   Holden, 'Nursing sisters', p. 18.

Although distribution patterns to different destinations varied, Africa and the Caribbean were among the most frequent countries of destination cited. Normally a tour of duty would last for three years, but many nurses did several tours and made the colonial nursing service an important part of their careers. A small minority were entered onto a roll of merit for long service.

The colonial nursing service

The CO seems to have taken very little active role in influencing the work of the Association until relatively far into the interwar period. A report to the Secretary of State in 1939 recommended the creation of a unified nursing service in the colonies and, typically, saw nursing as an important cultural conduit into the local population:

> through nursing the sick in native hospitals, training local nurses and welfare work among the mothers' babies, she [the European nurse] is brought closely in touch with the life of the people and her value to the colony increases as she becomes familiar with the language and customs and wins the confidence of the native people, especially of the women.[35]

From 1930, colonial policy in East Africa in particular was recommending the spread of education as a means of promoting the economic advancement of the country:

> As in the political sphere so in the social, it should be the aim to train the natives themselves to take on an ever increasing part, not only in the work of the educational, medical, administrative and other services alike, by filling in such services any posts for which individuals may increasingly become qualified, but also in the local direction of these services through the native councils already referred to.[36]

Such councils were the professional registration bodies responsible for the regulation of training standards, and the vehicles for reciprocal recognition of qualifications between Britain and its colonies. The Rushcliffe Committee on the Training of Nurses in the Colonies (1943–5) endorsed the need for a unified colonial nursing service in which a policy of recruitment from local people was to be supported by a policy of local training provision with the prospect of attaining a standard that would 'merit reciprocal registration with the Nursing Councils in the

---

35   Cited in *ibid.*, p. 6.
36   Memo on native policy in East Africa, 1930, cited by J. Welch, *Nursing Education related to the Cultural Background in East and Southeast African Colonies* (Carneigie Corporation, New York, 1941), p. 1.

UK'.[37] These would be the vehicles through which mobility and migration could be endorsed and mediated.

International recruitment to the UK

Having sketched out some aspects of recruitment to the colonial nursing service, it is worth considering the pattern of international recruitment of nurses to the UK within the same time period. Data are sparse, but census sources demonstrate that there is very little evidence of recruitment from the colonies prior to the period after the Second World War. This underlines the low-profile role that the CO played in recruitment until after the inception of the NHS. Interestingly, however, measures to facilitate the recruitment of foreign probationers to the UK had been in place since 1902. The Aliens Act 1902 enabled the recruitment of probationers under certain restricted conditions where (a) the foreigner came from a country in which the hospital provision was poor and there was no opportunity for proper training; (b) there was definite evidence that the hospital in Britain could not obtain British applicants, and (c) such trainees returned to their native countries after completing training.

It is not known how many hospitals took advantage of this opportunity before the establishment of the Ministry of Health in 1919, but presumably the mechanism was a response to a demand. There are few available data on numbers of so-called foreign nurses working in the UK during the interwar period because census returns linking occupation with nationality were only made erratically. In 1921, for example, there were 718 foreign-born nurses from 28 different countries, the majority coming from the USA (82 female nurses) and France (206 female nurses) while the largest single category of male nurses was Italian. How accurate these figures are is debatable but the flow of foreign nurses must have been sufficiently worrying to lead the Ministry of Labour in 1935 to limit permits for foreign probationers to 3 per cent of probationer posts, on the understanding that the foreigner would return to her own country after training had been completed.[38]

The situation changed with the Second World War and the introduction of the NHS. The demand for recruitment rose during and after the war. Again there is very little evidence of recruitment from the colonies. The major source of recruits in 1947 was from Ireland. The Wood Committee, set up to consider the nursing needs of the new NHS, estimated that some 15,000 (12 per cent) of the total hospital nursing workforce had been born in Eire.[39] Recruitment of nurses from

37 PRO, CO998, Committee on the Training of Nurses for the Colonies: Minutes and Papers 1943–1945, para. 30, p. 11.
38 PRO, MH55/447, Letter, Ministry of Labour to the Secretary, Ministry of Health, 6 September 1935.
39 Ministry of Health, Department of Health for Scotland, Ministry of Health and National Labour, *Working Party on the Recruitment and Training of Nurses* (London, 1947), para. 40.

Eire had been intensified throughout the war: the Ministry of Labour had a recruitment liaison office staffed by technical nursing officers in Dublin. The numbers peaked in 1946 at 2,561 female recruits, and fell to 80 in 1954.[40]

By contrast, recruitment of European foreign nationals for training steadily increased from 584 in 1946 to 2,234 in 1957. Perhaps surprisingly, given the prevailing anti-German sentiment after the war, it was German nurses who consti- tuted the largest single group of overseas workers during this period.[41] Those accepted could enter on a permit valid for only three years, register with the police, and enter employment specified by the Ministry of Labour and National Service. They were not allowed to leave their assigned employment without the consent of the Ministry. This was *de facto* direction of labour, which had operated during the war and had been feared by some nurse leaders as the price of the introduction of the NHS.[42]

In 1957 the Ministry of Labour handed its recruitment and 'placing' functions in nursing over to the Ministry of Health which then became responsible for statistics on the nursing services, recruitment campaigns, and matters related to publicity. Only in the late 1960s and early 1970s did the 'marriage of convenience' between the nursing shortage in the NHS and Commonwealth citizens keen to enter the UK to train as nurses become established.[43] By 1971 there were 15,000 overseas student nurses in the UK, of whom 40 per cent were West Indian, 29 per cent Asian and 27 per cent African.[44]

Conclusion

The above account attempts to locate the current dilemmas associated with the international recruitment of nurses to the UK within a wider historical context. I have suggested that current recruitment trends have their roots in a longer set of historical practices which have received only passing attention from historians. Further research is needed to explore the association between patterns of recruit- ment to Britain in the post-NHS period, and the mobility and migration patterns of British nurses to the colonies before World War Two. In particular, the records of the CO itself are crucial to examining the interaction between the two, the dynam- ics, directional flow, source, and countries of destination of recruits in particular. The international recruitment of nurses reflects longer-standing problems of work- force planning and 'push' and 'pull' factors which have tended to favour richer industrialized countries. Nurse migration can be seen as a symptom of wider

40   Ministry of Labour and National Service, *Annual Reports* (London, 1939–47).
41   Ministry of Labour and National Service, *Annual Reports* (London, 1947–57).
42   R. Dingwall, A.M. Rafferty and C. Webster, *An Introduction to the Social History of Nursing* (London, 1988), p. 105.
43   M. Thomas and J. Morton-Williams (1972), cited by S. Beishon, S. Virdee and Ann Hagell, *Nursing in a Multi-ethnic NHS* (London, 1995), p. 100.
44   *Ibid.*

systemic problems in planning for nursing workforces in either domestic or destination countries. It reflects a failure to 'grow one's own' by recruiting and retaining sufficient numbers of appropriately skilled nurses. A key consideration is the ethical dilemma of exacerbating 'brain drain' in skill-depleted countries. Buchan and others note that England and Ireland have introduced guidelines, but the impact of these is difficult to evaluate in the short time since they have been in operation. In any case they refer in the main to the mechanisms of recruitment *per se*, rather than to the underpinning rationale. Moreover a distinction needs to be drawn between aggressive actions by government to recruit, and individual decisions to migrate.[45] Ultimately there is an interesting historical irony to the debate over international recruitment within the UK. For it was to their dominions, such as South Africa and New Zealand, that early reformers of British nursing looked to justify the granting of state registration within the UK at the turn of the twentieth century. Britain, they argued, was falling behind the rest of the world.[46] Nurse historians played their part and applauded the export of British-trained nurses as part of Britain's 'civilizing' mission to the world. Failure to secure progressive measures such as registration, it was argued, would have an adverse impact on Britain's imperial fortunes.[47] It is not just governments who need to consider the policy implications of international recruitment. Nurses and their organizations need to acknowledge the degree to which they may have colluded with and benefited from overseas recruitment in the expansion of their own professional 'empire'.[48] Many challenges lie ahead as we wrestle with the complex challenges of expanding the delivery capacity of the NHS and matching the characteristics of the workforce with the population served. Migration and mobility are complex issues and the effects may not be entirely negative. The policy challenge is complex, requiring concerted action across different countries to resolve. The challenge for governments is to work towards a managed policy which creates a win-win situation for both the domestic and destination countries concerned.[49]

45 Buchan, Parkin and Sochalski, *International Nurse Mobility*.
46 *Ibid.*
47 Rafferty, *Politics of Nursing Knowledge*.
48 S. Tooley, *The History of Nursing in the British Empire* (London, 1906), p. i.
49 Beishon, Virdee and Hagell, *Nursing in a Multi-ethnic NHS*, p. 10.

Chapter 17

Professional Status and Professional Regulation in the 1970s: The Case of the Briggs Committee on Nursing and the Merrison Committee on the Regulation of the Medical Profession

Jane Lewis

The early 1970s are commonly acknowledged to have been the high point of post-war professional power. As Hafferty and McKinlay have pointed out, Freidson's influential work on the professional dominance of medicine was formulated at a time that many now regard as the golden age of medicine.[1] By the end of the 1970s the radical critique of medicine was well under way.[2] In Britain, the early 1970s was also marked by the first major reorganization of the National Health Service (NHS) since its foundation in 1948. The report of the Briggs Committee on Nursing was published in 1972 and that of the Merrison Committee on the Regulation of the Medical Profession in 1975.[3] The Committees recommended the reform of the statutory bodies charged with regulating nursing (the General Nursing Councils for England and Wales and for Scotland, the Central Midwives Boards

The research for this chapter was carried out as part of a larger project on the history of the UKCC (see C. Davies and A. Beach, *Interpreting Professional Self-Regulation. A History of the United Kingdom Central Council for Nursing, Midwifery and Health Visiting* (London, 2000)). I am grateful to Abigail Beach for research assistance and to Celia Davies for her comments.

1   F.W. Hafferty and J.B. McKinlay, 'Introduction', in *The Changing Medical Profession. An International Perspective*, ed. F.W. Hafferty and J.B. McKinlay (Oxford, 1993), pp. 3–7; E. Freidson, *Profession of Medicine: A Study of the Sociology of Applied Knowledge* (New York, 1970).
2   For example, I. Illich, *Limits to Medicine: Medical Nemesis* (London, 1976); and I. Kennedy, *The Unmasking of Medicine* (London, 1981).
3   *Report of the Committee on Nursing* (Cmnd. 5115, London, 1972); *Report of the Committee of Inquiry into the Regulation of the Medical Profession* (Cmnd. 6018, London, 1975).

for England and Wales and for Scotland, and the Northern Ireland Council for Nurses and Midwives) and medicine (the General Medical Council). This was legislated for in 1978 for medicine and in 1979 for nursing.

It is possible to interpret these measures as part of the 'modernization' of the legislation regulating health professionals, which took place against the economic and career demands of health professionals and the backdrop of rapid changes in the NHS.[4] However, the differences between the approaches taken by the two committees are more striking than any similarities. The circumstances of their appointment were rather different: Briggs was billed as a large-scale review of a nursing profession in crisis (nurses and midwives submitted a 'massive revaluation claim' early in 1973 and were not at all satisfied with the outcome[5]), while Merrison was an altogether smaller affair, intended to lay to rest long-running discontent within the medical profession about the General Medical Council (GMC). But the reports of the Committees and the subsequent debate and legislation provide a valuable opportunity to compare the relative power of the two professions and the nature of their relationship with the state, in particular, the extent to which professional issues in respect of nursing were subordinated to government's concerns about the needs of the health service (particularly for cheap labour) in a way that would have been unthinkable for medicine.

The recent literature on the medical profession has been sternly critical of earlier occupation-centred approaches,[6] stressing the importance of considering the relationships between professions, and the relationship between professions, markets and the state. In particular, it has been suggested that the state has tended to be left out of discussions of professionalization.[7] Moran and Wood have stressed the importance of distinguishing between professional self-regulation and state-led self-regulation.[8] The GMC has derived its being and its authority from state legislation. However, as Stacey has cautioned, state regulation on its own does not confer professional prestige, as the example of nursing shows.[9] A key issue would therefore seem to be the precise nature of the relationship between a profession and the

4   This is how R. Dingwall, A.M. Rafferty and C. Webster, *An Introduction to the Social History of Nursing* (London, 1988), p. 205, interpret Briggs.

5   C. Webster, *The Health Services since the War. Volume 2, Government and Health Care: The British National Health Service 1958–1979* (London, 1996), p. 435.

6   R. Dingwall, 'Professions and social order in a global society', unpublished plenary paper given to the IS Working Group 02 Conference, Nottingham, Sept. 1996; R. Dingwall and P. Fenn, 'A "respectable profession"? Sociological and economic perspectives on the regulation of professional services', *International Review of Law and Economics*, 7 (1987), 51–64.

7   J. Frenk and L. Duran-Arenas, 'The medical profession and the state', in Hafferty and McKinlay, *The Changing Medical Profession*, pp. 25–42.

8   M. Moran and B. Wood, *States, Regulation and the Medical Profession* (Buckingham, 1993). See also M. Moran, *Governing the Health Care State* (Manchester, 1999), pp. 99–135.

9   M. Stacey, 'Collective therapeutic responsibility. Lessons from the GMC', in *The Healing Bond*, ed. S. Budd and U. Sharma (London, 1994), p. 110.

state. An analysis of the Briggs and Merrison Committees and their consequences reveals that while they had issues in common, the way in which it was assumed that professional regulation would work and the way in which the legislative changes were decided were radically different, reflecting above all differences in the professional status and power of nursing *vis à vis* medicine.[10]

Briggs and Merrison: context

The Briggs Committee was set up against a background of uncertainty over the consequences of the planned reorganization of the National Health Service, growing government pressure for cost containment in the delivery of health care, and prolonged industrial unrest among nurses and other public staff. In addition, a number of reports published since 1964 had argued for the reform of particular aspects of nursing. The Royal College of Nursing (RCN) published a report, *Administering the Hospital Nursing Service* in 1964, which made the case for greater recognition to be accorded nurse administrators.[11] The government's Committee on Senior Nursing Staff (the Salmon Report), published in 1966, accepted the need to integrate nurses into the NHS management structure, especially in view of the proposed reorganization of the hospital service around the district general hospital. The Report outlined a new structure of nursing grades based on three tiers of management responsibility and recommended the organization of nursing services around distinct 'spheres of authority', identified as sections, units, areas, and divisions.[12] For nurses at the top level, the new structure promised access to the hospital's policy-making committees and the hope of parity with other professionals in the NHS, but for others, particularly the more junior grades of nurse and those who chose to focus their career on a clinical specialty or nurse education, the Salmon changes seemed less beneficial.[13] Indeed, nurse tutors in particular saw themselves as positively disadvantaged by the new career

---

10   These in turn have of course been determined in large measure by the way in which nursing and medicine are gendered, something that is not part of the discussion in this chapter, but see C. Davies, *Gender and the Professional Predicament in Nursing* (Buckingham, 1995).

11   Royal College of Nursing, *Administering the Hospital Nursing Service* (London, 1964).

12   Ministry of Health, *Report of the Committee on Senior Nursing Staff Structure* (London, 1966).

13   The Salmon Committee was concerned with hospital nursing only. A parallel review for local authority nursing services was established at the end of 1968 under the chairmanship of E.L. Mayston (Department of Health and Social Security [DHSS], *Report of Working Party on Management Structure in the Local Authority Nursing Services* (London, 1969)).

structure, compared with their colleagues in administration and with teachers in technical colleges.[14]

Their dissatisfaction grew as it became clear that government was not inclined to address a second Report published by the RCN in 1964 on nurse education (the Platt Report). This report was a strong statement of the need for radical change in the way in which nurses were educated. It called for full 'student' status for nurses, higher educational qualifications for entrants, a lower age of entry and fewer, more independent schools of nursing.[15] These recommendations were viewed askance by Ministers, who feared their cost implications. The system of nurse training provided above all a cheap labour force for the hospitals. Nevertheless, support was given to the need to address the issue of nurse education (although not to all the recommendations of the RCN) by the 1968 Report of the National Board for Prices and Incomes on the pay of nurses and midwives.[16] Finally, the Departmental Committee on Nurse Tutors, set up in 1968 by the Ministry of Health, the RCN and the General Nursing Council (GNC) was perceived by government to be on course to repeat the approach of the Platt Committee by focusing on long-term and unrealistic objectives in respect of nurse education.[17] It is worth noting that all these programmes for reform by-passed the GNC, which felt somewhat aggrieved at the Platt Report's deliberate and pointed criticism of its own attempts to improve the standard of nurse education.[18]

Only a major review of nursing could stop nurse leaders' pursuit of root and branch educational reform, which was particularly threatening to government given the huge costs it represented at a time of strong public pay demands.[19] The RCN wanted to see the appointment of a Royal Commission to explore the future of nursing education, just as the 1968 Todd Commission had addressed the organization and content of medical education.[20] While it had been asked informally to hold back its request, the Department of Health and Social Security (DHSS) recognized

14   Webster, *Government and Health Care*, pp. 249–59.

15   Royal College of Nursing, *A Reform of Nursing Education* (London, 1964).

16   National Board for Prices and Incomes, Report no. 60: *Pay of Nurses and Midwives in the National Health Service* (Cmnd. 3585, London, 1968).

17   Webster, *Government and Health Care*, p. 261. For the DHSS viewpoint on Platt, see Kew, Public Record Office (PRO), MH165/152, memo by D. Somerville on the establishment of a committee on nurse training, 25 October 1968. The working party on nurse tutors was established in 1968 and chaired by the Chief Nursing Officer, Dame Kathleen Raven. It was allowed to fall into abeyance following the issue of its report in 1970.

18   General Nursing Council for England and Wales, *Platt Report on a Reform of Nursing Education: Memorandum from the General Nursing Council for England and Wales* (London, 1965); E. Bendall and E Raybould, *A History of the General Nursing Council for England and Wales, 1919-69* (London, 1969), pp. 200–2.

19   Webster, *Government and Health Care*, pp. 260–1.

20   *Report of the Royal Commission on Medical Education* (Cmnd. 3569, London, 1968).

that the College could not be restrained for long.[21] The case for a detailed review was strong but, in the DHSS's opinion, could not be divorced from an examination of manpower and service implications. Taking the Platt Report as an example, the Department doubted that the profession, whether in the form of the RCN or the GNC, had the inclination or the capabilities to address these issues. It did not trust the RCN and while the GNC had tended to put the needs of the NHS before those of the profession (it had, after all, opposed the Platt Report for being unrealistic in its demands), it had not shown any conspicuous leadership. The DHSS felt that the GNC was 'quite incapable of making any real effort to deal with the problems we see'.[22] Thus government failed to take responsibility for the long-deferred issue of nurse education, which had effectively been sacrificed to the goal of producing a cheap hospital labour force, and blamed the nursing profession either for inaction, or for making 'unrealistic' proposals.

In the summer of 1969, after considerable deliberation, the DHSS took the pre-emptive step of recommending the establishment of a committee of inquiry. By this time, growing agitation over nursing pay and conditions had made a wide-ranging review politically expedient. At the beginning of the 1970s, the government faced another huge pay demand of 27 per cent on behalf of the nurses, which had to be managed alongside movement towards profoundly reorganizing the NHS and attempts to shift the balance of care away from the hospital and towards the 'community'. In seeming recognition of the apparent stalemate that beset nursing, Richard Crossman, the Secretary of State for Social Services, told the Department in October that the Prime Minister, Harold Wilson, wished to see 'a completely new study of nursing' which would embrace such issues as 'the nurse's place in society, her status, training, pay and working conditions'.[23] The Prime Minister also insisted on the importance and urgency of these deliberations.[24]

Professor Asa Briggs, Vice-Chancellor of the University of Sussex, was approached by the Minister of State for Health, Baroness Serota, in December 1969 and agreed to accept the Chair, provided that a satisfactory settlement of the nurses' pay claims could be reached.[25] The establishment of the committee was announced in the House of Commons in March 1970. The Committee consisted of sixteen members, the Chair included; two more were added later. Nine of these were women and nine were also nurses and midwives. Government wanted all levels of nursing experience represented, but local authority nurses, that is, district

---

21   PRO, MH165/146. Meeting on the proposed department enquiry into nurse training, 20 October 1968. The Royal Commission on Medical Education had been established in 1965 and reported in 1968.
22   PRO, MH165/152, Memo by D. Somerville, 25 October 1968.
23   PRO, MH 165/146, Policy meeting on nurse training, 24 October 1969. In his diaries, Crossman acknowledged the threat that nurses posed to the government's prices and incomes policy, see Dingwall, Rafferty and Webster, *An Introduction to the Social History of Nursing*.
24   Webster, *Government and Health Care*, p. 263.
25   PRO, MH165/146, 19 December 1969.

nurses and health visitors, were given only one representative, as were midwives. Three non-nursing members were clinicians, one was an educationalist, one an economic human resources expert, one a chair of the Whitley Council staff side, one a hospital administrator and one a representative of the consumer interest. The sensitivities involved in securing nursing members who were representative of the profession signalled the deep divisions within nursing that were to bedevil the debates over the Briggs Report. Indeed, it was in some measure the very different voices of what have been called the 'managers' and the 'professionalizers' within nursing,[26] together with the lack of any firm steer from the GNC, that prompted government to seize the initiative and appoint a committee of inquiry, although the main impetus undoubtedly came, as was usual in the case of nursing, from the need to manage a crisis.

In many respects the Merrison Committee was similarly constituted to Briggs. It consisted of 15 members, of whom seven were medical and five were women. The General Secretary of the Royal College of Nursing was a member and was counted as one of the 'lay' members. Whereas the terms of reference for the Briggs Committee were broad, requiring a review of the role of nurses and midwives and their education and training in order to make the best use of available manpower and to meet the needs of the soon-to-be integrated NHS,[27] those for Merrison were much more narrowly focused on the changes that were needed in the provisions for regulating the profession, the functions of the body charged with responsibility for regulation (the GMC) and composition of that body. In fact (as the next section will show) this did not stop the Committees covering some very similar ground.

However, the Merrison Committee was appointed not because of any perception of general crisis in the medical profession, as had been the case with the Todd Commission, where the demand and supply of doctors was one of the chief issues. Rather, the issue was the acute dissatisfaction within the medical profession with the GMC. Both junior hospital doctors and general practitioners in particular perceived the GMC as an elitist, elderly, out-of-touch body.[28] In 1970 a Special Representative Meeting of the BMA demanded that a majority of the GMC should be elected by the profession, while the medical press in the shape of *Pulse* and *World Medicine* led the rebellion against paying the annual retention fee levied by the GMC for the medical register. Three working parties appointed by the profession, chaired by Brynmor Jones, Dr S. Wand and Sir Ronald Tunbridge reported in March 1971, March 1972 and November 1972 respectively, but failed to resolve the dispute. At the end of 1972, the GMC voted to strike off the dissident doctors who had not paid their retention fee and government stepped in with the appointment of a committee under the chairmanship of Sir Alec Merrison, Vice-

26 R. White, 'From matron to manager: the political construction of reality', in *Political Issues in Nursing: Past, Present and Future*, ed. R. White (Chichester, 1986), pp. 45–68.

27 'Integration' referred to bringing local authority health services into the NHS.

28 M. Stacey, *Regulating British Medicine: the GMC* (Chichester, 1992), p. 30; Webster, *Government and Health Care*, p. 706.

Chancellor of the University of Bristol, and not a medical man. Recalling the events of 1972 as he introduced the legislation to implement Merrison in 1977, Lord Wells-Pestell said that government intervened in order to avert a serious situation 'for the NHS and the profession generally'.[29] As in the case of nursing, government intervention was linked to service as much as to professional issues. In many respects the divisions within medicine were even more explicit in respect of the Merrison Committee than they were in the case of Briggs, which makes the way in which they ceased to be a decisive factor in the debates following the publication of the Merrison Report all the more interesting.

Briggs and Merrison: text[30]

In their organization the Briggs and Merrison Reports appear almost as mirror images of each other. Briggs begins with educational issues, proceeds to discuss the utilization of resources and *ends* with recommendations regarding what it calls 'organizational frameworks', by which it means the machinery for professional regulation. Merrison *begins* with a discussion of professional regulation and what it entails and then considers educational matters, including the standards that should be applied in the case of overseas doctors, disciplinary issues and comes finally to the way in which the GMC should be structured. In part, this contrast may be held to follow naturally from the different circumstances prompting the setting up of the Committees and the difference in their terms of reference. Certainly issues to do with discipline were outside Briggs's remit. However, it is striking that Briggs never referred directly to the issue of professional regulation as such, and never explicitly considered the nature of professional regulation and its relation to the state and to society, as did Merrison in its opening chapter.

The Merrison Report began with the clear assumption as to the desirability of professional self-regulation: 'We take the view that the medical profession should be largely self-regulating' (paragraph 11), while recognizing that the GMC derived its authority from legislation (paragraph 10). The assumption was that the medical profession could carry out the work of regulation in the interests of the public at large.[31] In Merrison's view, the key to regulation lay in the GMC's keeping of the professional register. The GMC had to make sure that only 'competent' doctors were admitted to the register and that those 'unfit to practise' were excluded from it (paragraph 1). Thus the whole approach of the Report was to make recommendations that would ensure that the GMC was in a position to do this successfully. Its main recommendations were that the GMC be restructured; that it revamp its disciplinary procedures and set up a committee to deal with disciplinary procedures for sick doctors; that it take over responsibility for overseeing the

29   *House of Lords Debates*, 29 November 1977, c. 1148.
30   The notes in brackets in this section refer to paragraphs in the Briggs and Merrison Reports.
31   Davies and Beach, *Interpreting Professional Self-Regulation*, p. 189.

whole of medical training, post-graduate as well as undergraduate; that it test and register overseas doctors; and that it take responsibility for the maintenance of standards by issuing guidance to doctors. In short, the GMC was to move on to more 'active' regulation.

The position of the General Nursing Councils and Central Midwifery Boards was not central to the Briggs Committee in the same way. It did not start, as did the Merrison Committee, with the aim of making recommendations for legislative change that would enable the profession to better regulate itself, that is, to improve the system of state-sponsored self-regulation. The Briggs Committee's consideration of the machinery for regulation came late, both in the deliberations of the Committee itself and in the Report. When considering the draft Report in April 1972, the Chairman found great disparity in the amounts of material on different topics and, while there was plenty on the role and function of the nurse, there was plainly 'insufficient on statutory frameworks'.[32]

The main recommendations of the Briggs Committee were as follows: firstly, to lower the age of entry into nursing from 18 to 17 by 1975; secondly, to make entry requirements dependent on a flexible system designed to test motivation and aptitude, rather than on specifically formal training; thirdly, to restructure training, introducing an eighteen-month general training leading to a first statutory qualification (the Certificate in Nursing Practice) and a further (optional) eighteen-month course leading to full registration; fourthly, to replace the four specialized parts of the existing register by a single, undifferentiated register and to introduce improvements in the career structure in order to achieve a clearer identification of nurses and midwives with advanced clinical qualifications; fifthly, to discontinue the statutory certification of health visitors, thereby eliminating the need for the Council for the Education and Training of Health Visitors (CETHV); sixthly, to establish Area Committees for Nursing and Midwifery (in line with the anticipated reorganization of the NHS) that would supervise and finance local colleges of nursing and midwifery for the education of all nurses and midwives, and to establish manpower and personnel departments at Area level to oversee recruitment; and finally, to replace the five separate statutory regulatory bodies by a single Central Nursing and Midwifery Council for Great Britain with responsibility for standards of statutory qualifications and for discipline, supported by three Nursing and Midwifery Education Boards for England, Scotland and Wales, supervising the detail of education with a Standing Midwifery Committee of the Central Council to 'control' and 'advise' (the language was ambiguous) on midwifery practice.

It is clear that Briggs saw the lead in all this being taken by government. The new statutory bodies were seen more as administrative than professional agencies. Briggs's starting point was not the profession, as it was in the case of Merrison, but the health service. An integrated NHS, such as would be achieved by the

32   PRO, MH165/170, CN (72), Minutes of 19th meeting of Briggs Committee, 28–9 April 1972, p. 2.

forthcoming reorganization (in 1974), would require 'a more flexible and co-operative deployment of nursing and midwifery staff' (paragraph 12), which in turn required a more flexible approach to nurse education. Briggs was at pains to insist that the nursing profession be recognized as separate from and as complementary to medicine (paragraph 142). The nurse 'is not one of the doctor's means of treating patients. She is the person who cares for and co-ordinates the care of the people who are her patients' (paragraph 151). Briggs made a passionate plea for nursing as the premier caring profession: 'nurs'ng and midwifery is more than a workforce. It is a profession' (paragraph 520). However, the whole organization of the Report effectively subordinated professional to service concerns.

The issue of education, which was also central to the Merrison Report, is a good example of this. The RCN had campaigned for higher entry requirements for nursing, based on 'O' and 'A' levels, a firm differentiation of the different routes into nursing, and a clearer distinction between the Roll (state-enrolled nurses who underwent a two-year training) and the Register (state-registered nurses who trained for three years). Minimum standards for entry to nursing had been set as recently as 1962 and the Royal College was anxious to improve these. However, the Briggs Committee was convinced that the reorganized NHS would need a more flexible approach to nurse training. Early on in its deliberations the Chairman of the Sub-Committee on Education criticized the traditional early specialization in nurse training.[33] As the boundaries between hospital and community began to break down in the newly-integrated NHS, nurses would need experience of both care environments. Thus the Committee promoted the advantages of a single port of entry and a comprehensive initial training, with specialization following registration or enrolment.[34] The aim, it was argued, should be the training of 'nurses who were all-rounders with a good enough basic education to enable them to function satisfactorily within the nursing team at basic level and to progress from basic to specialized nursing skills with further education'.[35] The committee thus recommended an eighteen-month training period for a certificate that would be common to all nurses, followed by a further 18 months in order to qualify as a registered nurse. The 'comprehensive' model of learning, with goals reached through different tracks and at a varied pace, strongly influenced both the substance and rhetoric of the Briggs Committee's recommendations.[36] The Committee was conscious of the growing importance of the SEN grade nurse to overall manpower: between 1962 and 1970 the proportion of 'pupil' (training for entry to the roll) to 'student' (training for entry to the register) nurses had increased from

33 PRO, MH165/156, CN (70) 49: note by Professor Ivor Batchelor, 'The Role and Education of the Nurse', 5 September 1970.
34 PRO, MH165/149, 6th meeting of Briggs Committee, 13–15 November 1970.
35 PRO, MH165/168, CN (71), 'The Future of Nurse Education', 17th meeting of the Briggs Committee, 3–4 December 1971.
36 PRO, MH165/163, Minutes of the 15th meeting of Briggs Committee, 8–9 October 1971; Dingwall, Rafferty, and Webster, *An Introduction to the Social History of Nursing*, p. 207.

13 per cent to 42 per cent. This meant that entry requirements for training had to reflect the significance of this source of recruits. Briggs rejected the RCN's desire to increase the formal qualifications required of recruits: 'Suitability should not be determined by O-levels alone. We know less about how to identify "motivation" than we know about how to measure "academic ability"' (paragraph 259 (e)).

In contrast, Merrison was anxious to work with the profession's concerns about the dilution of standards as a response to service needs. It reported in particular that training received during the pre-registration year (the year between graduation and full registration) was particularly heavily criticized by young doctors. Among the junior staff of a London hospital only 5 per cent felt that it was satisfactory; the vast majority felt that service needs took precedence over education. Merrison concluded that 'any registration system must ineluctably involve the registering body in the control of the standards of the education conferring a right to registration' (paragraph 131). This was a rather different position to the one adopted by Briggs, which, while it fully recognized the problem posed by the nurse's position as 'learner and worker' (paragraph 212 (a)), was not prepared to endanger the needs of the NHS by endorsing the RCN's wish that all trainee nurses be treated as students.

The focus on nursing as a labour force may also explain the lack of attention in Briggs to overseas nurses. The question of the standards of overseas doctors occupied a whole chapter in the Merrison Report, which was profession-focused. The response of the *British Medical Journal* and the *Lancet* to the publication of the Merrison Report was above all to welcome the boost it promised to give standards in medicine.[37] The issue in respect of overseas doctors was both the level of their qualifications, including their ability to speak English, and their willingness to put up with poor conditions of work in the NHS. The *British Medical Journal* deplored the way in which overseas doctors were prepared to work in sub-standard hospitals and thus to keep the NHS going. One third of doctors on the register were from overseas in 1972. The number of doctors entering British medical schools (and hence the cost of training) was controlled by government quota, but issues regarding medical education were subject to consultation between the GMC, the Royal Colleges and Faculties and government departments in a way that nursing education was not.

In the non-teaching hospitals of the Greater London area, the same hospitals that relied heavily on overseas doctors, 62 per cent of all trainee nurses were born overseas (paragraph 416). Yet 'immigrant nurses' only warranted a few paragraphs in the Briggs Report. This was in part because the issue of standards in nursing was entirely different from medicine. Nurses were not only split between the 'Roll' and 'Register' in a manner entirely different from doctors, but as many as 19 per cent of acute hospital nurses in England and Wales in 1971, and 37 per cent of nurses in hospitals other than mental illness/handicap and acute, were untrained auxiliaries

37   'Towards a reborn GMC', *The Lancet*, 305 (1975), 901–2; 'A good report', *British Medical Journal*, 270 (1975), 155–6.

(Table 33, p. 135). Thus the issue of standards of qualifications for nurses from overseas was not as visible and anxieties were not so acute. In addition, it was clear that the main anxieties of the Briggs Report related to shortages of nursing staff and problems of recruitment and retention. It was therefore unlikely that reliance on overseas nurses would be made an issue. As Webster has pointed out, immigrant nurses had strengthened the hand of the Minister of Health (Enoch Powell) in resisting claims for higher pay in the early 1960s; immigrant nurses provided a plentiful supply of cheap labour.[38]

The priority given by the Briggs Committee to the issue of the nursing labour force may also explain the linkage that it was keen to make between education and management in nursing. Its concern about service needs led to recommendations regarding the management of nursing and midwifery resources, and was bolstered by the idea that nursing management could not be separated from nursing practice (paragraphs 479 (b) and 538 (a)). Nursing was the premier caring profession and its work necessarily included the organization of caring. Behind this justification lay the large amount of evidence collected by Briggs as to inefficiencies in the deployment of the nursing labour force.

In terms of the statutory bodies themselves, there appear to be some interesting similarities in respect of the position of the nursing Councils and the GMC in regard to the central issue of education. However, on closer examination their meaning is rather different. Many of the powers of the bodies for the two professions were similar. For example, neither the nursing Councils nor the GMC had oversight of specialist education. For nursing, the Joint Board of Clinical Nursing Studies had been established in England and Wales in 1966 to advise on post-certificate training, while for medicine, the Joint Committees on Higher Training emerged after the Todd Commission on medical education and provided accreditation in the different specialties. Both Briggs and Merrison recommended that oversight of specialist education come under the statutory regulatory bodies. In respect of the education leading to registration, both the nursing councils and the GMC had the power to lay down syllabuses and to inspect and to approve the schools. However, it seems that neither exercised its power of inspection to any great extent. In the case of nursing, this was largely because service requirements and the large number of training schools made it almost impossible for the Councils to take strong action. In contrast, when asked why it made so little use of its direct supervisory powers, the GMC told the Merrison Committee that it:

> felt some doubt whether the formal kind of visitation and inspection which the Act contemplates would, if carried out generally, be a useful exercise in contemporary conditions. It appears unlikely that Medical Schools of Universities in the United Kingdom would be found insufficient in respect of their curricula and examination, unless the council had previously become aware of the development of a potentially unsatisfactory situation [paragraph 35].

38 Webster, *Government and Health Care*, p. 173.

The Committee concluded that the main work of the GMC in undergraduate medical education was to be found 'in this work of discussion, advice, and encouragement rather than in the exercise of its formal powers' (paragraph 36). In other words, the GMC exercised its powers informally, something the Merrison Committee endorsed: '[we] have no doubt of the value of this method of working' (paragraph 83). Indeed, the key to understanding the power of the GMC lies in its ability to consult and negotiate informally with other medical bodies – the Royal Colleges, the medical schools and the BMA – and government departments.

The GMC was thus at the centre of a web of regulation and was able to work in large measure informally in a way that the nursing Councils were not. Merrison emphasized the importance of self-regulation, which, given the fact that regulation of medicine was by definition state-sponsored, meant ensuring that the profession was *enabled* to take the initiative in regulatory matters. As Stacey has observed, the basis for self-regulation rested on the idea of clinical autonomy. The doctor's responsibility was to the patient for diagnosis and treatment and only his/her peers could comment on matters of clinical judgement.[39] Merrison thus conceptualized regulation as 'a contract between public and profession' (paragraph 4), with considerable trust accorded to the profession by the state. The GMC was able to operate informally because of government's trust in its power to induct its new members and to ensure that they behaved in the public interest. Nursing and midwifery, with their long-standing subordination to medicine, have not succeeded in securing the same kind of self-regulation. Rather, nurses and midwives have been more stringently regulated in the formal sense, for example midwives have been subject to inspection (by non-midwives) and have been required to register their intention to practise each year. This may be seen as, in essence, a form of re-registration, something that Merrison considered (paragraph 162), but concluded that it would be for the GMC to decide whether to implement.

Nurses and midwives were not opposed to the formal controls exercised over their practice by their Councils, but this formal supervision negated clinical autonomy, the very basis on which the more powerful professional control exercised by the medical profession was predicated. The issue of re-registration for doctors was raised again by the radical critics of professional dominance in medicine by the end of the decade.[40] For as Stacey has argued, notwithstanding Merrison's idea of a contract between public and profession, regulation of medicine worked more in the interests of the profession than in the interests of the patient.[41] This was why the GMC's role in judging 'fitness to practise' was such a large issue for the Merrison Committee. The Committee was deciding how government should legislate to update the regulation of medicine, while accepting the primacy of the role played by the profession. Thus the Committee also recommended that the GMC take more

39   Stacey, *Regulating British Medicine*, p. 12.
40   E.g. Kennedy, *The Unmasking of Medicine*, p. 123.
41   Stacey, *Regulating British Medicine*.

responsibility in advising on ethical issues, but again in a more informal than formal manner. Guidelines were preferred to a code of practice.

Thus, paradoxically, the nursing Councils exercised considerably more formal control over some aspects of nursing practice than did the GMC over medical practice, and yet they were much less powerful. The power of the GMC derived from the extent to which it was able informally to influence, negotiate, consult and control. State-sponsored regulation meant something entirely different in respect of medicine than it did in the case of nursing. Rudolf Klein has characterized the relationship between medicine and the state as the politics of 'the double-bed'.[42] The aptness of this description for medicine becomes more striking when the implementation of the Reports is considered. Medicine was able to wield an influence that was absent in the case of nursing.

Briggs and Merrison: from reports to legislation

Whereas legislation followed the Merrison Report after three years, it took seven years to begin the process of legislating on Briggs, something that was resented by nurses and which was indeed related to the power that each profession was able to wield.

The main problem for government in respect of the Briggs Report was the cost implications. Towards the end of the Report it was acknowledged that its recommendations for a new education programme would require 14,500 extra staff for the non-psychiatric hospitals in Britain over a seven-year period to replace the work contribution of students on secondment or undergoing theoretical education (paragraph 662). The Treasury was concerned that the Report 'might arouse hopes and encourage pressures for increased expenditure' which, given the 'bleak' outlook for public expenditure, 'may not be able to be achieved', and advocated delaying publication.[43] The Treasury was also worried about the cost implications of the Merrison Report, and the DHSS had some difficulty in persuading it that the Merrison Bill did not have hidden consequences for public expenditure.[44] But the Briggs recommendations were obviously much more open to criticism on public expenditure grounds because they focused much more firmly on restructuring education and training. This carried inevitable costs because of the nurse's position as 'learner and worker' in the NHS and because of the sheer size of the nursing labour force. It seems also to have been the case that the DHSS was anxious to placate the medical profession in advance of the BMA's Annual Representative Meeting in 1977 by announcing a Bill. The dispute that had prompted the Merrison enquiry had been internal to the profession, but also threatened to disrupt the NHS. Arguably, any threat on the part of nurses to disrupt the NHS would have been just

42   R. Klein, 'National variations on international trends', in Hafferty and McKinlay, *The Changing Medical Profession*, p. 205.

43   PRO, MH165/208, Memo on Treasury reaction, c. September 1972.

44   Webster, *Government and Health Care*, p. 708.

as serious, but it soon became obvious that the divisions among nurses over Briggs were widening rather than contracting, which provided ample justification for government to delay.

Initial responses from nurses to the Briggs Report were on the whole favourable. Most expressed relief that a major review had finally been undertaken and the *tone* of Briggs also had much appeal for the profession. The Report took considerable pains to highlight 'the unique caring role of nurses and midwives' (paragraph 39): the nurse was a complement to the doctor rather than part of his armoury. Because of Briggs's almost passionate defence of nursing and the space devoted to the need for educational reform, much was expected. However, as different groups within the profession absorbed Briggs 'in the round', reservations began to be expressed. The RCN welcomed the Report, but had reason to fear the dilution of nursing standards, having fought hard to achieve a minimum entry requirement in the early 1960s. The Briggs recommendations made it possible that nursing would be the only profession that did not insist on minimum entry qualifications. Briggs's attention to service needs was fundamentally at odds with the RCN's stress on student status for nurses.

However, the fundamental tensions over the Briggs Report arose from the professional divisions within nursing and from the different national identities. The most biting criticism came from the Health Visitors' Association, which submitted its comments on the Report early in 1973. It charged that the nature of health visiting had been misunderstood, which it suggested was perhaps not surprising as only one member of the committee 'had any direct personal experience of health visiting and of the community nursing service'.[45] Nurses employed by the local authorities saw in Briggs the makings of a take-over by hospital nursing via the idea of a comprehensive education designed to suit the needs of an integrated NHS. Health visitors felt that their traditions had been ignored. While the 1979 legislation did not change the name of health visitors to 'family health sisters', as Briggs had recommended, health visitors remained unhappy at the disappearance of their own training body. Midwives were also suspicious, also fearing the loss of their own statutory body and hence parity with nurses. Scottish midwives asked for an 'assurance' that 'a degree of autonomy would be given to the Board for Scotland to plan and execute policy relative to Scottish conditions and to allow for experimentation'.[46]

Opposition from Scotland in particular to the formation of one central regulatory board was strong, fuelled and complicated by the contemporary political

---

45   PRO, MH165/204, comments from the Health Visitors' Association, 15 January 1973. The Council for the Education and Training of Health Visitors and the Society of Chief Nursing Officers (Public Health) had similar concerns, but were less dogmatic in their opposition. See also MH165/206, Brief for Secretary of State's meeting with health visitors, 10 May 1973.

46   PRO, MH165/206, Comments from the Royal College of Midwives (Scottish Board), n.d.

debate on devolution.[47] Briggs had given very little guidance on the constitution of the new statutory bodies and on the relationship between the Central Council and the National Education Boards it recommended.[48] Long debates ensued on the issues of where responsibility for disciplinary procedure should rest, at national or central level, and, by 1974, whether the Central Council should not be restricted to more of a co-ordinating role.[49] Wales did not have its own statutory body and therefore did not stand to lose anything with the establishment of a Central Council; nevertheless in the charged atmosphere of the wider debate on devolution Welsh officials stood by Scotland.[50]

Legislation on Briggs failed to reach the reserve list for the 1975/6 and 1976/7 parliamentary sessions because of the exigencies of the parliamentary timetable, the lack of agreement between the nursing organizations, geographical tensions and increasing anxiety about the public expenditure implications as the economic crisis worsened. As uncertainty grew, divisions within the nursing profession became worse. Other specialist groups, primarily the district nurses and mental health and handicap nurses, grew more vocal in the defence of their particular concerns.[51] Protest by district nurses continued right up until the last phase of the legislative process, despite opposition from the nursing Councils, which began to fear that professional unity would be completely eroded. The 1979 Nurses, Midwives and Health Visitors Act set up the UK Central Council to regulate nursing, midwifery and health visiting and a single centralized register for all qualified nurses. The interests of midwifery were to be protected through a Midwifery Standing Committee of the Council, and health visiting through a (less powerful) Health Visiting Joint Committee. In a sense, the legislation addressed only the easy parts of Briggs; the controversial education reforms were not touched.

The story of the Merrison legislation was very different. The GMC itself was broadly in favour of the Report, although it was defensive in respect of the issue of

47 Following the publication of the Royal Commission on the Constitution in October 1973 (Cmnd. 5460) and especially after the success of nationalist parties in the general elections of February and October 1974, devolution occupied a significant place on the political agenda. The strength of the nationalists in a precariously balanced parliament encouraged Labour to develop proposals for Scottish and Welsh devolution.

48 PRO, MH165/79, Note of meeting with statutory bodies, 24 June 1974. Representatives from the two General Nursing Councils, the two Central Midwives Boards, and the Council for the Education and Training of Health Visitors were invited to this meeting with officials from the DHSS, the Scottish Home and Health Dept. and the Welsh Office. An observer from Northern Ireland was also present. See also MH 165/79, Note of meeting with statutory bodies, 29 October 1974.

49 PRO, MH165/80, Letter to R.B. Hodgetts, DHSS from I. Sharp, SHHD, 5 December 1974.

50 PRO, MH165/85, Letter from R.H. Jones, Welsh Office, to I. Sharp, SHHD, 13 December 1974.

51 PRO, MH165/111, Meeting notes and papers of working group 4 of the Briggs Co-ordinating Committee (set up late in 1977).

overseas doctors' registration and its conduct of disciplinary hearings, and resistant to the proposals for graduate training.[52] In 1977 a bill was introduced that promised to implement only two of the five major recommendations of the Merrison Report: the composition of the GMC, making it bigger and giving a majority to elected members, and the establishment of a health committee to deal with the problem of the sick doctor and his fitness to practise (one of the GMC's own proposals). According to David Ennals, the Secretary of State, lack of agreement within the medical profession meant that it was not possible to proceed further than this.[53] Disunity was not the prerogative of nurses. However, at this point Lord Hunt of Fawley, a London general practitioner, stepped in to negotiate with the different medical interests and to table amendments to the legislation. Lord Hunt began by invoking, in the manner of Merrison, the right of the medical profession to 'set its own standards'.[54] Speaking in the House of Lords in December 1977, Lord Hunt read a letter from Sir Alec Merrison giving broad support to his endeavours. Opposition from the Royal Colleges and Faculties to Merrison's recommendation regarding the establishment of an indicative specialist register by the GMC remained strong,[55] but by early in 1978 Lord Hunt had secured agreement on a clause giving the GMC the power to give guidance on ethical issues, and on the registration of overseas doctors. As Stacey has remarked, this represented a 'remarkable feat on the part of Lord Hunt and the BMA, all of whose PR resources were used. Lay involvement in the debates in both Houses was minimal'.[56] The contrast with the position of nursing is striking. Nurses did not have the kind of medico-political forces that were at the disposal of doctors and could not operate the kind of sophisticated informal negotiations and consultations undertaken by Lord Hunt. Medicine showed itself to be dominant within the political process (just as the GMC was at the centre of the machinery of regulation that included the NHS and government as well as the GMC) and this was crucial to securing the passage of the legislation.

Conclusion

The Merrison Report defined professional regulation in terms of a contract between public and profession, a position that has also been adopted by Dahrendorf in his defence of the English professions' contract with society rather than with the state.[57] However, this is to miss the way in which, first, the power of the medical

52   Stacey, *Regulating British Medicine*, pp. 62–3.
53   House of Commons, Debates, 2 August 1977, written answer, c. 347.
54   House of Lords, Debates, 29 November 1977, c. 1166.
55   E.g., M.D. Vickers, 'Specialist registration: a critical look at the proposals of the Merrison Report', *British Medical Journal*, 272 (1976), 328–31.
56   Stacey, *Regulating British Medicine*, p. 65.
57   R. Dahrendorf, 'In defence of the English professions', *Journal of the Royal Society of Medicine*, 77 (1984), 178–85.

profession has been upheld by the nature of its relationship with the state. By endorsing professional self-regulation, the state also tipped the balance in the contract between profession and public firmly in favour of the profession. Medicine was trusted to regulate itself in the public interest. The Merrison Committee began by recognizing this form of regulation as desirable. Doctors were, relative to nurses, a small, homogeneous and elite community and were assumed by the Merrison Committee (and by government) to be reasonable people who would act in the public interest. Furthermore, the passing of the legislation following the Merrison Report showed the extent to which the medical profession had sufficient status to be able to exert informal political influence.

The position of nursing was very different. The Briggs Report did insist on nursing's status as a separate profession, but as the divisions that opened up over the Report showed, nurses were both a large and heterogeneous body. Nursing had never been trusted to regulate itself in the same way as medicine; its regulatory structure had always been more rule-based. Furthermore, nursing lacked the power and status to exercise the kind of informal influence exerted by medicine. Dahrendorf's characterization of the relationship of the professions with state and society also misses the extent to which the favourable balance of relations with the state achieved by medicine helped it to retain its dominant position over other health care professions, particularly nursing. As Davies has remarked: 'A subordinated profession cannot secure the same level of institutional self-sufficiency and closure as a dominant one'.[58] The idea of professional self-regulation had never been accepted in respect of nursing and was not by the Briggs Committee, whereas it underpinned the whole structure of the Merrison Report on medicine.

Of course, the trust to behave in the public interest that underlay the idea of professional self-regulation for doctors has been severely undermined by medical scandals during the past decade. Thus the Labour Government stated in 1998 that 'the organization of professional self-regulation...owes more to history than to the needs of patients in a modern NHS' and gave notice of its intention to turn once more to the work of 'modernizing' the framework of regulation for clinical professionals.[59] Ian Kennedy's characterization of the kind of professional self-regulation enjoyed by doctors as 'an odd paternalistic kind of consumerism, in which the professional presumes to be the sympathetic advocate of the consumer's interests'[60] seems to be more in tune with today's than Dahrendorf's views, despite being written over twenty years ago. In the world of the 'new public management' and performance indicators, but also of more demand for a voice for lay people and patients, it seems unlikely that *self*-regulation will be an option for any profession.

---

58   C. Davies, 'What about the girl next door? Gender and the politics of professional self-regulation', in G. Bendelow, M. Carpenter, C. Vauier and S. Williams, eds, *Gender, Health and Healing: The Public/Private Divide* (London, 2002), pp. 91–107.

59   Department of Health, *A First Class Service: Quality in the new NHS* (London, 1998), paragraph 3.47.

60   Kennedy, *The Unmasking of Medicine*, p. 123.

Chapter 18

New Social Movement or Government-Funded Voluntary Sector? ASH (Action on Smoking and Health), Science, and Anti-Tobacco Activism in the 1970s

Virginia Berridge

The change after the Second World War from infectious to chronic disease as a major concern for health policy was epitomized by the rise of smoking as a health issue. The connection between smoking and lung cancer had been discussed pre-war, both as a putative connection and more definitely in research and health policy in Nazi Germany.[1] But the publication, by Doll and Hill in the UK, and by Wynder and Graham in the US, of epidemiological research demonstrating the link, marked the beginning of smoking's post-war health policy career. Webster has pointed to the initial reluctance of the British government to take up this issue in the 1950s and has commented that the 'powerful and complex' advisory machinery which operated between the Medical Research Council (MRC) and the newly established National Health Service (NHS) served to bring about a cautious response, aided by close relationships between government and industry and the smoking habits of senior politicians.[2]

The reports produced subsequently by the Royal College of Physicians (RCP), in particular the first report, *Smoking and Health*, published in 1962, and the second report, *Smoking and Health Now* (1971) changed this situation. They placed smoking more centrally on both the public and the policy agenda and were important forces in the initiation of a new style of public health.[3] It was during the 1970s

I am grateful to the Wellcome Trust who funded the original research on which this work was based. Thanks are due to Margaret Pelling, for editorial comments, and to Ingrid James for secretarial assistance.

1   R.N. Proctor, *The Nazi War on Cancer* (Princeton, 1999); G.D. Smith, S.A. Strobele, and M. Egger, 'Smoking and health promotion in Nazi Germany', *Journal of Epidemiology and Community Health*, 48 (1994), 220–3.
2   C. Webster, 'Tobacco smoking addiction: a challenge to the National Health Service', *British Journal of Addiction*, 79 (1984), 7–16.
3   V. Berridge, 'Post-war smoking policy in the UK and the redefinition of public

that this new public health agenda, stressing the role of lifestyle and of individual behavioural factors, fully emerged. Of particular importance for this new agenda and for smoking policy was an anti-tobacco organization, Action on Smoking and Health (ASH), which was founded in 1971 in the wake of the publication of the second RCP report. This chapter aims to trace the history of ASH and of its leading participants during the 1970s.

It is surprising how little has been written about post-war health activism. The importance of self-help groups in health has been acknowledged in general health histories and distinctions have been drawn between 'inwardly' and 'outwardly' focused groups, those catering for their members, and those with a wider campaigning function.4 The continued importance of voluntary organizations has been stressed by studies of the 'moving frontier' between post-war governments, the welfare state and traditions of voluntarism.5 One problem, which is addressed in this chapter, is how to characterize the nature of activist effort, including which set of theoretical and analytical frameworks is appropriate. Can this be set within new social movement theory, which, with some exceptions, has had little of an historical dimension?6 Or is this a study of the voluntary/state relationship, currently of interest in studies of service provision and health policy?7 Is it a study of consumerism in health? Or of the media, and 'agenda setting'?8 It is one of the arguments of this chapter that no one set of concepts, by itself, can fully explain the type of organizational style which ASH embodied and which became the norm for public health issues. Much existing theory also tends to skirt around the policy significance of activism – which, for an organization like ASH, was crucial. Here the use of concepts of policy networks and communities is helpful and will be drawn on in this chapter.

The origins of ASH

ASH was by no means the first anti-tobacco organization. Such groupings came and went in the nineteenth century. Like the temperance, inebriety, anti-opium and anti-alcohol movements, they drew on a crucial mix of medicine and morality. The issue of juvenile smoking saw more anti-smoking organizations established at the

   health', *Twentieth Century British History*, 14 (2003), 61–82.
4 C. Webster, *Caring for Health: History and Diversity* (3rd edn, Milton Keynes, 2001), pp. 227–8.
5 G. Finlayson, *Citizen, State and Social Welfare in Britain, 1830–1990* (Oxford, 1993).
6 N. Crossley, 'Transforming the mental health field: the early history of the National Association for Mental Health', *Sociology of Health and Illness*, 20 (1998), 458–88.
7 J. Mohan and M. Gorsky, *Don't Look Back? Voluntary and Charitable Finance of Hospitals in Britain, Past and Present* (London, 2001).
8 D.W. Greenberg, 'Staging media events to achieve legitimacy: a case study of Britain's Friends of the Earth', *Political Communication and Persuasion*, 2 (1985), 347–62; M. McCarthy, *Campaigning for the Poor. CPAG and the Politics of Welfare* (Beckenham, 1988).

end of the nineteenth century.[9] ASH's main predecessor in the twentieth century was the National Society of Non-Smokers (NSNS), founded in 1926. Its secretary for much of its existence after the Second World War was Tom Hurst, an Edinburgh hospital administrator; the NSNS concentrated on the 'clean air' and environmentally harmful aspects of smoking, but its appeal was based on moral endeavour rather than on science. It argued that it was selfish to smoke near others. Of the initial 146 promoters of the society, only 38 were active scientists and the rest were moralists, evangelists and social critics.[10] At its inception, the Society gained two thousand members in a few months, organized in local branches. The main aim was to protect the rights of non-smokers, not to stop all smoking, although the Society did oppose young people's smoking. Its campaign to secure premises with smoke-free areas had little success. The NSNS did not use science in its arguments at all and in general it regarded smoking as quite legitimate as long as it did not offend the sensibilities of others.

The appeal of ASH was rather different. It was founded in 1971, at the time of the publication of the second RCP report, *Smoking and Health Now*. But the need for some kind of external pressure group, although not necessarily on the ASH model, had been foreseen in the Ministry of Health long before ASH's foundation. If we look back ten years to the early 1960s, an exchange of views within the health department made this point clearly. During the discussions on what policy line should be followed in response to the first RCP report in 1962, various options – legal, fiscal and publicity – were on the agenda. The central problem was the widespread social acceptability of the habit, and the perceived fluidity of the 'scientific facts' surrounding smoking risk. What could justify action? Enid Russell-Smith of the Ministry of Health wrote perceptively:

> There is at present very little in the way of an anti-smoking lobby and it may well be that at the present intermediate stage, when the nature of the connection between smoking and lung cancer has still not been fully established, the most effective measure to limit smoking would be the promotion of a voluntary anti-smoking movement. It would be much easier for the Government and the local authorities to take regulatory measures against smoking if there were a body of opinion pressing them to do so.[11]

9   R.B. Walker, 'Medical aspects of tobacco smoking and the anti-tobacco movement in Britain in the nineteenth century', *Medical History*, 24 (1980), 391–402; M. Hilton and S. Nightingale, '"A microbe of the devil's own make": religion and science in the British anti-tobacco movement, 1853–1908', in S. Lock, L. Reynolds and E.M. Tansey, eds, *Ashes to Ashes: The History of Smoking and Health* (Amsterdam, 1998), pp. 41–77; J. Welshman, 'Images of youth: the problem of juvenile smoking', *Addiction*, 91 (1996), 1379–86.

10   M. Hilton, 'Constructing tobacco: perspectives on consumer culture in Britain, 1850–1950', unpublished University of Lancaster Ph.D. thesis (1996), p. 238.

11   Public Record Office, Ministry of Health papers, MH 55/2204: Minute from Enid Russell-Smith, 5 February 1962.

The setting up of ASH, some nine years later, illustrated this interaction between anti-smoking sentiment among civil servants and public health activists outside. It was an example of the political science concept of the policy community, linking interests in and outside government.[12] The initial planned focus for the organization was the dissemination of information. In 1969, after an internal departmental group had reviewed progress on smoking and health, the Central Health Services Council decided to advise the Secretary of State for Social Services to encourage the establishment of a body comparable to the US Inter-Agency Council and to establish a section in the Department of Health and Social Security (DHSS) able to collate the large amount of information coming forward about smoking and health. After some delay, the internal section was set up under a Senior Medical Officer, Dr Julia Dawkins, who had previously been in the Department of Education dealing with drugs and sex education. But the Minister, presumably Crossman at this stage, was doubtful about the value of setting up a body comparable to the Inter-Agency Council and so the initiative did not come directly from government.[13]

Doctors with public health interests had been having similar discussions since the late 1960s. There was a need for a 'central information point', and also a body which, as a group of doctors independent of the Ministry, would be able to exert more pressure.[14] The eventual initiative for the founding of ASH came from Dr Charles Fletcher, secretary of the first two RCP committees, and Dr Keith Ball, a doctor with a strong interest in public health. Ball worked at the Central Middlesex Hospital, a powerhouse of social medicine sentiment.[15] However, Dr Dawkins was also closely involved. ASH's foundation was central to moves by anti-smoking interests to secure government action and to publicize the risks of smoking to the public in the wake of the 1971 report. There was some discussion initially about what the new organization should be called. Names suggested at a steering committee in October 1970 included National Council on Smoking and Health (NCSH), British Association on Smoking and Health (BASH), Council or Commission for Action on Smoking and Health (CASH) and the subsequently adopted ASH.[16] The form the organization might take was also fluid at this stage. Dawkins saw it as 'a group of members of the various professions, including industry, who were concerned with tobacco', while Fletcher and Max Rosenheim, President of

12 D. Marsh and R.A.W. Rhodes, *Policy Networks in British Government* (Oxford, 1992).
13 Public Record Office, Ministry of Health papers, MH 154/619,1969–1971; London, Royal College of Physicians, Working party proposals for a national council, Registration, membership and organization of ASH (Action on Smoking and Health Ltd).
14 London, Wellcome Library for the History and Understanding of Medicine, ASH archive, SA/ASH/C.8, Box 7: Letter from Keith Ball to Charles Fletcher, 5 February 1968.
15 Webster, 'Tobacco smoking addiction', p. 11.
16 Wellcome Library for the History and Understanding of Medicine, ASH archive, Box 70, SA/ASH/Q. 3/2/1: Meeting of steering committee, 19 October 1970.

the RCP, initially saw it as a 'very large group of people representing all sorts of organizations', which was to be sponsored by the College. The American model of an Inter-Agency Council was clearly influential, along with similar Australian organizations, although it was subsequently agreed that those models would not be applicable in the UK.

Sir George Godber, Chief Medical Officer, had already stimulated action through the RCP in the 1960s in order to goad government into action.[17] He saw ASH as fulfilling a similar ongoing irritant function, in alliance with the newly established (1968) Health Education Council (HEC). In a 1969 minute, he commented:

> If the RCP will start it and the HEC also take part we would have something very different from the interdepartmental committee. A voluntary group may be a thorn in our flesh – but only if we are inert and deserve it. This is one of our biggest health problems. We made a start five years before the Americans and they are really doing something now while we are in the doldrums. We really must show we are in earnest.[18]

The initial aims of the proposed national council were a mixture of risk reduction and risk elimination; to maintain pressure on government to bring in legislation; to increase efforts to discourage smoking among all sections of the population; but also to encourage less hazardous forms of smoking and to consider the economic problems related to a reduction of cigarette smoking.[19] This risk reduction objective was part of the public health agenda for smoking at the time; but later drafts of ASH's aims dropped the explicit commitment to it. This was a portent of the future stance of the organization.

The launch of ASH in January 1971 was attended by between 150 and 200 people representing around 75 organizations. The Council of the new body was primarily medical, but with input from both new-style (advertising and the media) organizations, and traditional voluntary bodies: Lady Anglesea, past chair of the National Federation of Women's Institutes, represented women's interests. (She thought there should be pipes suitable for women.) Dr John Dunwoody, a former junior Minister in the Department of Health and ex-MP, was part-time secretary. In a letter enclosing a launch leaflet which he sent to Dawkins in 1971, he clearly envisaged a media and public opinion role for ASH:

> ASH intends to examine the problem very thoroughly; it will not be just a clearing house for posters. ASH will sponsor research into why people smoke and into

17   C.C. Booth, 'Smoking and the gold-headed cane', in C.C. Booth, ed., *Balancing Act: Essays to Honour Stephen Lock* (London, 1991), pp. 49–55.

18   Public Record Office, Ministry of Health papers, MH 154/169: Minute from George Godber, 18 June 1969.

19   Public Record Office, Ministry of Health papers, MH 154/169: Aims of proposed national council, 2 June 1970.

patterns of smoking. It will also act as a pressure group and as a centre for information on smoking and health...the most important activity that ASH will undertake will be an advertising campaign to discourage people from smoking.

Dunwoody wanted to drop the 'Black Widow' approach of the road accident campaigns, which had aimed to shock drivers into responsible behaviour. Instead, he envisaged marketing social acceptability. Financial and material incentives were to be encouraged, with group therapy on the lines of Weight Watchers, and a focus on children and young people. 'Primarily the campaign will attempt to take the social cachet that surrounds smoking and turn it on its head.'[20] But Dunwoody's proposals initially ruffled feathers. Dawkins had seen ASH as a high-powered professional body, but these ideas infringed on the territory of the Health Education Council. The HEC was annoyed at the overlap with its role. Max Rosenheim apologized and ASH's launch leaflet was hastily withdrawn.

The arrival of Daube and the media agenda

This initial contretemps left the organization without much of an activist role. For the first year or two its activities centred on a group of supporting doctors, writing letters to the *Lancet*. The harm reduction focus of the 1960s continued. In 1973, the organization set up an expert group to look at the issue of the safety of pipes and cigars, about which it had received many enquiries. Switching to a pipe or smoking cigars instead of cigarettes were widely advocated as harm/risk reduction strategies. The expert group came up with no clear answer, although it concluded that it was likely that risk was reduced. There was, however, a risk to others from 'so called "passive smoking"'. But this risk was minute. This report was reproduced as a leaflet by the HEC.[21]

Dunwoody's departure in 1973 and the arrival of Mike Daube as Director brought a change of emphasis and style. Daube brought with him a campaigning stance from his previous work at the housing charity Shelter, which had pioneered a media and publicity-conscious approach to social issues. He was strongly influenced by the new style of campaigning which the Director of Shelter, Des Wilson, had introduced. He also had a background in student politics. A letter he wrote to Charles Fletcher in 1973 about a funding application gives a flavour of this style:

20   Public Record Office, Ministry of Health papers, MH 154/169: Letter from Dunwoody to Dawkins, 5 January 1971.
21   Health Education Council (later Authority, now Health Development Agency), Leaflet archive, 14950.1, 'Pipe and cigar smoking: report of an expert group appointed by ASH'. Reprinted from *The Practitioner*, 210 (1973). The current location of the HEA archive is unknown.

I have tried to define the areas of commitment fairly widely, while also conforming to the requirement that they be controversial. I suspect that one of the reasons for ASH's failure has been that it has been to a large extent a reacting organization, rather than one that has set out to create news...so the suggestions that I have made in this application...are concerned with creating news in a way that could have a fair impact on the anti-smoking campaign.[22]

In an interview he gave to an Australian journalist, William Norman, in the mid-1970s, he argued in a similar way:

It seemed to me when I came into ASH that here was a pressure campaign that was ripe. It hadn't been properly used. You had your villain. You had your St. George and the dragon scenario, you had your growing ecology bandwagon, growing interest in consumerism. It seemed there were a lot of prospects of making something out of it.[23]

An indication of this new approach came shortly after Daube's appointment when he wrote a piece for the journal *Adweek*, attacking the textile firm Courtaulds for 'irresponsible action' in marketing Planet, a tobacco substitute, before it had been reviewed by the Department's Independent Scientific Committee on Smoking and Health (ISCSH). Courtaulds threatened a libel action, although this was never ultimately brought to court. In Daube's view, the furore was a good thing. 'The first thing it did was to show that we had teeth. I think if I were being a little honest and a little arrogant, I would say Courtaulds established ASH as a pressure group.'[24]

This was the tone of ASH's activities throughout the 1970s. It was intensely media-conscious. The organization bought shares (or one share) in tobacco companies and would then turn up to ask awkward questions at the AGM. It collaborated on a Thames TV, *This Week* programme; it worked with journalists like Peter Taylor whose anti-smoking programmes had a clear impact. Daube operated according to the American activist text, *Rules for Radicals*: 'rule one is to personalize the problem – the people running the major companies are responsible for those deaths.'[25]

The medical and health correspondents, a newly emergent occupational group, – Ronnie Bedford at the *Daily Mirror*, Nicholas Timmins at the Press Association, Oliver Gillie and Christine Doyle – were vital allies. A major aim was to keep tobacco on the front pages; the story did not matter, but the media coverage did. Daube favoured ASH's move to new offices at the Family Planning Association in

22 Wellcome Library for the History and Understanding of Medicine, ASH archive, SA/ASH/0.4/3, Box 71: Letter from Mike Daube to Charles Fletcher, 3 August 1973.
23 Wellcome Library for the History and Understanding of Medicine, ASH archive, SA/ASH, William Norman collection, R. 12, Box 77: Interview with Mike Daube, no date but c.1975–6.
24 *Ibid.*
25 Author's collection, Mike Daube, interview with Virginia Berridge, 11 March 1999: Notes of interview.

Mortimer Street mainly because the organization would be closer to the BBC in Portland Place. The organization did not just react to news, but also created it in a way which has become more familiar since. Daube described to Norman how he set up a media storm over the production of a low-tar cigarette called Westminster Abbey. He got onto a journalist and suggested:

> 'I wonder what Westminster Abbey think about that, why don't you ask them.' She phoned up W.A. and they said, no, we don't know about it. Ten minutes later I phoned up as Mike Daube from ASH and they said, 'Funny, we have just had a journalist on to us asking about this'. I said, 'really, well it shows how wide the interest is'.[26]

Then a piece was brought out in *Adweek*, and Westminster Abbey sent Daube a copy. He wrote to the Dean of the Abbey complaining, the Dean consulted lawyers, and he and the journalists were phoning up and keeping in touch. It was what Daube called the 'rapier and stiletto' approach – now better known as 'spin'.

Remembered by Keith Ball twenty years later as 'a young man with long hair and a purple suit', Daube made ASH important as a political force in the 1970s.[27] The political climate helped. Edward Heath was a non-smoker who made Cabinet meetings non-smoking and initiated a cross-departmental study of smoking policy options. Daube helped to set up the Commons All Party group on smoking in 1976, which, although chaired by the Labour MP Laurie Pavitt, had active members from the Conservative Party, among them the MPs Lynda Chalker and Sir George Young.

Relations with government: Owen and the Medicines Act Initiative

Perhaps the greatest period of influence came during the Labour government of 1974–9 during David Owen's tenure as Minister of Health from 1974–6. Owen was a keen non-smoker whose moves to do something about smoking were tolerated by the overall Departmental Minister, the smoker, Barbara Castle.[28] Owen spoke at a joint ASH/HEC conference on smoking in 1974, 'Smoking – Whose Problem?'[29] He had plans to bring tobacco substitutes, being tested under the aegis of the ISCSH, under the regulatory provisions of the 1968 Medicines Act so that they would be controlled like medicines. The implication was that tobacco would eventually go down that route, too. The ISCSH would be upgraded into the

26   ASH Archive, Norman interview with Daube.
27   Comment at witness seminar at 'Ashes to Ashes' conference on smoking at Wellcome Institute, 26–7 April 1995: author's notes.
28   B. Castle, *The Castle Diaries, 1964–1976* (London, 1990), entry for Tuesday, 5 August 1975, p. 641.
29   Wellcome Library for the History and Understanding of Medicine, ASH Archive, SA/AHS/M.1/6, Box 51.

licensing body on the model of the Committee on the Safety of Drugs. The sequence of events in 1976 showed ASH's insider/outsider relationship clearly. The MP Robert Kilroy-Silk, a close friend of David Owen, came top of the ballot for a ten-minute bill and asked Owen what he should do with it. Owen wanted action on tobacco, so Kilroy-Silk's motion, as eventually put to the House on 16 January 1976, proposed action under section 105 of the 1968 Medicines Act. If passed, this would bring 'tobacco and smoking substances which are not themselves medicinal products, but if used without proper safeguards are capable of causing damage to the health of the community', under the regulatory provisions of the Act.[30] Tobacco and tobacco substitutes would be controlled just like medicines.

In the interview conducted at the time with William Norman, Daube described how ASH was a vital conduit in the process. Owen could not offer Kilroy-Silk any direct DHSS help for his bill, but there was nothing to stop the Minister asking his department to brief Daube and ASH on a hypothetical situation which related to its content. A 'very senior civil servant' discussed the terms with Daube, for reference to Kilroy-Silk. Kilroy-Silk's intervention, aided by ASH, brought matters to a head and secured Owen the leverage he needed to go ahead against the various competing interests. At the same time, ASH maintained its oppositional role, selectively leaking information to urge the Minister on to more significant action.[31] Owen himself referred to this role (although not to the behind-the-scenes moves concerning Kilroy-Silk) in an interview at the time. He was 'orchestrating his moves' round the Medicines Act option – he used the Commons, ASH attacked him, and there were also informal contacts with sympathetic parts of industry.[32] ASH was also in discussion with the Treasury, helping to secure the higher cigarette taxation policies of the Labour Chancellor, Denis Healey.[33] A similar relationship operated over the answering of Parliamentary Questions (PQs), where Daube would be rung up from within government for help in answering them; and sometimes he encouraged the 'planting' of PQs.

But there was always a limit to the overt opposition:

> With several PQs I have discussed with them what the terms of the PQ should be. Because I want to embarrass them, obviously, in some ways, but I don't want to ask the kind of really embarrassing question. It is not my job just to make life difficult.[34]

---

30 Hansard, *House of Commons Debates*, 16 January 1976, Vol. 93–4, cols 785–871.
31 Norman interview with Daube.
32 Wellcome Library for the History and Understanding of Medicine, ASH archive, SA/ASH, William Norman collection, R.24, Box 79: Interview with David Owen, 20 January 1976.
33 M. Daube, 'The politics of smoking: thoughts on the Labour record', *Community Medicine*, 1 (1979), 306–14.
34 ASH archive, Norman interview with Daube.

This was, indeed, as two ASH activists recalled in an interview in the 1990s, the 'golden age' so far as the organization was concerned.[35] ASH fulfilled an important facilitating role within the political process, with networks between government and this outside organization. It achieved this role within politics while at the same time becoming a high-profile public presence. In fact, its media profile was part of its attraction to politicians because it made it appear a 'force to be reckoned with' and therefore useful as a counterweight to the stance of industry and of other government departments. 'Doctors weren't good at publicity', said one of the ASH pioneers.[36] This was not entirely the case, since Charles Fletcher himself had been a pioneer in the medical use of the media with his programme, *Your Life in Their Hands*, in the 1950s.[37] The 1962 report had been launched by the Royal College of Physicians with great media flair. ASH remained an organization in which doctors were important. Doctors remained in a majority on the Council and Daube himself never went further than those in overall charge wanted. His role was that of a useful stalking horse. For example, he told Norman of an exchange where Charles Fletcher had called him and reported on a lunch with Robert Hunter, chairman of the ISCSH. Hunter had been at a meeting with Owen and the industry and had told Fletcher that Owen was proposing a pact with industry. Fletcher could not do anything with the story – but Daube could. He felt that the pressure put on Owen by this sort of selective leak was an important force, 'the best thing to happen for ten years'.[38]

ASH and the new public health agenda

Daube was a key mediator of the new science of anti-smoking. The role of public health science, the epidemiology of smoking, was of central importance in the organization. The scientists, Doll and Hill, did not see themselves as campaigners. Daube thought that, in a way, they were right. 'The researcher is seen to lose his objectivity as soon as he becomes a campaigner.' He was the pressure group tactical expert and this was his job within the organization. Yet ASH set up a research committee and the role of science was central to its mission.

However Daube was also instrumental in changing the policy agenda which had been developed since the 1950s. The new position was more opposed to industry and aimed at the elimination of the habit rather than its modification. There had always been those in the public health field who took this stance. Sir Robert Platt, for example, the President of the RCP who had encouraged the

35   Author's collection, interview with Ann McNeill and Patti White by Virginia Berridge, 10 November 1997.
36   Author's collection, interview with Keith Ball by Virginia Berridge, 5 December 1997.
37   K. Loughlin, '"Your Life in their Hands": the context of a medical-media controversy', *Media History*, 6 (2000), 177–88.
38   ASH archive, Norman interview with Daube.

publication of its first report, and Dr Keith Ball, one of ASH's founders, had always been opposed to links with industry. Charles Fletcher, in contrast, had favoured co-operation with industry, and there were industrial interests who took the same line. Fletcher was in contact with Geoffrey Todd, Director of the Tobacco Research Council, an industry-funded organization, who had provided valuable criticism of the statistics in the first RCP report.[39] He had also approached Sir John Partridge, Chairman of Imperial Tobacco, when ASH was launching an appeal for funds in 1972.[40] But this overall consensus for public health ended in the course of the 1970s.[41] The end of Owen's strategy of regulation (abandoned after he moved to the Foreign Office) and a feeling that ASH had 'marked time' while this strategy was in play politically also contributed to the new hostile public health stance.[42] ASH had submitted evidence to the Royal Commission on Civil Liability and Compensation in 1973–4 recommending that tobacco manufacturers be liable both for the harm caused by their cigarettes and for the establishment of a compensation fund. It was this hostility which was to develop further into a new agenda for public health by the end of the decade.

ASH had worked throughout the 1970s with the HEC, which was chaired by George Godber after his retirement as Chief Medical Officer. A briefing note for a meeting with Owen in 1975 showed that the earlier confusion about their respective roles had been resolved. The HEC was to pursue research, education and publicity activities; ASH was to act as a campaigning organization and catalyst, operating as a pressure group. At the end of the decade, the two organizations took a notably antagonistic stance to the launch of tobacco substitutes like New Smoking Material. They were concerned that part-substitute brands like NSM and Cytrel still contained 75 per cent tobacco and could be stronger than cigarettes already on the market.[43] The major press conference mounted by Imperial Tobacco to launch its part-substitute brands, held the day after the launch of the RCP's third report, *Smoking or Health*, effectively upstaged the Royal College. ASH was concerned, as letters from Daube to Jim Welch (a civil servant at the DHSS) make clear, that the publicity for substitutes would slow the downward trend in smoking which was becoming apparent in the 1970s.[44] The Council's advertisement in 1977 which said that smoking substitutes was like jumping from the 36th instead of the 39th floor of a tall building marked the end of any adherence to a harm-reduction

39   Wellcome Library for the History and Understanding of Medicine, ASH archive, Box 73, SA/AHS/Q.4/3: Letter from Fletcher to Harry Milt of American Cancer Society, 12 December 1973.

40   *Ibid.*, Letter from Fletcher to Partridge, 22 September 1972.

41   Although it continued as an objective in parts of the policy network. See Berridge, 'Post-war smoking policy', p. 2003.

42   Daube, 'The politics of smoking'.

43   Wellcome Library for the History and Understanding of Medicine, ASH archive, Box 23, SA/ASH/G.1: Letter from Daube to David Ennals, 24 June 1977.

44   Wellcome Library for the History and Understanding of Medicine, ASH archive, SA/ASH/G.3/1, Box 71: Letter from Daube to Jim Welch, DHSS, 6 July 1977.

approach. The aim, said the Council's report for 1978, was 'deterrence', a new terminology which epitomized the war between some public health interests and the industry.[45]

This new agenda for smoking was part of a larger agenda for public health and prevention encapsulated in the government's prevention documents at the end of the 1970s, and was part of a wider international movement.[46] The HEC itself, with its advertising campaigns formulated by the advertising agency, Saatchi and Saatchi, also showed a distinctively different approach. The 'new public health' concentrated on relationships and on the responsibility of the individual. Self-discipline, central publicity and habit-changing campaigns were central to its ethos. So far as smoking was concerned, the height of this new approach was to come in the 1980s with the elaboration of the science of passive smoking. But already, at the end of the 1970s, ASH was moving its policy agenda in this direction. The issue of the non-smoker was initially a moral one, one of human rights, as some of the activities at the end of the decade demonstrate. Fletcher had not been in favour of concentrating over-much on the 'nuisance' aspects of smoking – he saw this as a moral issue rather than a scientific one. By the end of the 1970s, Daube was moving ASH's focus towards the human-rights issues involved in smoking. Important in this respect was a conference held at the Kings Fund (date probably about 1977–8) on 'The Rights of the Non Smoker'.[47] The epidemiological case was to follow in the early 1980s.[48]

Centre and periphery: London and Scotland

ASH was new in its use of the media, and its organizational structure also made new departures for a pressure group. Its membership was around the 500-mark in the 1970s, but Daube did not wish to broaden it further. Such efforts would be pointless: a large membership, if it needed to be regularly serviced, would use up resources and be more of a hindrance than a help. ASH did develop some local branches in the 1970s, but these were few in number. The focus of the organization instead reflected its emphasis on London, the media and on political lobbying, as

45   Health Education Council, *Annual Report 1977–78* (London, 1978), p. 11.
46   C. Webster, *The Health Services since the War. Volume 2, Government and Health Care: The British National Health Service 1958–1979* (London, 1996), pp. 676–80; C. Webster and J. French, 'The cycle of conflict: the history of public health and health promotion movements', in L. Adams, M. Amos, and J. Munro, eds, *Promoting Health. Politics and Practice* (London, 2002), pp. 5–12.
47   ASH Box 36 (old system; currently untraceable): Letter from Daube to David Ennals, 18 February 1977.
48   V. Berridge, 'Passive smoking and its pre-history in Britain: policy speaks to science?', *Social Science and Medicine*, special historical issue, 'Science Speaks to Policy', 49 (1999), 1183–95.

for example through its involvement in the Commons All Party Group on Smoking.

But there was an important centre of activity outside London. This was Scottish ASH in Edinburgh. Founded in 1972 in a corner of the Royal College of Physicians of Edinburgh, it was originally local-authority funded, with the Scottish Office taking over after local government reorganization in 1975. Its work was different to that of ASH in London. It carried out projects and had project funding for action research: a dominant theme was to do something about advertising. The influence of Lady (Eileen) Crofton, who was the first Director, and her husband, Sir John Crofton, was considerable, as was that of the subsequent Director, Alison Hillhouse. They had close links into government and the Scottish health establishment. Scottish ASH was very much independent, but Crofton and Daube got on well, so the combination worked. The campaign initiated in 1985–6 against the chewing tobacco, Skoal Bandits, was highly successful and resulted in a ban.[49] The Scottish dimension to anti-smoking policy was an important one in many respects, and there were differences between Scottish and English activism on smoking, underlined by the differences between the two organizations. Scottish ASH ran community projects and also, through the work of Eileen Crofton and Alison Hillhouse, initiated work on children and smoking. Its activities gave the impetus to the growing interest in women and smoking in the anti-smoking field in the 1980s.[50] It, too, saw science as central and the Croftons set up a research committee for Scottish ASH.[51] The activities of the separate Scottish organization and its close links into Scottish public health policy emphasized the importance of the interest group in the Scottish as well as the English policy community.

ASH was not primarily a membership organization and increasingly in the 1970s its funding came, not from traditional voluntary sources, but from government. An ASH development committee chaired by the comedian Brian Rix, with support from Clement Freud, Spike Milligan and Norman Vaughan, launched a £200,000 appeal, but raised little.[52] Initial pump-priming funding from government was replaced by an ongoing DHSS grant. By 1978, it was reported that 90 per cent of ASH's income came from the DHSS. The organization expanded, with a deputy Director, an information officer and other posts. In 1977, the grant was £31,000 with donations standing at just over £5,000. In addition, there was a special government grant of £80,000 to enable ASH to deal with over half a million responses it had received to a television programme on stopping smoking.

49   M. Raw, P. White, and A. McNeill, *Clearing the Air. A Guide for Action on Tobacco* (London, 1990), pp. 100–12.

50   Author's collection, interview by Virginia Berridge with Eileen and John Crofton, 17 March 1999; E. Crofton, 'Some notes on the women's committee of ASH. A personal account by Eileen Crofton' (MS, 1999), copy in Virginia Berridge's possession.

51   Sir John Crofton, personal papers, autobiography: MS copies in Virginia Berridge's possession.

52   SA/ASH/5.7.

The later history of ASH is beyond the scope of this chapter. In the 1980s, under a Conservative government, it was less influential at the policy level. In the 1980s, too, the anti-tobacco alliance broadened with new players like the British Medical Association (BMA) joining in. ASH became one among several organizations and no longer the dominant force on the UK anti-smoking scene. The movement became an international one, stretching out to networks in Australia and the Far East, and it also developed local roots on a more extensive scale. The ASH model was used for other health-activist organizations in the UK like the Coronary Prevention Group (CPG); these also attracted government funding.

In the 1970s, ASH had pioneered a new style of health activism and voluntarism, centrally run and media-focused. It was a mediating organization also in another sense of that word. It mediated between health interests in government and those outside. Its funding by health interests in government and its use as a negotiating counterweight and 'stalking horse' showed how activists in these types of organizations formed part of the policy community round smoking, how they were locked into a relationship with government in which their assumed independence was one of their greatest assets. ASH was a useful organization for government, not least because of its high public profile. But it mediated in another way too, between scientists, their scientific claims and their possible policy and public context. Organizations like ASH were important in making scientific claims in both public and policy arenas. ASH helped stimulate that media role for science which has become so important in health policy-making in the subsequent decades.

How to make sense of these developments? In its combination of morality and science and its increasing focus on 'the trade', ASH recalled the older nineteenth-century models of temperance and the anti-opium movement.[53] In its funding relationship with government, it can be seen as both inheritor of earlier traditions of voluntarism, and harbinger of later close relationships between voluntarism and the state in the 1990s, in particular through the issue of government-funded voluntarism.[54] Commentators have ascribed the demise of the voluntary sector to the years after community care in the 1990s when government funding of such organizations altered their role and ethos. ASH was not a voluntary organization providing services.[55] Nevertheless the role of government funding of ASH and its successor campaigning organizations like the CPG can be seen as one precursor of the state-funded voluntary sector of the 1990s.

The tone and activity of ASH were also within the New Social Movement tradition. Here some parallels can be drawn with activism in respect of mental health. Crossley, in his examination of this phenomenon, has argued that anti-psychiatry was a New Social Movement, a top-down development from within

53   B. Harrison, *Drink and the Victorians* (reprinted edn, Keele, 1994).
54   R. Whelan, *Involuntary Action: How Voluntary is the 'Voluntary' Sector?* (London, 1999).
55   Some of its founders, Ball for example, had been active in setting up anti-smoking clinics. But generally these were peripheral in the 1970s and of small importance within the organization overall.

psychiatry, which was taken up and amplified by the New Left.[56] ASH in the 1970s also reflected this trajectory, although the parallels are not exact. The organization was initiated 'from above' by doctors, but carried forward by a radical, human rights style of campaigning by a PR expert with a background in left politics and in the new organizational style of pressure group epitomized by Shelter. ASH's Council was doctor-dominated, but also had members from campaigning backgrounds in general – for example Joan Ruddock of Oxford Housing Aid. It was a mixture of professional and campaigning activists. How did its subsequent influence compare with that of the mental health movement? Crossley comments that the influence of anti-psychiatry was exerted less within the profession and more on the subsequent development of the user movement. But ASH was different. It influenced the style of new public health campaigning organizations, and the agenda of public health more generally by the late 1970s. It was of course not the only animating force. The influences on the new public health agenda emerging at the end of the decade were many and various, but ASH's media-conscious, radical anti-industry style was important. It also influenced, as its later work on involuntary smoking illustrates, the 'non-user movement' of the 1990s, the activist organizations which coalesced round the 'scientific fact' of passive smoking. Writers on the NSM field have stressed the importance of science as a motivating force for such organizations and this also was the case for ASH.[57] Its public case rested on the technical and value-free agendas of science. It was essentially a professionalized case for action.

Some writers on NSM have located these movements within Bourdieu's concept of a 'field'; but theories of policy-making should also be considered. ASH was part of a network of interests within policy round the smoking issue which interacted in a pluralist way with government.[58] ASH was both an insider and an outsider organization. Its value to government in the 1970s rested on its outside image, while in reality its influence was exerted within government. ASH worked across the public health, parliamentary and media fields.

Its influence on the social positioning of smoking is more difficult to assess than its policy involvement. Smoking was beginning to decline by the end of the 1970s, even among women, where its prevalence had risen later than among men. The cross-class nature of smoking was beginning to shade into smoking as primarily a lower-class activity.[59] ASH contributed to this change of social positioning, but whether its policy influence or its public face and activities were most important is difficult to assess. It helped in media agenda-setting, but this in turn interacted with the changing beliefs and practices of media consumers, which were also influenced by government policies. Ultimately the importance of ASH

56   Crossley, 'Transforming the mental health field'.
57   R. Eyerman and A. Jamison, *Social Movements: A Cognitive Approach* (Cambridge, 1991).
58   C. Ham, *Health Policy in Britain* (Basingstoke, 1999).
59   Berridge, 'Post-war smoking policy', pp. 62–3. This class gradient was clearly in place by the 1990s.

was in its positioning as a boundary organization, as public and policy mediator of science into activism, as government-funded insider/outsider organization within policy-making networks, *and* as New Social Movement.

Select Publications of Charles Webster

Margaret Pelling

The bibliography is confined to published writing related to historical research. Annual reports on the work of the Wellcome Unit for the History of Medicine, for example, are omitted. Only longer book reviews, mainly essay reviews, have been included because of the numbers involved. Journals for which reviews are known to have been written are listed at the end of the bibliography. Some more recent short pieces (especially those on the National Health Service) may be missing. At least one short item, on local government and the National Health Service, was published in the 1980s under a variant of Webster's birth name of Karl Harrer; I have been unable to locate a source for this. Contributions to edited volumes are entered separately, but for untitled introductions see the entry for that volume. Later editions, or reprints, are listed under the date of first publication. Extracts from a number of publications were reprinted, with a short bibliography, in a collection on Puritanism, science and the Merton thesis edited in 1990 by I. Bernard Cohen; the section on Charles Webster's work was edited, with commentary, by Harold Cook. Details are entered separately below.

Most databases (including that of the Bodleian) include under Charles Webster's name a eulogium on the Italian historian Federico Chabod, published in 1960. I take responsibility for deciding that this is not by Webster. Some databases similarly include as his short pieces on nursing published in the 1970s and early 1980s by Colin Webster.

Ideally, the bibliography should include a section on 'other media', since Charles Webster has contributed extensively to radio and TV programmes. He was involved in at least one video project, the Institute of Historical Research's series, 'Interviews with Historians', c. 1988, in which he interviewed Margaret Gowing; this is still available commercially. However, given that such material is difficult to track down, and is generally not accessible to readers, I have not attempted to list it.

Archival and other materials relating to Charles Webster's work on the National Health Service are now on deposit at Oxford Brookes University.

I should like to thank my fellow editor, the contributors, Uffe Juul Jensen, and James Munro of *Health Matters* for helping to make this bibliography as complete as possible.

1963

'Richard Towneley and Boyle's law', *Nature*, 197 (1963), 226–8

1965

'The discovery of Boyle's law, and the concept of the elasticity of air in the seventeenth century', *Archive for History of Exact Sciences*, 2 (1965), 441–502
'William Harvey's conception of the heart as a pump', *Bulletin of the History of Medicine*, 39 (1965), 508–17

1966

'The recognition of plant sensitivity by English botanists in the seventeenth century', *Isis*, 57 (1966), 5–23
'Water as the ultimate principle of nature: the background to Boyle's Sceptical Chymist', *Ambix*, 13 (1966), 96–107
'Richard Towneley, 1629–1707, the Towneley group and seventeenth-century science', *Transactions of the Historic Society of Lancashire and Cheshire*, 118 (1966), 51–76. Extracts repr. in I.B. Cohen, K.E. Duffin and S. Strickland, eds, *Puritanism and the Rise of Modern Science: The Merton Thesis* (New Brunswick, NJ, Rutgers University Press, 1990), pp. 269–72.

1967

'English medical reformers of the Puritan Revolution: a background to the "Society of Chymical Physitians"', *Ambix*, 14 (1967), 16–41
'Harvey's *De generatione*: its origins and relevance to the theory of circulation', *British Journal for the History of Science*, 3 (1967), 262–74
'The College of Physicians: "Solomon's House" in Commonwealth England', *Bulletin of the History of Medicine*, 41 (1967), 393–412
'William Harvey's Biological Ideas' [essay review], *Ambix*, 14 (1967), 140–4
'Henry Power's experimental philosophy', *Ambix*, 14 (1967), 150–78
'The origins of the Royal Society' [essay review], *History of Science*, 6 (1967), 106–28

1969

'Henry More and Descartes: some new sources', *British Journal for the History of Science*, 4 (1969), 359–77

1970

(editor) *Samuel Hartlib and the Advancement of Learning* (Cambridge, Cambridge University Press, 1970). Introduction, pp. 1–72. Extracts from the Introduction repr. in Cohen, Duffin and Strickland, *Puritanism and the Rise of Modern Science* (1990) [see above], pp. 276–9.

'Macaria: Samuel Hartlib and the Great Reformation', *Acta Comeniana*, 26 (1970), 147–64

'Oxford's first revolutionaries', *Pelican*, 1 (1970), 75–7

1971

'Decimalization under Cromwell', *Nature*, 229 (1971), 463

'Science and the challenge to the scholastic curriculum 1640–1660', in *The Changing Curriculum*, History of Education Society Symposium (London, Methuen, 1971), pp. 21–35

'The Helmontian George Thomson and William Harvey: the revival and application of splenectomy to physiological research', *Medical History*, 15 (1971), 154–67

'The origins of blood transfusion: a reassessment', *Medical History*, 15 (1971), 387–92

(with C.B. Schmitt) 'Harvey and M.A. Severino: a neglected medical relationship', *Bulletin of the History of Medicine*, 45 (1971), 49–75. Reprinted in C.B. Schmitt, *Reappraisals in Renaissance Thought* (1989) [see below].

1972

(with C.B. Schmitt) 'Marco Aurelio Severino and his relationship to William Harvey: some preliminary considerations', in A.G. Debus, ed., *Science, Medicine and Society in the Renaissance: Essays to Honor Walter Pagel* (2 vols, New York, Science History Publications, 1972), ii, pp. 63–72

'The authorship and significance of *Macaria*', *Past and Present*, no. 56 (1972), 34–48. Reprinted in Webster, ed., *The Intellectual Revolution of the Seventeenth Century* (1974), pp. 369–85 [see below].

1973

'William Dell and the idea of university', in M. Teich and R. Young, eds, *Changing Perspectives in the History of Science: Essays in Honour of Joseph Needham* (London, Heinemann, 1973), pp. 110–26

1974

(editor) *The Intellectual Revolution of the Seventeenth Century* (London, Routledge and Kegan Paul, 1974). Introduction, pp. 1–22.

'New light on the Invisible College: the social relations of English science in the mid-seventeenth century', *Transactions of the Royal Historical Society*, 5th ser., 24 (1974), 19–42

'Science [and medicine]', in G. Watson, ed., *The New Cambridge Bibliography of English Literature, Vol. I: 600–1660* (Cambridge, Cambridge University Press, 1974), cols 2343–80

1975

The Great Instauration: Science, Medicine and Reform 1626–1660 (London, Duckworth, 1975). American edn (New York, Holmes & Meier Publishers, 1976); shortened Italian edn as *La grande instaurazione: scienza e riforma sociale nella rivoluzione puritana*, ed. P. Corsi (Milan, Feltrinelli, 1980); 2nd edn with new introduction (Oxford, Peter Lang, 2002). Extracts repr. in Cohen, Duffin and Strickland, *Puritanism and the Rise of Modern Science* (1990) [see above], pp. 280–8, 289–98.

'The curriculum of the grammar schools and universities 1500–1660: a critical review of the literature', *History of Education*, 4 (1975), 51–68

(with others) 'So you thought tutors couldn't read...', *Pelican*, 3 (1975), 22

1976

(editor) Special Issues on History and Education, *Oxford Review of Education*, 2, no. 3 (1976); 3, no. 1 (1977)

'Changing perspectives in the history of education' [introduction to previous entry], *Oxford Review of Education*, 2 (1976), 201–13

'The crisis of subsistence and health of the Puritan Revolution', *Bulletin of the Society for the Social History of Medicine*, 17 (1976), 8–10

'Health and hospital records', *Bulletin of the Society for the Social History of Medicine*, 18 (1976), 2–3

'Social history and medical science', *Bulletin of the Society for the Social History of Medicine*, 19 (1976), 1–3

1977

(editor, with F.R. Maddison and M. Pelling) *Linacre Studies: Essays on the Life and Work of Thomas Linacre c. 1460–1524* (Oxford, Clarendon Press, 1977). Introduction, pp. xiii–xlviii.

'Thomas Linacre and the foundation of the College of Physicians', in Maddison, Pelling and Webster, *Linacre Studies* [see previous entry], pp. 198–222

[preface to] J. Woodward and D. Richards, eds, *Health Care and Popular Medicine in Nineteenth Century England* (London, Croom Helm, 1977), p. [5]

'Chemical and industrial background to the work of John Jeyes', Appendix I in D. Palfreyman, *John Jeyes...the Making of a Household Name* (Thetford, Jeyes Group, 1977), pp. 97–102

1978

'The crisis of the hospitals during the Industrial Revolution', in E.G. Forbes, ed., *Human Implications of Scientific Advance*, Proceedings of the XVth International Congress of the History of Science, Edinburgh, 1977 (Edinburgh, Edinburgh University Press, 1978), pp. 214–23

1979

(editor) *Health, Medicine and Mortality in the Sixteenth Century* (Cambridge, Cambridge University Press, 1979). Introduction, pp. 1–7.

(with M. Pelling) 'Medical practitioners', in Webster, *Health, Medicine and Mortality* [see previous entry], pp. 165–235

'Alchemical and Paracelsian medicine', in Webster, *Health, Medicine and Mortality*, pp. 301–34

'Medical records', [introduction to] *The Preservation of Medical and Public Health Records*, Research Publications No. I (Oxford, Wellcome Unit for the History of Medicine, 1979), pp. 1–8

Utopian Planning and the Puritan Revolution: Gabriel Plattes, Samuel Hartlib, and Macaria, Research Publications No. II (Oxford, Wellcome Unit for the History of Medicine, 1979)

'William Harvey and the crisis of medicine in Jacobean England', in J.J. Bylebyl, ed., *William Harvey and his Age: The Professional and Social Context of the Discovery of the Circulation*, Henry E. Sigerist Supplement to *Bulletin of the History of Medicine*, new ser., no. 2 (Baltimore, Johns Hopkins University Press, 1979), pp. 1–27

'St Mark's Hospital, London; modern proctology was born here', *Proctology/Proktologie* [simultaneous English and German edns], 1 (1979), 46–51

'Sciences in cultures...*The Chemical Philosophy*' [essay review], *Isis*, 70 (1979), 588–92

1980

'Healthy or hungry Thirties?', *Bulletin of the Society for the Social History of Medicine*, 27 (1980), 22–4

'Medieval and renaissance interpretations of the cardio-vascular system', in C.J. Schwarz, N.T. Werthessen, and S. Wolf, eds, *Structure and Function of the Circulation* (3 vols, New York, Plenum Press, 1980–1), ii, pp. 1–45

1981

(editor) *Biology, Medicine and Society 1840–1940* (Cambridge, Cambridge University Press, 1981). Introduction, pp. 1–13.

1982

From Paracelsus to Newton: Magic and the Making of Modern Science [Eddington Memorial Lectures 1980] (Cambridge, Cambridge University Press, 1982). Italian edn as *Magia e scienza da Paracelso a Newton*, ed. P. Corsi (Bologna, Il Mulino, 1984); Spanish edn as *De Paracelso a Newton. La Magia en la Creación de la Ciencia Moderna* (Mexico, Fondo de Cultura Economica, 1988); Polish edn as *Od Paracelsus a do Newtona. Magia i powstanie nowozytnej nauki* (Warsaw, Polska Akademia Nauk Instytut Filozofii Socjologii, 1992); American edn (New York, Barnes & Noble, 1996); pbk edn (Mineola, NY, Dover Publications, 2005).

'Medicine as social history: changing ideas on doctors and patients in the age of Shakespeare', in L.G. Stevenson, ed., *A Celebration of Medical History* (Baltimore, Johns Hopkins University Press, 1982), pp. 103–26

'Paracelsus and demons: science as a synthesis of popular belief', in *Scienze Credenze Occulte Livelli di Cultura*, Istituto Nazionale di Studi sul Rinascimento (Florence, Leo S. Olschki, 1982), pp. 3–20

'Healthy or hungry Thirties?', *History Workshop Journal*, 13 (1982), 110–29

'Rewriting the National Health Service', *Oxford Medical School Gazette*, 33 (1982), 13–14

'Paracelsus and Paracelsianism: basic data', *Bulletin of the Society for the Social History of Medicine*, 30/31 (1982), 47–50

'Poverty' [essay review], *Bulletin of the Society for the Study of Labour History*, 45 (1982), 43–5

1983

'The historiography of medicine', in P. Corsi and P. Weindling, eds, *Information Sources in the History of Science and Medicine* (London, Butterworth, 1983), pp. 29–43. Italian edn as 'Storia della medicina: la storiografia della medicina', in P. Corsi and P. Weindling, eds, *Storia della scienza e della medicina: bibliografia critica* (Naples, Edizione Theoria, 1990), pp. 377–97.

'The health of the school child during the Depression', in N. Parry and D. McNair, eds, *The Fitness of the Nation – Physical and Health Education in the Nineteenth and Twentieth Centuries* (Leicester, History of Education Society, 1983), pp. 70–85

(with J. Gabbay) 'General introduction. Changing educational provision for the mentally handicapped: from the 1890s to the 1980s', *Oxford Review of Education*, Special Number on Mental Handicap and Education, 9 (1983), 169–75

'General practice under the panel – the last phase', *Bulletin of the Society for the Social History of Medicine*, 32 (1983), 20–3

'Joseph Needham' and 'Henry Ernest Sigerist', in A. Bullock and R.B. Woodings, eds, *The Fontana Biographical Companion to Modern Thought* (London, Collins, 1983), pp. 547, 704–5 [written as anon.] 'A National Health Service without democracy', *Medicine in Society*, 9, no. 4 (Winter 1983–4), 31–4

1984

Health: Historical Issues, CEPR Discussion Paper No. 5 (London, Centre for Economic Policy Research, 1984)

'Tobacco smoking addiction: a challenge to the National Health Service', in V. Berridge, ed., *British Journal of Addiction: Centenary Edition*, 79 (1984), 7–16

Back to the Thirties?, National Health Service Consultants' Association Paper [London, NHSCA, 1984]

1985

'Two-hundredth anniversary of the 1784 report on fever at Radcliffe Mill', *Bulletin of the Society for the Social History of Medicine*, 36 (1985), 65–70

Health, Welfare and Unemployment during the Depression, CEPR Discussion Paper No. 48 (London, CEPR, 1985)

'Nursing and the early crisis of the National Health Service', *History of Nursing Group Bulletin*, 7 (1985), 4–12

'Health, welfare and unemployment during the Depression', *Past and Present*, no. 109 (1985), 204–30

1986

'The Medical Faculty and the Physic Garden', in L.S. Sutherland and L.G. Mitchell, eds, *The History of the University of Oxford. Vol. V, The Eighteenth Century* (Oxford, Clarendon Press, 1986), pp. 683–723

'Puritanism, separatism, and science', in D.C. Lindberg and R.L. Numbers, eds, *God and Nature: Historical Essays on the Encounter between Christianity and Science* (Berkeley, University of California Press, 1986), pp. 192–217. Extracts repr. in Cohen, Duffin and Strickland, *Puritanism and the Rise of Modern Science* (1990) [see above], pp. 273–5.

'The origins of social medicine in Britain', *Bulletin of the Society for the Social History of Medicine*, 38 (1986), 52–5

(with J. Barry) 'The Manchester medical revolution', in B. Smith, ed., *Truth, Liberty, Religion: Essays Celebrating Two Hundred Years of Manchester College* (Oxford, Manchester College, 1986), pp. 167–83

'Il Lutero [Luther] della medicina', *Kos*, 4, 27 (1986), 14–19

'Medical Officers of Health – for the record', *Radical Community Medicine*, 27 (1986), 10–14

'Charles Bernard Schmitt (1933–86)', *Medical History*, 30 (1986), 468–9

1987

'*Eloge*, Charles Bernard Schmitt (1933–1986)', *Isis*, 78 (1987), 80–1

1988

The Health Services Since the War. Volume 1, Problems of Health Care: The British National Health Service Before 1957 (London, HMSO, 1988)

(with R. Dingwall and A.M. Rafferty) *An Introduction to the Social History of Nursing* (London, Routledge, 1988)

'The nineteenth-century afterlife of Paracelsus', in R. Cooter, ed., *Studies in the History of Alternative Medicine* (London, Macmillan, 1988), pp. 79–88

'Labour and the origins of the National Health Service', in N. Rupke, ed., *Science, Politics and the Public Good: Essays in Honour of Margaret Gowing* (Basingstoke and London, Macmillan, 1988), pp. 184–202

'Origins of the NHS: lessons from history', *Contemporary Record*, 2, 2 (1988), 33–6

'The National Health Service: the first 40 years' [conference report], *Social History of Medicine*, 1 (1988), 253–5

1989

(editor) C.B. Schmitt, *Reappraisals in Renaissance Thought* (London, Variorum Reprints, 1989)

'The Health Service', in D. Kavanagh and A. Seldon, eds, *The Thatcher Effect* (Oxford, Clarendon Press, 1989), pp. 166–82

'Is the Health Service safe?' [essay review], *Times Higher Education Supplement* (6 October 1989)

1990

'Conrad Gessner and the infidelity of Paracelsus', in J. Henry and S. Hutton, eds, *New Perspectives on Renaissance Thought. Essays in the History of Science, Education and Philosophy in Memory of Charles B. Schmitt* (London, Duckworth, 1990), pp. 13–23

The Victorian Public Health Legacy: A Challenge to the Future (Birmingham, Public Health Alliance and Institution of Environmental Health Officers, 1990)

'Conflict and consensus: explaining the British Health Service', *Twentieth Century British History*, 1 (1990), 115–51

'Doctors, public service and profit: general practitioners and the National Health Service', *Transactions of the Royal Historical Society*, 5th ser., 40 (1990), 197–216

'...Official history?' [rejoinder], *Social History of Medicine*, 3 (1990), 104–5

1991

(editor) *Aneurin Bevan on the National Health Service*, Research Publications No. X (Oxford, Wellcome Unit for the History of Medicine, 1991). Introduction, pp. xv–xvii.

'The elderly and the early National Health Service', in M. Pelling and R.M. Smith, eds, *Life, Death and the Elderly: Historical Perspectives* (London, Routledge, 1991), pp. 165–93

'Psychiatry and the early National Health Service: the role of the Mental Health Standing Advisory Committee', in G.E. Berrios and H. Freeman, eds, *150 Years of British Psychiatry: 1841–1991* (London, Royal College of Psychiatrists/Gaskell, 1991), pp. 103–16

'The golden age of Oxford medicine', *Oxford Medical School Gazette*, 42 (1991), 32–5

'Health advocacy in history', in A. Scott Samuel, ed., *Speaking Out for Public Health* (Birmingham, Public Health Alliance, 1991), pp. 10–20

1992

(with D. Hunter) 'Here we go again', *Health Service Journal,* 102, no. 5292 (5 March 1992), 26–7

'Public health in decline', *Health Matters*, 11 (Summer 1992), 10–11

'Beveridge after 50 years', *British Medical Journal*, 305 (1992), 901–2

1993

(editor) *Caring for Health: History and Diversity*, U205, Book 6 (Buckingham, Open University Press, 1993). Revised (3rd) edn (Milton Keynes, Open University Press, 2001).

'History and diversity', chapter 1 in *Caring for Health* [see previous entry], pp. 5–17. Revised 3rd edn (2001), pp. 11–29.

(with V. Berridge and G. Walt) 'Mobilisation for total welfare, 1948 to 1974', chapter 6 in *Caring for Health*, pp. 107–26. Revised 3rd edn (2001), pp. 167–96.

(with V. Berridge) 'The crisis of welfare, 1974 to the 1990s', chapter 7 in *Caring for Health*, pp. 127–49. Revised in 3rd edn (2001) as Webster, 'Caring for health in the UK, 1974 to 2001', pp. 197–252.

'Conclusions', chapter 10 in *Caring for Health*, pp. 193–7. Revised 3rd edn (2001), pp. 327–39.

'Inequalities in health: the failure of the NHS in postwar Britain', in *Health, Wealth and Poverty: Papers on Inequalities in Income and Health* (London, Medical World/Socialist Health Association, [1993]), pp. 1–2, 5

'The metamorphosis of Dawson of Penn', in D. Porter and R. Porter, eds, *Doctors, Politics and Society: Historical Essays*, Clio Medica 23 (Amsterdam, Rodopi, 1993), pp. 212–28

'Paracelsus: medicine as popular protest', in O.P. Grell and A. Cunningham, eds, *Medicine and the Reformation* (London, Routledge, 1993), pp. 57–77

'Worsley, Benjamin (1617/18–1677)', in *Dictionary of National Biography: Missing Persons*, ed. C.S. Nicholls (Oxford, Oxford University Press, 1993, 1994), pp. 732–3. Repr. in *The Oxford Dictionary of National Biography*, ed. H.C.G. Matthew and B. Harrison (60 vols and online, Oxford, Oxford University Press, 2004).

'Paracelsus, and 500 years of encouraging scientific inquiry', *British Medical Journal*, 306 (1993), 597–8

1994

'Benjamin Worsley: engineering for universal reform from the Invisible College to the Navigation Act', in M. Greengrass, M. Leslie and T. Raylor, eds, *Samuel Hartlib and Universal Reformation* (Cambridge, Cambridge University Press, 1994), pp. 213–35

'Paracelsus on natural and popular magic', in *Atti del Convegno Internazionale su Paracelso*, Goethe Institut, Rome, December 1993 (Rome, Edizioni Paracelso, [1994]), pp. 89–106

'Conservatives and consensus: the politics of the National Health Service, 1951–64', in A. Oakley and A.S. Williams, eds, *The Politics of the Welfare State* (London, UCL Press, 1994), pp. 54–74

'The National Health Service: the first forty years', in D. Light and A. May, eds, *Britain's Health System: From Welfare State to Managed Markets* (Washington, DC, Faulkner and Gray, 1994), pp. 13–20

'Saving children during the Depression: Britain's silent emergency, 1919–1939', *Disasters: The Journal of Disaster Studies and Management*, 18 (1994), 213–20

'Tuberculosis', in C. Seale and S. Pattison, eds, *Medical Knowledge: Doubt and Certainty*, U205, Book 1 (Milton Keynes, Open University Press, 1994), pp. 36–59. Revised edn, ed. C. Seale, S. Pattison and B. Davey (Milton Keynes, Open University Press, 2001), pp. 54–85.

'Medicine', in B. Harrison, ed., *The History of the University of Oxford. Vol. VIII, The Twentieth Century* (Oxford, Clarendon Press, 1994), pp. 317–43

1995

'Paracelsus confronts the saints: miracles, healing and the secularization of magic', *Social History of Medicine*, 8 (1995), 403–21

'The state and health care. The British National Health Service', in R.B.M. Rigter, ed., *Overheid en gezondheidszorg in de twintigste eeuw: verslag van het symposium ter gelegenheit van het vijfentwintigjarig bestaan van de Stichting Historia Medicinae...1993* (Rotterdam, Erasmus Publishing, 1995), pp. 127–35

'Overthrowing the market in health care: the achievements of the early National Health Service', *Journal of the Royal College of Physicians of London*, 29 (1995), 502–7

'The making of the National Health Service', *Modern History Review*, 6, 4 (1995), 11–13

'Local government and health care: the historical perspective', *British Medical Journal*, 310 (1995), 1584–7

'Goodbye to all that?' [regular column], *Health Matters*, 21 (Spring 1995), 5

'The battle for the health centre', *Health Matters*, 22 (Summer 1995), 5

'Will New Labour restore old democracy?', *Health Matters*, 23 (Autumn 1995), 5

'A spirit of healthy competition', *Health Matters*, 24 (Winter 1995/6), 5

1996

The Health Services since the War. Volume 2, Government and Health Care: The National Health Service 1958–1979 (London, The Stationery Office, 1996)

'Sundhed versus marked – det skaebnesvangrre dilemma for et offentligt sundhedsvaesen' [Health versus market – the fatal dilemma for a public health care system], in U. Juul Jensen, J. Quesel and P. Fuur Andersen, eds, *Forskelle og Forandring – Bidrag til Humanistisk Sundhedsforskning* (Aarhus, Philosophia, 1996), pp. 231–49

'When will governments put public health first?', *Health Matters*, 25 (Spring 1996), 5

'Why has it taken so long to achieve so little?' [complaints procedures], *Health Matters*, 26 (Summer 1996), 5

'Where is Labour's vision for the NHS of 1997?', *Health Matters*, 27 (Autumn 1996), 5

'A case of "tragic incoordination"?', *Health Matters*, 28 (Winter 1996/7), 5

1997

'Government policy on school meals and welfare foods 1939–1970', in D.F. Smith, ed., *Nutrition in Britain: Science, Scientists, and Politics in the Twentieth Century* (London, Routledge, 1997), pp. 190–213

'Le reinvenzione di Robert Boyle', *Rivista Storica Italiana*, 109 (1997), 298–306

'NHS charges. Light on the charge brigade', *Health Service Journal*, 107, no. 5562 (17 July 1997), 26–8

'Ministers matter to the NHS', *Health Matters*, 29 (Spring 1997), 5

'NHS: charging ahead with Labour?', *Health Matters*, 30 (Summer 1997), 5

'Eugenic sterilisation: Europe's shame', *Health Matters*, 31 (Autumn 1997), 14–15

'Launching the new NHS – on a tight budget', *Health Matters*, 32 (Winter 1997/8), 5

1998

The National Health Service: A Political History (Oxford, Oxford University Press, 1998). Revised edn (Oxford, Oxford University Press, 2002).

(editor, with J. Horder and I. Loudon) *General Practice under the National Health Service 1948–1997* (London, Clarendon Press, 1998)

'The politics of general practice', in Loudon, Horder and Webster, eds, *General Practice under the National Health Service* [see previous entry], pp. 20–44

'Bare heads against red hats: a portrait of Paracelsus', in K. Bayertz and R. Porter, eds, *From Physico-theology to Bio-technology: Essays in the Social and Cultural History of Biosciences: A Festschrift for Mikuláš Teich*, Clio Medica 48 (Amsterdam, Rodopi, 1998), pp. 54–75

National Health Service Reorganisation: Learning from History? (London, Office of Health Economics, 1998)

'Nursing and the early crisis of the NHS', *International History of Nursing Journal*, 3 (1998), 36–43

'20 questions' [Aneurin Bevan 'interviewed' by Webster], *Nursing Times*, 94, no. 26 (1 July 1998), 28

'In Bevan's name', *Nursing Times*, 94, no. 26 (1 July 1998), 34–5

'The BMA and the NHS', *British Medical Journal*, 317 (1998), 45–7

'Blair and Bevan: more than 50 years apart', *Health Matters*, 33 (Spring 1998), 5

'A little of old Labour does good', *Health Matters*, 34 (Summer/Autumn 1998), 5

'The very long history of the PCG [Primary Care Groups]', *Health Matters*, 35 (Winter 1998/9), 5

'50 years of the NHS', *History Today*, 48 (1998), 2–5

1999

'Paracelsus, the Jews, and the magic of the Orient', *Acta Comeniana*, 13 (1999), 11–26

'Community care: older than the NHS', *Health Matters*, 36 (Spring 1999), 5

'Time to breach the contract', *Health Matters*, 37 (Summer 1999), 5

'New Labour promises but old Tory policies', *Health Matters*, 38 (Autumn 1999), 5

'Look back in wonder', *Health Matters*, 39 (Winter 1999/2000), 5

'Margaret Gowing, 1921–98', *History Workshop Journal*, 47 (1999), 327–30

2000

'Medicine and the welfare state 1930–1970', in R. Cooter and J. Pickstone, eds, *Medicine in the Twentieth Century* (Amsterdam, Harwood Academic, 2000), pp. 125–40

'Note A [to chap. 21]. The Medical School under Osler', in M.G. Brock and M.C. Curthoys, eds, *The History of the University of Oxford. Vol. VII, Nineteenth-Century Oxford, Part 2* (Oxford, Clarendon Press, 2000), pp. 504–7

'The year of the NHS Plan: a review of 2000', *British Journal of Health Care Management*, 6 (2000), 561–3

'The early NHS and the crisis of public health nursing', *International History of Nursing Journal*, 5 (2000), 4–10

'Can we have some more?', *Health Matters*, 42 (Autumn 2000), 19

'Patients' friends pushed aside by Labour's PALS [Patient Advisory and Liaison Service]', *Health Matters*, 43 (Winter 2000/1), 5

2001

(with I. Loudon) 'Limits to demand for health care...' [letter], *British Medical Journal*, 322 (2001), 734

'Knowing members of the Advisory Board: Charles Webster' [intellectual autobiography], *History of Psychiatry*, 12 (2001), 375–9

2002

'Investigating inequalities in health before Black', *Contemporary British History*, 16 (2002), 81–103 (Special Issue, 'Poor Health. Social Inequality Before and After the Black Report', ed. V. Berridge and S. Blume; repr. as separate volume, London, Frank Cass, 2003)

'Paracelsus, Paracelsianism, and the secularization of the worldview', *Science in Context*, 15 (2002), 9–27

(with J. French) 'The cycle of conflict: the history of the public health and health promotion movements', in L. Adams, M. Amos, and J. Monro, eds, *Promoting Health: Politics and Practice* (London, Sage Publications, 2002), pp. 5–12. Reprinted in M. Sidell et al., *Debates and Dilemmas in Promoting Health: A Reader* (2nd edn, London, Palgrave, 2003), pp. 9–19.

'The parable of the incompetent steward', *British Journal of Health Care Management*, 8 (2002), 113–14

(contributor) 'And did they "save the NHS"?', *Health Matters*, 49 (Autumn 2002), 12

Journals in which reviews have appeared include:

Ambix
American Historical Review
American Journal of Epidemiology
Annals of Science
British Journal of Addiction
British Journal for the History of Science
British Journal for the Philosophy of Science
British Medical Journal
Bulletin of the History of Medicine
Bulletin of the Society for the Study of Labour History

Contemporary Physics
Durham Research Review
English Historical Review
Health Services Journal
History
History and Archaeology Review
History of Education
History of Science
History of Universities
International Journal of the History of Sport
International Studies in the Philosophy of Science
Isis
Journal of Ecclesiastical History
Journal of Educational Administration and History
Journal of Modern History
Journal of Tropical Medicine and Hygiene
Labour History Review
Listener
Medical History
Nature
New Statesman
Notes & Queries
Nuncius: Annali di Storia della Scienza
Oxford Magazine
Pharmacy in History
Psychological Medicine
Review of English Studies
Social History
Social History of Medicine
Society for the Study of Labour History Bulletin
Sociology of Health and Illness
Speculum
Times Health Supplement
Times Higher Education Supplement
Times Literary Supplement
Twentieth Century British History
Update: The Journal of Postgraduate General Practice
Urban History Yearbook
Welsh History Review

Index

Index

Printed and bound by CPI Group (UK) Ltd, Croydon, CR0 4YY

17/10/2024

01775685-0019